The CMT Review Guide

Developed by the American Association for Medical Transcription

Betty Honkonen, CMT, FAAMT
Lea M. Sims, CMT, FAAMT, Editor
Laura Bryan, CMT, Associate Editor
Diane Heath, CMT, Associate Editor

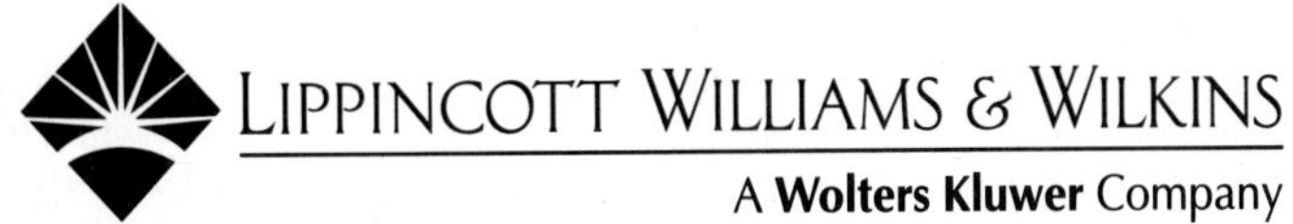

Philadelphia • Baltimore • New York • London
Buenos Aires • Hong Kong • Sydney • Tokyo

Publisher: Julie K. Stegman
Senior Product Manager: Eric Branger
Associate Managing Editor: Amy Millholen
Copyeditor: Diane Heath
Production Coordinator: Jason Delaney
Editorial Assistant: Pete Devereaux
Interior Design: Melissa Olson
Frontmatter Design: Hearthside Publishing Services
Compositor: Maryland Composition
Printer: Quebecor World Taunton

100 Sycamore Avenue
Modesto, CA 95354-0550
www.aamt.org

Lippincott Williams & Wilkins
A Wolters Kluwer Health Company
351 West Camden Street
Baltimore, MD 21201-2346
www.stedmans.com
stedmans@lww.com

Printed in the United States of America

Library of Congress Cataloging-in-Publication Data

Honkonen, Betty.
The CMT review guide / developed by the American Association for Medical Transcription ; Betty Honkonen, Lea M. Sims, editor.
p. ; cm.
Includes bibliographical references.
ISBN 0-7817-6000-3
1. Medical transcription—Examinations—Study guides. I. Sims, Lea M. II. American Association for Medical Transcription. III. Title. [DNLM: 1. Medical Records—Examination Questions. 2. Certification—Examination Questions. WX 18.2 H773c 2006]
R728.8.H655 2006
653'.18—dc22

2005005803

The publishers have made every effort to trace the copyright holders for borrowed material. If they have inadvertently overlooked any, they will be pleased to make the necessary arrangements at the first opportunity.

To purchase additional copies of this book, call our customer service department at **(800) 638-3030** or fax orders to **(301) 824-7390**. International customers should call **(301) 714-2324**. *or*

Visit Stedman's on the Internet: http://www.stedmans.com.

Visit American Association for Medical Transcription on the Internet: http://www.aamt.org

05 06 07 08 09 10
1 2 3 4 5 6 7 8 9 10

Preface

"Education is an ornament in prosperity, and a refuge in adversity."
Aristotle

Obviously, Aristotle recognized the shifting sands upon which most of us live our lives, particularly when it comes to our professional growth and development. These words, uttered by the famous Greek philosopher who is also referred to as the great observer, are a startlingly accurate description of modern-day education, professionalism, and credentialing.

In times of prosperity, a professional credential and the education it represents *can* be an ornament, something that adorns our names and lends credibility and stature to the professional skill-set we already possess. It can be argued during those prosperous times, that the credential is quite simply a *bonus*, that *something extra*, but not necessarily critical to survival.

Many would say that this was true of the CMT credential in years past. With so few skilled workers in the industry and such a critical demand for them, the CMT credential was deemed not that important to finding or retaining employment or securing a niche in the future. But, as Aristotle reminds us, those sands upon which we stand can quite rapidly and without announcement shift beneath our feet, and we can find ourselves on new and unpredictable ground.

Within a short time, the evolution of technologies in healthcare documentation (i.e., speech recognition, EMR systems, etc.) and the emergence of global competition have shifted the paradigm upon which we operate within the industry. There is significant pressure in the healthcare delivery system to lower costs, and many within that system are highly motivated to eliminate transcription from the expense equation. Inarguably, those times of *adversity* to which Aristotle refers above are now upon us, and it is education—and the credentialing that verifies it—that must now become the *refuge* we seek to secure our future in healthcare.

If you have invested in this review guide, then you have undoubtedly recognized this critical need for yourself and are taking those important steps that will ensure your viability in the electronic healthcare future. And like many, you are probably overwhelmed with the concept of preparing for a formal exam of this magnitude.

It is the goal of this review guide to assist you in approaching the preparation for this exam in an organized and informed manner. This guide will provide clear objectives based on the CMT exam outline that you will need to consider and topically address when evaluating your own readiness to sit for the exam. It will also give you the chance to do practice questions written in the style of the exam and dictation exercises.

The chapters follow a specific format and include objectives, resources for study, and review questions. In addition, the medical specialty chapters also have sample reports and proofreading exercises.

The CMT Review Guide also includes a CD-ROM with an additional 20 multiple-choice questions for all the medical specialty chapters and approximately 10 dictation excerpts for each medical specialty to assist you in preparing for the practical portion of the exam.

As indicated above, a checklist of objectives is provided at the beginning of every chapter, and we encourage you to utilize this book as a workbook, checking those objectives off one by one when you are confident that you have studied that content sufficiently. While this text will not expand on those objectives nor provide you the detailed content you need to study, it will provide a *Resources for Study* section that outlines the chapters and pages in our recommended texts to assist you in studying the suggested content in that chapter.

Given the fact that so many MTs already possess these texts (many are required in most MT educational programs), we have selected the following suggested texts to which we will continually refer throughout this book:

1. Chabner D-E. *The Language of Medicine*, 7th ed. Philadelphia: Saunders, 2004. ISBN#: 1416001263.

2. Dirckx JH. *H & P: A Nonphysician's Guide to the Medical and History Examination.* Modesto, CA: Health Professions Institute, 2001. ISBN#: 0934385343.

3. Dirckx JH. *Human Diseases.* Modesto, CA: Health Professions Institute, 2003. ISBN#: 0934385386.

4. Dirckx JH. *Laboratory Tests & Diagnostic Procedures in Medicine.* Modesto, CA: Health Professions Institute, 2004. ISBN#: 0934385491.

5. Hughes P (ed). *The AAMT Book of Style for Medical Transcription*, 2nd ed. Modesto: AAMT, 2002. ISBN#: 0935229388.

6. Sabin WA. *The Gregg Reference Manual.* Burr Ridge, IL: McGraw-Hill/Irwin, 2004. ISBN#: 0072936533.

7. Turley SM. *Understanding Pharmacology for Health Professionals.* Upper Saddle River, NJ: Prentice Hall, 2002. ISBN#: 0130417424.

There is so much content that could be potentially encountered on the

CMT exam that it would be impossible to try and cover it all in one text. To cover only some of it would likewise be confusing and misleading. The streamlined, concept-focused guide you now possess reflects our intent to provide you with a resource to help you identify areas in which you may need additional preparation and to give you practice answering questions similar to the ones on the actual exam.

Ultimately, the burden of exhaustive study will fall on your own shoulders. This book is not designed to be a "cram" text for test preparation, which is why we are pointing you to the content you should be familiar with and review in order to pass the exam rather than providing content. The real benefit of this text lies in its organizational approach to study. Often, having a resource that maps it out for you can be just the help you need to tackle such an overwhelming warehouse of information. Additionally, every candidate preparing for the exam needs practice with questions. Certainly, no one can get enough of those when studying for an exam like this one, and this text and CD are full of them.

Finally, it is important to note that this text is best combined with other CMT exam preparatory objectives, like participating in AAMT's online CMT prep courses or getting involved in a mentoring or exam prep study group where this text can be utilized with others for maximized results.

Congratulations on making the decision to register your skills through the CMT credentialing process and for choosing this text to assist you in making that happen.

Good luck!

Lea M. Sims, CMT, FAAMT
Director of Publications & Communications, AAMT
lea@aamt.org

User's Guide

This User's Guide shows you how to best use *The CMT Review Guide* by highlighting the features of the chapters.

OBJECTIVES CHECKLIST

A checklist of objectives to assist you in self-evaluation.

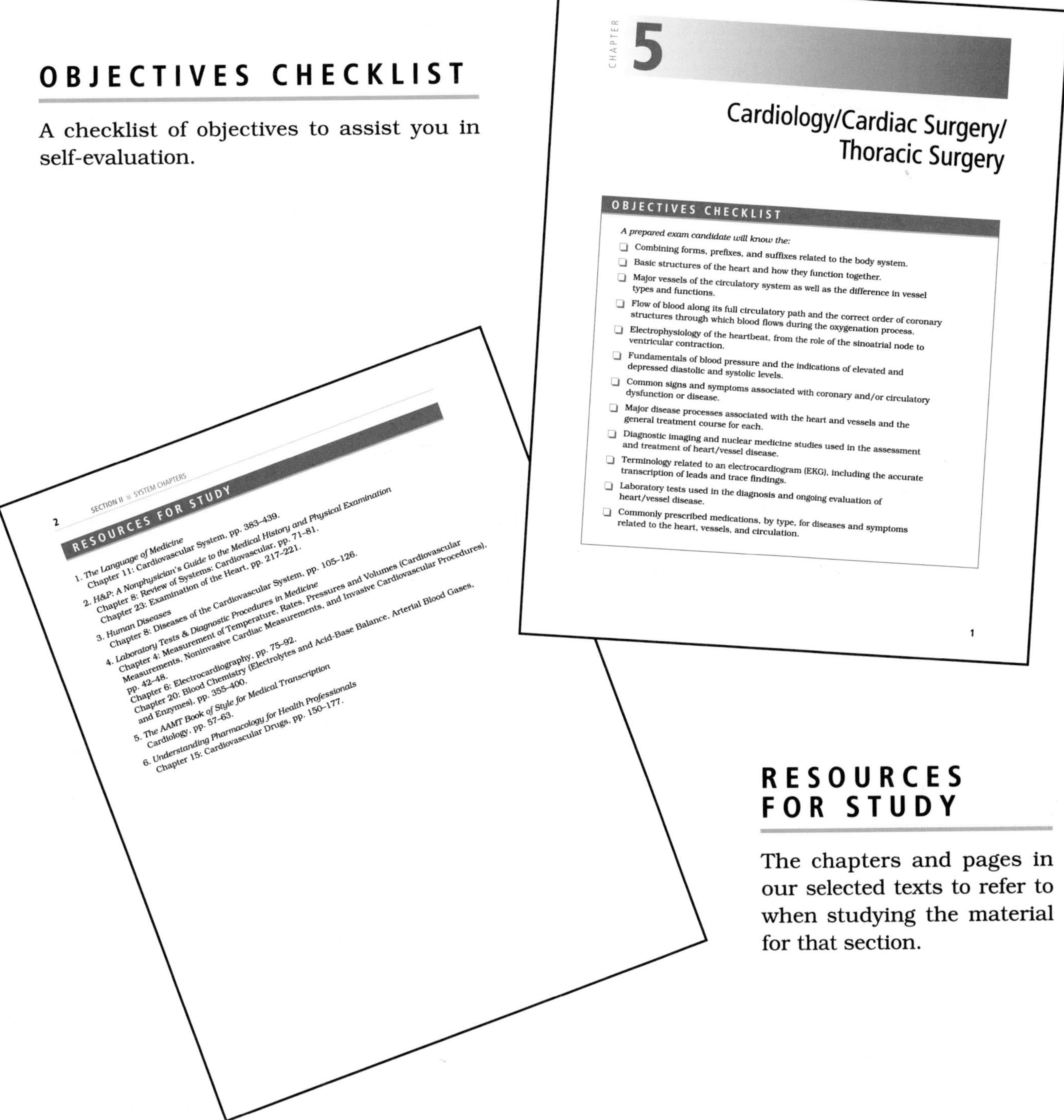

CHAPTER 5

Cardiology/Cardiac Surgery/ Thoracic Surgery

OBJECTIVES CHECKLIST

A prepared exam candidate will know the:

- ❑ Combining forms, prefixes, and suffixes related to the body system.
- ❑ Basic structures of the heart and how they function together.
- ❑ Major vessels of the circulatory system as well as the difference in vessel types and functions.
- ❑ Flow of blood along its full circulatory path and the correct order of coronary structures through which blood flows during the oxygenation process.
- ❑ Electrophysiology of the heartbeat, from the role of the sinoatrial node to ventricular contraction.
- ❑ Fundamentals of blood pressure and the indications of elevated and depressed diastolic and systolic levels.
- ❑ Common signs and symptoms associated with coronary and/or circulatory dysfunction or disease.
- ❑ Major disease processes associated with the heart and vessels and the general treatment course for each.
- ❑ Diagnostic imaging and nuclear medicine studies used in the assessment and treatment of heart/vessel disease.
- ❑ Terminology related to an electrocardiogram (EKG), including the accurate transcription of leads and trace findings.
- ❑ Laboratory tests used in the diagnosis and ongoing evaluation of heart/vessel disease.
- ❑ Commonly prescribed medications, by type, for diseases and symptoms related to the heart, vessels, and circulation.

1

2 SECTION II ■ SYSTEM CHAPTERS

RESOURCES FOR STUDY

1. *The Language of Medicine*
   Chapter 11: Cardiovascular System, pp. 383–439.
2. *H&P: A Nonphysician's Guide to the Medical History and Physical Examination*
   Chapter 8: Review of Systems: Cardiovascular, pp. 71–81.
   Chapter 23: Examination of the Heart, pp. 217–221.
3. *Human Diseases*
   Chapter 8: Diseases of the Cardiovascular System, pp. 105–126.
4. *Laboratory Tests & Diagnostic Procedures in Medicine*
   Chapter 4: Measurement of Temperature, Rates, Pressures and Volumes (Cardiovascular Measurements, Noninvasive Cardiac Measurements, and Invasive Cardiovascular Procedures), pp. 42–48.
   Chapter 6: Electrocardiography, pp. 75–92.
   Chapter 20: Blood Chemistry (Electrolytes and Acid-Base Balance, Arterial Blood Gases, and Enzymes), pp. 355–400.
5. *The AAMT Book of Style for Medical Transcription*
   Cardiology, pp. 57–63.
6. *Understanding Pharmacology for Health Professionals*
   Chapter 15: Cardiovascular Drugs, pp. 150–177.

RESOURCES FOR STUDY

The chapters and pages in our selected texts to refer to when studying the material for that section.

SAMPLE REPORTS

Located in all of the systems chapters, the samples are representative of common reports encountered in medical specialties.

SAMPLE REPORTS

The following four reports are examples of reports you might encounter while transcribing emergency medicine.

OPERATIVE NOTE

DATE OF OPERATION
02/21/2004

SURGEON OF RECORD
John Smith, MD

PREOPERATIVE DIAGNOSIS
Left index finger cellulitis.

POSTOPERATIVE DIAGNOSIS
Left index finger cellulitis.

PROCEDURE PERFORMED
Hickman catheter placement.

ANESTHESIA
Monitored anesthesia care.

COMPLICATIONS
None noted.

ESTIMATED BLOOD LOSS
Minimal.

INTRAVENOUS FLUIDS
200 mL of Crystalloid.

INDICATIONS FOR PROCEDURE
The patient is a 33-year-old Haitian male who had a gunshot wound to his left index finger and subsequently underwent surgery by the orthopedic hand service. This included having a piece of hardware placed. The patient presented to the surgical emergency room today with purulent drainage from his finger and underwent incision and drainage of his left index finger. The patient will require long-term antibiotics and, for this reason, a Hickman catheter was requested by the orthopedic team.

PROCEDURE IN DETAIL
The patient was given intravenous sedation and then prepped and draped in the usual sterile fashion, still in the surgical emergency room. We then proceeded to cannulate the left subclavian vein and passed a guide wire through the needle.

Then we made a tunnel under the skin with an exit approximately 4 cm below our initial cannulation site. After that, we measured the Hickman catheter, making sure the cuff would be at the level of the skin of the lower incision and the tip would be at the level of the superior vena

(continued)

OPERATIVE REPORT

DATE OF OPERATION
01/06/2004

SURGEON OF RECORD
John Jones, MD

PREOPERATIVE DIAGNOSIS
Gunshot wound to the abdomen.

POSTOPERATIVE DIAGNOSES
1. Gunshot wound to the abdomen.
2. Laceration of the duodenum.
3. Injury to the head of the pancreas.
4. Injury to the inferior vena cava.
5. Injury to the right renal artery.

PROCEDURES PERFORMED
1. Closure of stomach laceration.
2. Closure of duodenal laceration.
3. Drainage of pancreas.
4. Repair of renal artery.
5. Repair of inferior vena cava.

ANESTHESIA
General endotracheal anesthesia.

JUSTIFICATION FOR PROCEDURE
This is an 18-year-old known gang member who presented to the trauma center with a gunshot wound to the abdomen.

PROCEDURE IN DETAIL
The patient was brought to the operating room in the trauma center, placed in the supine position, and prepped and draped in the usual sterile fashion. The abdomen was entered through a long midline incision. Upon entering the abdomen, the abdomen was packed to control bleeding.

Examination of the abdomen revealed the following injuries: There was a long laceration of the greater curvature of the stomach. There was a hole through-and-through on the head of the pancreas and a small laceration of the duodenum. The bullet projectile also caused a large right retroperitoneal hematoma. The right side of the colon was mobilized and the duodenum was kocherized. Kocherization of the duodenum revealed the through-and-through injury to the head of the pancreas and also revealed the small hole through the duodenum mentioned previously.

After the right side of the colon was mobilized, it was evident that the bullet had gone through the hilum of the right kidney, and exploration of that area revealed that the renal artery had been lacerated and there was also a small hole in the inferior vena cava. The small hole in the inferior vena cava was closed with figure-of-8 sutures of 5-0 Prolene. The renal artery was controlled proximally and distally and was completely divided and débrided. Following this, a primary anastomosis was performed with 6-0 Prolene interrupted stitches.

(continued)

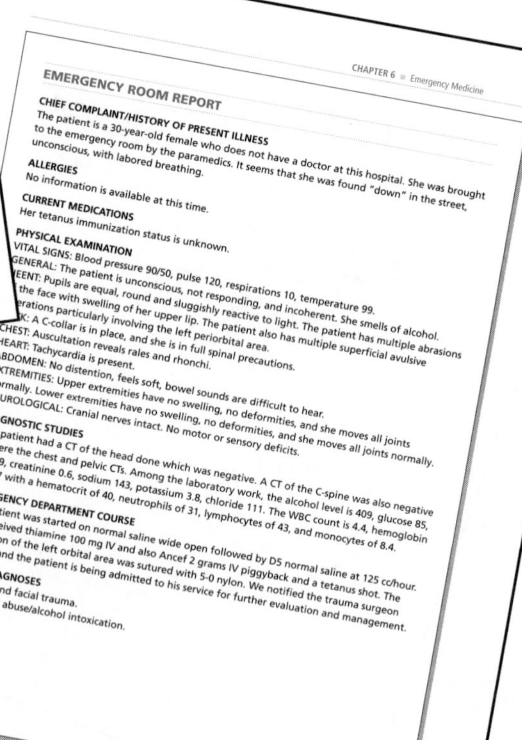

EMERGENCY ROOM REPORT

CHIEF COMPLAINT/HISTORY OF PRESENT ILLNESS
The patient is a 30-year-old female who does not have a doctor at this hospital. She was brought to the emergency room by the paramedics. It seems that she was found "down" in the street, unconscious, with labored breathing.

ALLERGIES
No information is available at this time.

CURRENT MEDICATIONS
Her tetanus immunization status is unknown.

PHYSICAL EXAMINATION
VITAL SIGNS: Blood pressure 90/50, pulse 120, respirations 10, temperature 99.
GENERAL: The patient is unconscious, not responding, and incoherent. She smells of alcohol.
EENT: Pupils are equal, round and sluggishly reactive to light. The patient has multiple abrasions the face with swelling of her upper lip. The patient also has multiple superficial avulsive erations particularly involving the left periorbital area.
K: A C-collar is in place, and she is in full spinal precautions.
CHEST: Auscultation reveals rales and rhonchi.
HEART: Tachycardia is present.
ABDOMEN: No distention, feels soft, bowel sounds are difficult to hear.
EXTREMITIES: Upper extremities have no swelling, no deformities, and she moves all joints normally. Lower extremities have no swelling, no deformities, and she moves all joints normally.
NEUROLOGICAL: Cranial nerves intact. No motor or sensory deficits.

DIAGNOSTIC STUDIES
The patient had a CT of the head done which was negative. A CT of the C-spine was also negative as were the chest and pelvic CTs. Among the laboratory work, the alcohol level is 409, glucose 85, BUN 9, creatinine 0.6, sodium 143, potassium 3.8, chloride 111. The WBC count is 4.4, hemoglobin is 13.7 with a hematocrit of 40, neutrophils of 31, lymphocytes of 43, and monocytes of 8.4.

EMERGENCY DEPARTMENT COURSE
The patient was started on normal saline wide open followed by D5 normal saline at 125 cc/hour. She received thiamine 100 mg IV and also Ancef 2 grams IV piggyback and a tetanus shot. The laceration of the left orbital area was sutured with 5-0 nylon. We notified the trauma surgeon on-call, and the patient is being admitted to his service for further evaluation and management.

FINAL DIAGNOSES
1. Head and facial trauma.
2. Alcohol abuse/alcohol intoxication.

REVIEW QUESTIONS

Multiple-choice exam-style questions for exam practice.

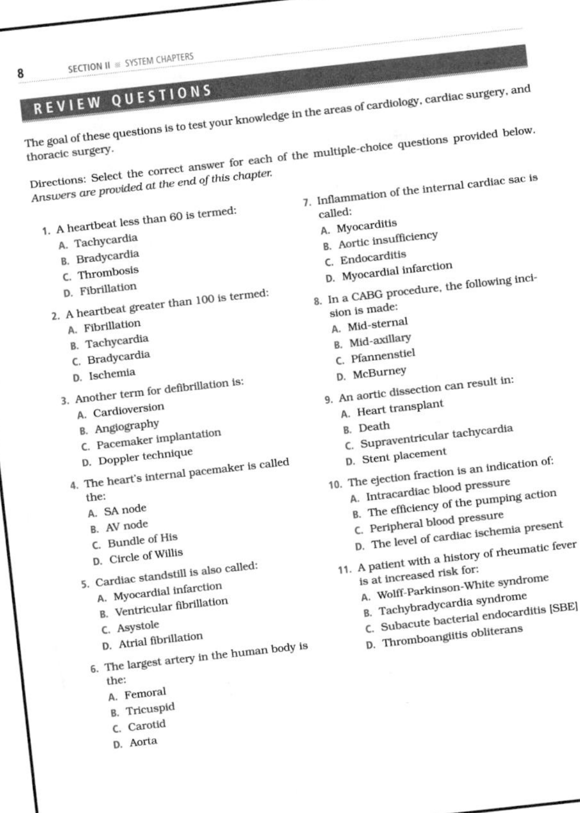

8 SECTION II ■ SYSTEM CHAPTERS

REVIEW QUESTIONS

The goal of these questions is to test your knowledge in the areas of cardiology, cardiac surgery, and thoracic surgery.

Directions: Select the correct answer for each of the multiple-choice questions provided below. *Answers are provided at the end of this chapter.*

1. A heartbeat less than 60 is termed:
   A. Tachycardia
   B. Bradycardia
   C. Thrombosis
   D. Fibrillation
2. A heartbeat greater than 100 is termed:
   A. Fibrillation
   B. Tachycardia
   C. Bradycardia
   D. Ischemia
3. Another term for defibrillation is:
   A. Cardioversion
   B. Angiography
   C. Pacemaker implantation
   D. Doppler technique
4. The heart's internal pacemaker is called the:
   A. SA node
   B. AV node
   C. Bundle of His
   D. Circle of Willis
5. Cardiac standstill is also called:
   A. Myocardial infarction
   B. Ventricular fibrillation
   C. Asystole
   D. Atrial fibrillation
6. The largest artery in the human body is the:
   A. Femoral
   B. Tricuspid
   C. Carotid
   D. Aorta
7. Inflammation of the internal cardiac sac is called:
   A. Myocarditis
   B. Aortic insufficiency
   C. Endocarditis
   D. Myocardial infarction
8. In a CABG procedure, the following incision is made:
   A. Mid-sternal
   B. Mid-axillary
   C. Pfannenstiel
   D. McBurney
9. An aortic dissection can result in:
   A. Heart transplant
   B. Death
   C. Supraventricular tachycardia
   D. Stent placement
10. The ejection fraction is an indication of:
    A. Intracardiac blood pressure
    B. The efficiency of the pumping action
    C. Peripheral blood pressure
    D. The level of cardiac ischemia present
11. A patient with a history of rheumatic fever is at increased risk for:
    A. Wolff-Parkinson-White syndrome
    B. Tachybradycardia syndrome
    C. Subacute bacterial endocarditis [SBE]
    D. Thromboangiitis obliterans

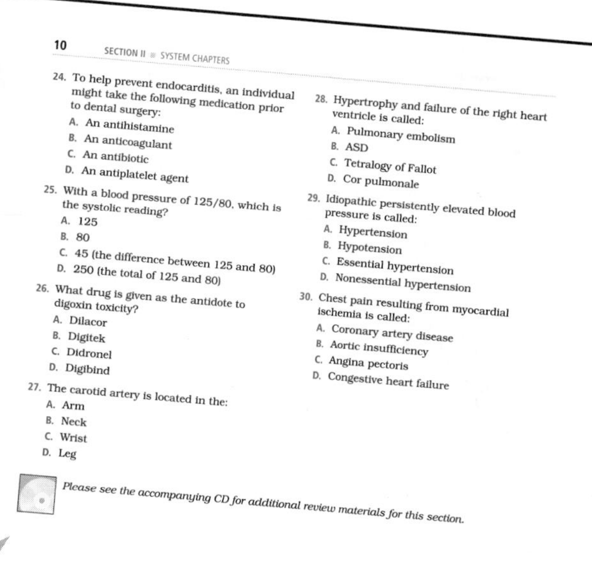

10 SECTION II ■ SYSTEM CHAPTERS

24. To help prevent endocarditis, an individual might take the following medication prior to dental surgery:
    A. An antihistamine
    B. An anticoagulant
    C. An antibiotic
    D. An antiplatelet agent
25. With a blood pressure of 125/80, which is the systolic reading?
    A. 125
    B. 80
    C. 45 (the difference between 125 and 80)
    D. 250 (the total of 125 and 80)
26. What drug is given as the antidote to digoxin toxicity?
    A. Dilacor
    B. Digitek
    C. Didronel
    D. Digibind
27. The carotid artery is located in the:
    A. Arm
    B. Neck
    C. Wrist
    D. Leg
28. Hypertrophy and failure of the right heart ventricle is called:
    A. Pulmonary embolism
    B. ASD
    C. Tetralogy of Fallot
    D. Cor pulmonale
29. Idiopathic persistently elevated blood pressure is called:
    A. Hypertension
    B. Hypotension
    C. Essential hypertension
    D. Nonessential hypertension
30. Chest pain resulting from myocardial ischemia is called:
    A. Coronary artery disease
    B. Aortic insufficiency
    C. Angina pectoris
    D. Congestive heart failure

Please see the accompanying CD for additional review materials for this section.

CD-ROM

The CD icon indicates areas in which the reader should consult the CD included with the book for additional review materials. The CD contains hundreds of additional review questions, PLUS approximately 10 dictation exercises for each of the systems chapters.

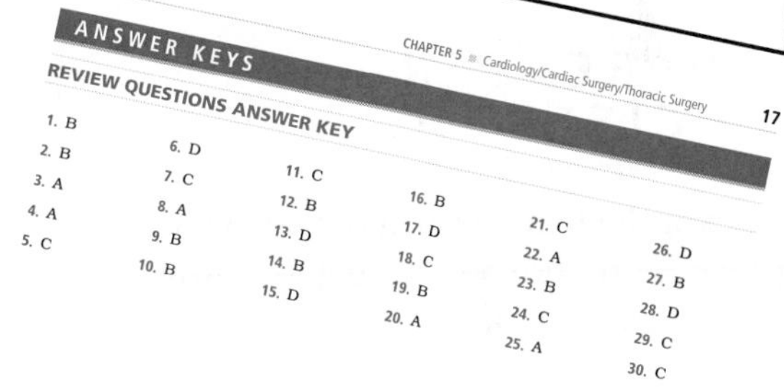

CHAPTER 5 ■ Cardiology/Cardiac Surgery/Thoracic Surgery 17

ANSWER KEYS

REVIEW QUESTIONS ANSWER KEY

1. B
2. B
3. A
4. A
5. C
6. D
7. C
8. A
9. B
10. B
11. C
12. B
13. D
14. B
15. D
16. B
17. D
18. C
19. B
20. A
21. C
22. A
23. B
24. C
25. A
26. D
27. B
28. D
29. C
30. C

REVIEW QUESTIONS ANSWER KEY

Answers are provided to all multiple-choice questions at the end of each chapter.

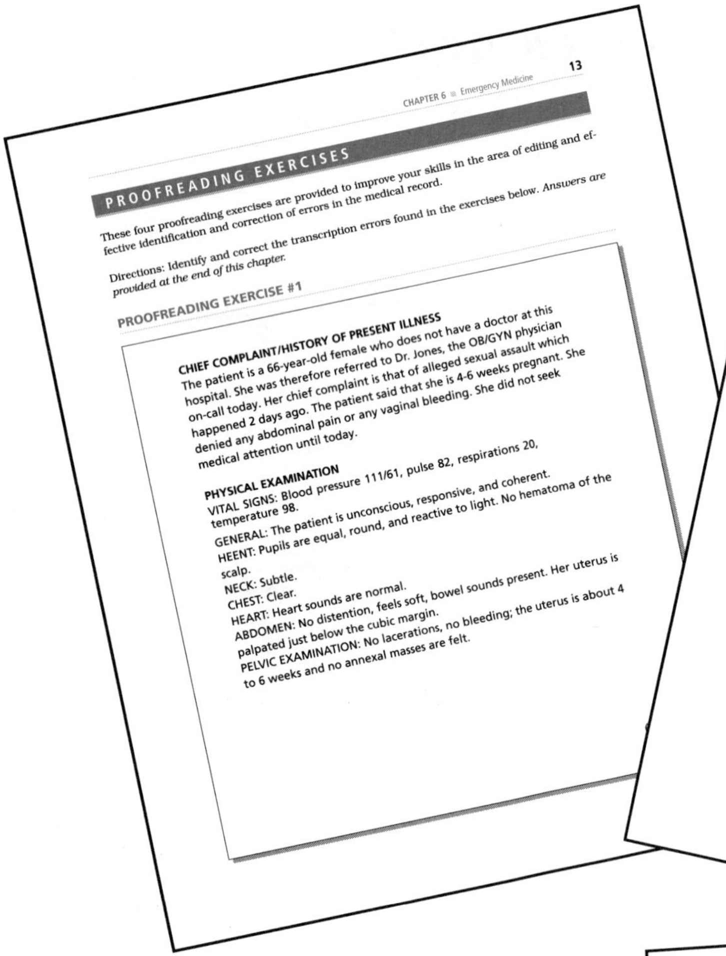

13

CHAPTER 6 ■ Emergency Medicine

PROOFREADING EXERCISES

These four proofreading exercises are provided to improve your skills in the area of editing and effective identification and correction of errors in the medical record.

Directions: Identify and correct the transcription errors found in the exercises below. *Answers are provided at the end of this chapter.*

PROOFREADING EXERCISE #1

CHIEF COMPLAINT/HISTORY OF PRESENT ILLNESS
The patient is a 66-year-old female who does not have a doctor at this hospital. She was therefore referred to Dr. Jones, the OB/GYN physician on-call today. Her chief complaint is that of alleged sexual assault which happened 2 days ago. The patient said that she is 4-6 weeks pregnant. She denied any abdominal pain or any vaginal bleeding. She did not seek medical attention until today.

PHYSICAL EXAMINATION
VITAL SIGNS: Blood pressure 111/61, pulse 82, respirations 20, temperature 98.
GENERAL: The patient is unconscious, responsive, and coherent.
HEENT: Pupils are equal, round, and reactive to light. No hematoma of the scalp.
NECK: Subtle.
CHEST: Clear.
HEART: Heart sounds are normal.
ABDOMEN: No distention, feels soft, bowel sounds present. Her uterus is palpated just below the cubic margin.
PELVIC EXAMINATION: No lacerations, no bleeding; the uterus is about 4 to 6 weeks and no annexal masses are felt.

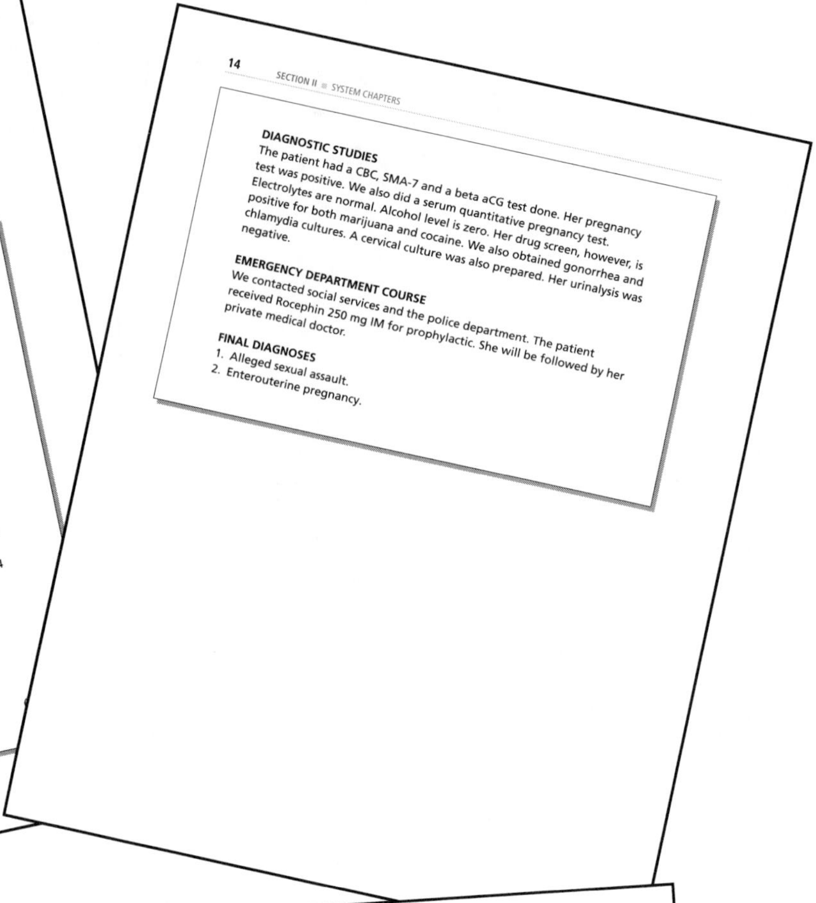

14 SECTION II ■ SYSTEM CHAPTERS

DIAGNOSTIC STUDIES
The patient had a CBC, SMA-7 and a beta aCG test done. Her pregnancy test was positive. We also did a serum quantitative pregnancy test. Electrolytes are normal. Alcohol level is zero. Her drug screen, however, is positive for both marijuana and cocaine. We also obtained gonorrhea and chlamydia cultures. A cervical culture was also prepared. Her urinalysis was negative.

EMERGENCY DEPARTMENT COURSE
We contacted social services and the police department. The patient received Rocephin 250 mg IM for prophylactic. She will be followed by her private medical doctor.

FINAL DIAGNOSES
1. Alleged sexual assault.
2. Enterouterine pregnancy.

PROOFREADING EXERCISES

These exercises at the end of the systems chapters help sharpen your QA editorial and proofreading skills.

PROOFREADING EXERCISES KEY

Answers to the proofreading exercises in the systems chapters feature call-out boxes that show and explain the correct answers.

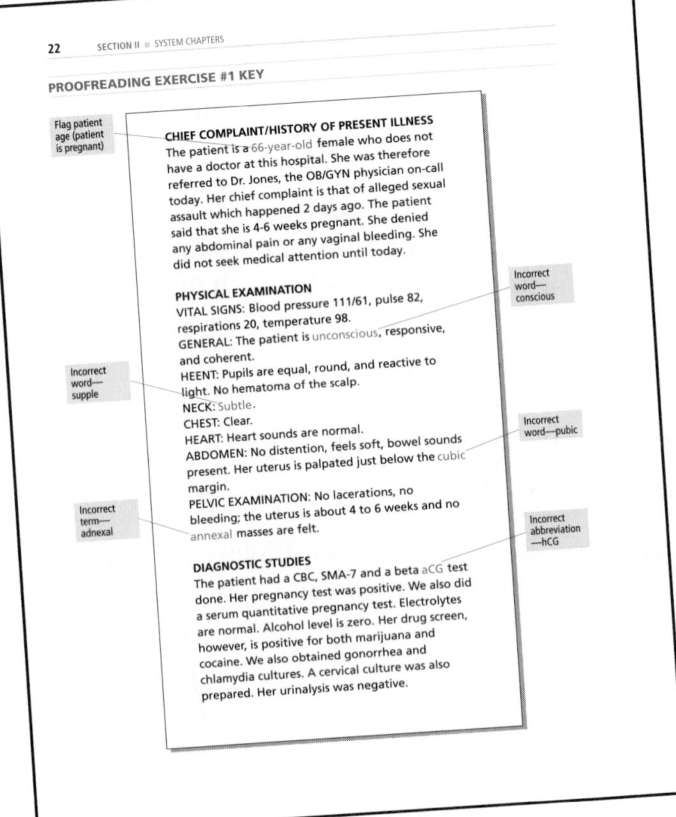
22 SECTION II ■ SYSTEM CHAPTERS

PROOFREADING EXERCISE #1 KEY

CHIEF COMPLAINT/HISTORY OF PRESENT ILLNESS
The patient is a 66-year-old female who does not have a doctor at this hospital. She was therefore referred to Dr. Jones, the OB/GYN physician on-call today. Her chief complaint is that of alleged sexual assault which happened 2 days ago. The patient said that she is 4-6 weeks pregnant. She denied any abdominal pain or any vaginal bleeding. She did not seek medical attention until today.

Flag patient age (patient is pregnant)

PHYSICAL EXAMINATION
VITAL SIGNS: Blood pressure 111/61, pulse 82, respirations 20, temperature 98.
GENERAL: The patient is unconscious, responsive, and coherent.
HEENT: Pupils are equal, round, and reactive to light. No hematoma of the scalp.
NECK: Subtle.
CHEST: Clear.
HEART: Heart sounds are normal.
ABDOMEN: No distention, feels soft, bowel sounds present. Her uterus is palpated just below the cubic margin.
PELVIC EXAMINATION: No lacerations, no bleeding; the uterus is about 4 to 6 weeks and no annexal masses are felt.

Incorrect word—conscious

Incorrect word—supple

Incorrect word—pubic

Incorrect term—adnexal

DIAGNOSTIC STUDIES
The patient had a CBC, SMA-7 and a beta aCG test done. Her pregnancy test was positive. We also did a serum quantitative pregnancy test. Electrolytes are normal. Alcohol level is zero. Her drug screen, however, is positive for both marijuana and cocaine. We also obtained gonorrhea and chlamydia cultures. A cervical culture was also prepared. Her urinalysis was negative.

Incorrect abbreviation—hCG

Acknowledgements

I would like to thank the following individuals who were instrumental in the writing of the CMT Review Guide.

My primary contributing authors include: Sherry Roth, PA, CMT, FAAMT, who assisted in too many areas to list here, and Peggy Beck, RHIA, CMT, FAAMT, who assisted in writing the HIM section as well as the psychiatry/psychology section.

Others who provided material or wrote questions include: Suzanne Gallivan, CMT, for the plurals and foreign words section, Sharon Walcott, CMT, for some questions in the ENT section, Phyllis Gursky for some questions in the hematology/oncology section, and Patricia McCoy for some questions in the dermatology section.

I would also like to thank the following people for their guidance, wisdom, and overall support: Alfred G. Smith, MD, for his assistance with the ophthalmology chapter, Kenneth Schafer, of Expert Medical Transcription, Inc., for his understanding when my daily production dropped due to "pressing book issues," and my husband, Carter Honkonen, for picking up my spirits on a daily basis and just for listening when I needed to "vent."

Others who provided sample reports and without whom this project would have been much more difficult, include: Kathy Martin, CMT; Mary Beth Evans, CMT; Laura Bryan, CMT; Linda Merino; Joanne Griffin, CMT; Challis Kelchner; Janet Distefano; and one very good "mystery" friend, who wishes to remain anonymous (you know who you are).

I would be remiss if I failed to thank Ann Donnelly, MS, CMT, FAAMT, for asking me to take on this project in the first place, and Peter Preziosi, PhD, CAE, Executive Director of AAMT, who was supportive and motivational throughout the course of this project. I also appreciate the guidance provided by Julie Stegman and Eric Branger of Lippincott Williams & Wilkins.

Finally, I would like to thank Lea Sims, CMT, FAAMT, Director of Publications for AAMT and overall coordinator of this project for AAMT. In addition to her assistance with writing in the English language section, Lea entered management of this project very late but took the reins and led it through many changes in order to provide the best possible product to assist medical transcriptionists who need a place to start when studying for the CMT examination.

Betty Honkonen, CMT, FAAMT

Reviewers

The publishers, author, and editors gratefully acknowledge the valuable contributions made by the following professionals who reviewed this text:

Catherine Baxter
Plantersville, Texas

Ruth Chaney, CMT, FAAMT
Mosinee, Wisconsin

Susan Lucci, CMT, RHIT
Parker, Colorado

P.J. Posey, CMT
Coppell, Texas

Kathy Schleis, CMT, RHIT, CHP
Manitowoc, Wisconsin

Janet Stiles, BSN
Richardson, Texas

Pat Vargo, CMT
Abingdon, Maryland

Sharon Walcott, CMT
Miami, Florida

Kristin Wall
Orange Park, Florida

Table of Contents

SECTION I

Medical Language

CHAPTER 1

Medical Language Fundamentals

OBJECTIVES CHECKLIST

A prepared exam candidate will know the:

- ❑ Common prefixes and suffixes utilized in medical language.
- ❑ Latin and Greek roots used in the formation of medical terms.
- ❑ Role and function of combining vowels in the formation of medical terms.
- ❑ Fundamentals of word formation with affixes, roots, and combining vowels.
- ❑ Methods for deconstructing words based on these fundamental parts for the purpose of identification and definition.

RESOURCE FOR STUDY

The Language of Medicine
Chapter 1: Basic Word Structure, pp. 1–30.
Chapter 3: Suffixes, pp. 75–107.
Chapter 4: Prefixes, pp. 109–138.

PREFIXES AND SUFFIXES

Prefixes with Variant Meanings

PREFIX	MEANING	EXAMPLES
ab-	from, away, off	abnormal, abdicate
ad-	to, toward	adhere, adjoin
ante-	before, in front of, earlier than	antecedent, antecubital
anti-	opposite of, hostile to	antibiotic, antisocial
be-	make, against, to a great degree	belittle, bemoan
bi-	two, twice	bicycle, bivalve
de-	away, opposite of, reduce	deactivate, devitalize
dia-	through, across	diameter, diagonal
dis-	opposite of, apart, away	dissatisfy, disjointed
en-	cause to be, put in or on	enable, engulf
syn-	with, together	synchronize, synthesis
trans-	across, beyond, through	transabdominal, transaction
ultra-	beyond in space, excessive	ultraviolet, ultramodern
un-	not, the opposite of	unable, unwind

Prefixes/Suffixes with Invariant Meanings

PREFIX	MEANING	EXAMPLES
anthropo-	man	anthropoid
auto-	self	autonomous
biblio-	book	bibliography
bio-	life	biology
centro-	center	centrofacial
centri-	center	centrifuge
cosmo-	universe	cosmonaut
heter-/hetero-	different	heterosexual
homo-	same	homosexual
hydro-	water	hydroplane
iso-	equal	isometrics
lith-/litho-	stone	lithography
micro-	small	microscope
macro-	large	macrophage
mono-	one	monocyte
neuro-	nerve	neurologist
omni-	all	omnipotent
pan-	all	panchromatic
penta-	five	pentagram
phil-/philo-	love	philanthropist
phono-	sound	phonograph

SUFFIX	MEANING	EXAMPLES
-fication/-ation	action of, process of	classification, dramatization
-gram	written or drawn	diagram
-graph	writing, recording, or drawing	telegraph, lithograph
-graphy	description of a subject or field	oceanography
-ics	the science or art of	athletics
-itis-	inflammation	tonsillitis
-latry	the worship of	idolatry
-meter	measuring device	thermometer
-metry	process of measuring	photometry
-ology/-logy	the study of	cardiology
-phore	bearer or producer	semaphore
-phobia	illogical fear	claustrophobia
-scope	observing instrument	microscope
-scopy	seeing or observing	microscopy
-ance	These noun suffixes are used to form abstract nouns with the meaning of "quality, state, or condition," and action or result of an action.	tolerance
-ation		adoration
-ion		incision
-ism		truism
-dom		kingdom
-ery		monastery
-mony		matrimony
-ment		government
-tion		sanction
-er	These noun suffixes pertain to living or non-living agents.	helper
-eer		engineer
-grapher		photographer
-ess		princess
-ier		courier
-ster		monster
-ist		Marxist
-stress		mistress
-trix		executrix

GREEK AND LATIN ROOTS

Greek Root Words

ROOT	MEANING	EXAMPLES
aero	air	aerial, aerodynamics
aesthet	perception	anesthetic
amphi	both ways	amphibious, amphitheater
anthro	man	anthropologist
archaeo	primitive, ancient	archaeology
ast	star	asterisk, astrophysics
atmo	vapor, steam	atmosphere
auto	self	automatic, autobiography
baro	pressure	barometer
biblio	book	bibliography, bible
bio	life	biology, biography
card/cardio	heart	cardiac, cardiology
chrono	time	chronological
cosmo	world, universe	cosmopolitan
crypto	hidden, secret	cryptography

cyclo	wheel	cycle, bicycle
deca	ten	decade
demo	people	democracy
dont	teeth	orthodontist
electro	electric	electricity
ethno	race, nation	ethnicity
gam	marriage	polygamy
geo	earth	geography
graph/gram	write	telegraph, telegram
gyn	woman	gynecologist
gyro	circle	gyroscope
helio	the sun	helioscope
hema/hemo	blood	hematoma, hemophilia
hemi	half	hemisphere, hemiparesis
hetero	different	heterogeneous
holo	whole	holocaust
homo	same	homogeneous
hydro	water	hydroplane
hypno	sleep	hypnosis
hypo	under, below	hypodermic
iatry	medical treatment	psychiatry, podiatry
ideo	idea	idealogy
iso	equal, alike	isometric, isobar
kilo	one thousand	kilogram
kine/cine	move	kinetic, cinema
litho	stone	monolith, lithography
log	word	dialogue, apology
macro	large	macrocephaly
mania	madness	maniac
mech	machine	mechanical
mega	great	megaphone
meter	measure	barometer, thermometer
micro	small	microscope, microbe

Latin Root Words

ROOT	MEANING	EXAMPLES
act	do	action, reaction
agri	field, soil	agriculture
alt	high	altimeter, altitude
ambi	both ways	ambidextrous, ambiguous
amo/ami	love	amiable, amorous
ang	bend	angle, rectangle
anim	feeling	animosity, animation
ann/enn	year	annual, anniversary
apt/ept	suitable	aptitude, ineptitude
aqua	water	aquatic, aquarium
art	skill	artistic, artisan
aud/audit	hear	auditorium, audition
bene	good	benefit, benediction
brev	short	brevity, abbreviate
cap	head	cap, captain, capitol
cede/ceed	go	proceed, exceed
ceive/cept	seize	receive, receptacle
centi	100	century, centipede
cent	center	centrifuge
cert	sure	certain, certified
cide/cise	cut, kill	suicide, scissor, incise

circ	around	circle, circular
clam/claim	shout	proclaim, clamor
clar	clear	clarity, declare
cline	lean	incline, recline, decline
clud/clos/clus	shut	include, closet, seclusion
cogn	know	recognize, cognition
corp	body	corporal, corporation
counter/contra	against	counteract, contradict
cranio	skull	craniology, cranium
cred	believe	credit, incredible
curr	run	current, occurrence
dict	speak	dictate, predict
domin	master	dominate, predominate
deci	one-tenth	decibel
don/donat	give	donation, donor
duct	lead	conduct, conductor
equ	equal	equality, equilibrium
fac/fec	make, do	manufacture, affect
fic/fy	make, do	suffice, classify
fer	carry	ferry, transfer
fibor	fiber	fibrous, fibrovascular
fict	pretend	fiction, fictitious
fid	faithful	fidelity, confidence
firm	fixed	infirm, confirm
flect/flex	bend	reflection, reflex
form	shape	conform, formula
fract/frag	break	fracture, fragment
frater	brother	fraternity
fuga/fugi	flee	fugitive, refugee
grad/gress	by steps	gradually, progress
grat	pleasing, thankful	grateful, congratulate
plic/plex	interweave, fold	complicated, perplex
plur	more	plural
pop	people	population, popular
port	carry	portable, transport
pos/pon	place, put	position
post	after	postmortem, postscript
prehend	seize	comprehend
prehens	seize	comprehension
prim/princ	first	primitive, principle
pugn	fight	pugilist
put	think	reputation, disreputable
quadri/quad	four	quadrilateral, quadruplet
quer/ques/quis	seek	query, question, inquisitive
rad/ray	spoke, ray, root	radius, radiate
rect	straight	erect, rectify, direction
reg	king	regal, reign
rid	laugh	ridicule, deride
rupt	break	rupture, abrupt, bankrupt
san	healthy	sanitary, sane
scend	climb	ascend, descendant
scribe/script	write	inscribe, scripture
sect	cut	dissect, intersect
sept	seven	septuplets
sens	feelings	sensible, sensitive
serv	serve	servant, service
sess/set	sit	session, settle
sex	six	sextet
sign	mark	signature, signal
sim	like	similar, simultaneous

sist/stat	stand	insist, status
sol	alone	solo, solitary
solv/solu	loosen	dissolve, solution
spec/spic	see	spectator, suspicion
spir	breathe	spirometry, respiration
stell	star	stellate, stellar
stimu	whip	stimulation
strict	tighten	restrict, constriction
struct	build	construct, instructor
sum/sup	superior	supreme, summit
tact/tang	touch	intact, tangible
temp	time	temporary, temporal
ten/tend	hold, stretch	retentive, intend
term	end	terminal, determine
terr	land	terrain, territory
tex	weave	textile, texture
tort	twist	torture, contortion
tract	pull, drag	tractor, attraction
trans	across	transport, transdermal
trib	give	contribute, tributary
trud/trus	push	intrude, protrusion
turb	confusion	disturb, turbulence
vag	wander	vagabond, vagrant
var	different	variant, varied
ven/vent	come	convention, intervene
vert	turn	convert, reverse
vict/vince	conquer	victory, convince
vis/vid	see	vision, evidence
viv/vit	live	vivid, vitamin
voc	voice	vocal, advocate
volv	roll	revolver, revolutionary

COMBINING FORMS

When a suffix beginning with a consonant is added to a root word, a vowel (usually an o) is inserted to aid in pronunciation. Some examples are:

neur + o + logy = neurology (study of the nervous system)

cardi + o + logy = cardiology (study of the heart)

gastr + o + enterology = gastroenterology (study of the stomach and intestines)

In many textbooks, the **combining vowels** are separated from the root words with a virgule (/) such as: nephr/o, cephal/o, and hyster/o.
In this format, the root is usually referred to as the *combining form.*

A combining vowel is not necessary if the ending begins with a vowel as follows:

cyst + itis = cystitis (inflammation of the urinary bladder)

gastr + itis = gastritis (inflammation of the stomach)

card + itis = carditis (inflammation of the heart)

Some exceptions to this rule do occur in order to make medical terms easier to pronounce. These will be obvious to you as you encounter them. It is important to note in the examples above that you must often start with the suffix when attempting to define a word based on its constructed forms. Once the suffix has been defined, you should begin at the front of the word and work to the right in breaking the word down by parts.

REVIEW EXERCISES

I. For each of the combining forms, prefixes, or suffixes below, select the correct definition.

1. erythr/o
   A. blood
   B. red
   C. swelling
   D. rash

2. kary/o
   A. nucleus
   B. potassium
   C. hard, cornea
   D. humpback

3. furc/o
   A. luminous
   B. resembling
   C. fungus
   D. forking

4. ipsi-
   A. same
   B. contralateral
   C. transverse
   D. process

5. nos/o
   A. nose
   B. hospital
   C. disease
   D. none

6. –physis
   A. to grow
   B. plant
   C. role, function
   D. to bear

7. thec/o
   A. spine
   B. vertebra
   C. sheath
   D. membrane

8. hol/o
   A. heart
   B. whole
   C. hollow
   D. natural

9. myx/o
   A. mixed, combined
   B. muscle
   C. genetically altered
   D. mucus

10. eu-
    A. new
    B. good; normal
    C. out, away from
    D. inward

II. For each definition based on word parts, provide the correct formed term. *Hint: Word parts will not always be arranged in the same order as the definition provided.*

11. (pertaining to) + (the study of) + (bacteria)
12. (incomplete) + (dilation/expansion)
13. (person who) + (records) + (words/phrases)
14. (pertaining to) + (many) + (form/shape) + (nuclear)
15. (condition of) + (lung) + (dust)
16. (condition of) + (all) + (deficient) + (pituitary)
17. (stimulating the function of) + (adrenal) + (cortex)
18. (deficiency of) + (granules) + (cells)
19. (condition of) + (varied/irregular) + (cells)
20. (pertaining to) + (mind) + (body)

ANSWER KEY

REVIEW EXERCISES

1. B
2. A
3. D
4. A
5. C
6. A
7. C
8. B
9. D
10. B
11. bacteriologic
12. atelectasis
13. lexicographer
14. polymorphonuclear
15. pneumoconiosis
16. panhypopituitarism
17. adrenocorticotropin
18. granulocytopenia
19. poikilocytosis
20. psychosomatic

CHAPTER 2

Foreign Influence on Medical Language

OBJECTIVES CHECKLIST

A prepared exam candidate will know the:

- ❑ Greek alphabet, particularly those letters that are commonly used alone or in conjunction with other terms in medical language.
- ❑ Rules for pluralizing Greek and Latin terms.
- ❑ Common French terminology encountered in medical language.
- ❑ Common German terminology encountered in medical language.

RESOURCE FOR STUDY

The AAMT Book of Style for Medical Transcription
Foreign terms, p. 174.
French, p. 182.
Greek letters, pp. 197–198.
Latin abbreviations, pp. 237–238.
Plurals, pp. 318–323.

OVERVIEW

The current lexicography of medical language is vast and complex. This living and constantly evolving language has been profoundly influenced over time by a diverse number of cultural and linguistic sources, many of which are still evident in the language today. While certainly the English medical terms with which we are familiar can be etymologically traced to earlier language forms, there are quite a few foreign terms that remain unaltered in circular usage today. It is important for an MT to be aware of their use and application as well as the appropriate way to document them.

GREEK LANGUAGE

Greek Alphabet

α	alpha
β	beta
χ	chi
δ	delta
ε	epsilon
η	eta
γ	gamma
ι	iota
κ	kappa
λ	lamda
μ	mu
ν	nu
ω	omega
ο	omicron
φ	phi
π	pi
ψ	psi
ρ	rho
ς, σ	sigma
τ	tau
θ	theta
υ	upsilon
ξ	xi
ζ	zeta

The Greek alphabet appears frequently in laboratory data and sometimes elsewhere. Some examples are:

alpha-fetoprotein

beta blockers

gamma knife

delta wave

Omega compression hip screw

Greek plurals are fairly simple, if you know the rules, as follow:

-a changes to –ata:

stigma to *stigmata*

condyloma to *condylomata*

-on changes to –a:

phenomenon to *phenomena*

criterion to *criteria*

-s changes to –des:

iris to *irides*

epididymis to *epididymides*

arthritis to *arthritides*

EXCEPT for:

–osis which changes to –oses:

anastomosis to *anastomoses*

diagnosis to *diagnoses*

-x changes to –ces or –ges:

varix to *varices*

phalanx to *phalanges*

LATIN TERMINOLOGY & USAGE

"Vox audita perit; litera scripta manet"

Latin proverb meaning: *"The spoken word perishes; the written word remains."*

Some commonly misspelled (and mispronounced) Latin terms:

et al. *et alia—and other individuals*

etc. *et cetera—and other things*

vice versa—with the order reversed

LATIN PLURALS

The most common plural formations include the following:

-a to –ae:

ulna to *ulnae*

concha to *chonchae*

-us to −i:

radius to *radii*

musculus to *musculi*

-um to −a:

acetabulum to *acetabula*

atrium to *atria*

Examples of other Latin plurals:

SINGULAR	PLURAL	SINGULAR	PLURAL
adnexa	no plural—collective noun	*labium*	*labia*
carpus	*carpi*	*matrix*	*matrices*
corpus	*corpora*	*naris*	*nares*
coxa	*coxae*	*os (mouth)*	*ora*
crus	*crura*	*os (bone)*	*ossa*
genu	*genua*	*sequela*	*sequelae*
hallux	*halluces*	*vomer*	plural not used

NOMINA ANATOMICA

Some of the most difficult Latin terminology to master is included in the Nomina Anatomica (noted as N.A. in your medical dictionary). The Nomina Anatomica is the collection of formal names given to parts of the anatomy by an official (universal) organization of scientists. Forming plurals from these names can be a challenge, and here is why:

Latin nouns require different endings for different uses in sentences, for differences in number (singular/plural), and even for differences in gender.

Some of the uses in sentences include the following:

Subject (nominative)
Possessive form (genitive)—basically a modifier
Indirect object (dative)
Object of verb (accusative)
Object of preposition (ablative)

Latin verbs are rarely seen in medical terminology, except for the participial (participle) form, which is used as an adjective. The endings for adjectives (including participles) change to agree with the noun modified, including the gender of that noun.

Examples:
curriculum vitae (course of one's career/life)—singular noun plus possessive singular form of noun

lupus erythematosus (red wolf)—masculine singular noun, masculine singular adjective

flexor digitorum longus (N.A.)—masculine singular noun, genitive plural noun, masculine singular form of adjective

(tendo) dorsalis pedis—masculine singular noun, masculine/feminine singular form of adjective, possessive singular form of noun

valvulae conniventes (N.A. plicae circulares)—feminine plural noun, masculine/feminine plural adjective, probably a participle

Some medical phrases combine Greek and Latin (or Latinize the Greek).

Examples:
Condylomata acuminata—appears to contain two similar word endings, but it is actually the plural of condyloma acuminatus. *Condyloma* needs the Greek –*a* to –*ata* rule, and *acuminatus* needs the Latin –*um* to –*a* rule.

You can see why it would be easy for the MT novice to use the wrong Latin ending inadvertently, thus creating a form which says the wrong thing.

It is recommended that MTs memorize and/or print a list of the correct spellings for commonly used Latin words and phrases, and use a reliable medical dictionary for the others.

The information above will, hopefully, help you to do effective research into Latin forms and endings. It will also relieve confusion due to Latin endings that are not the same (or not different) when you expect them to be.

SINGULAR AND PLURAL OF SOME LATIN NOUNS

Typical declension of noun or adjective ending in –a:

	SINGULAR	PLURAL
Nominative	vertebra	vertebrae
Genitive	vertebrae	vertebrarum
Dative	vertebrae	vertebris
Accusative	vertebram	vertebras
Ablative	vertebra	vertebris

Typical declension of noun or adjective ending in –us:

	SINGULAR	PLURAL
Nominative	humerus	humeri
Genitive	humeri	humerorum
Dative	humero	humeris
Accusative	humerum	humeros
Ablative	humero	humeris

Typical declension of noun or adjective ending in –um:

	SINGULAR	PLURAL
Nominative	ovum	ova
Genitive	ovi	ovorum
Dative	ovo	ovis
Accusative	ovum	ova

Ablative	ovo	ovis

Declension of another kind of noun:

	SINGULAR	PLURAL
Nominative	corpus	corpora
Genitive	corporis	corporum
Dative	corpori	corporibus
Accusative	corpus	corpora
Ablative	corpore	corporibus

*There are many variations in type of noun. There are also irregular nouns, which do not follow any of the rules.

FRANCO-PRUSSIAN INFLUENCES (FRENCH AND GERMAN)

FRENCH

(Definitions given here are the most common ones. Please refer to your medical dictionary for other related definitions.)

café au lait	pigmented spots seen on skin in neurofibromatosis
cerclage	encircling with a ring or loop, as in an incompetent cervix
curettage	removal of material from a wall or a cavity
déjà vu	the illusion that a new situation has been experienced before
debridement	removal of foreign matter and unhealthy tissue, as from a wound
en bloc	in a lump
en face	head on
fourchette	posterior union of labia minora
gavage	forced feeding by tube, superalimentation
grand mal	major seizure with aura, sudden loss of consciousness, and generalized convulsion
jamais vu	the illusion that a familiar situation is being experienced for the first time (opposite of déjà vu)
lavage	washing out or irrigating, especially the stomach or bowel
mal de mer	seasickness
peau d'orange	dimpling of the skin, as seen in breast cancer
petit mal	minor seizure with only momentary loss of consciousness
torsade de pointes	a ventricular tachycardia with waxing and waning QRS amplitudes. It produces an EKG pattern resembling a ballet step. Translates as "twist on the toes."

GERMAN

blitz	bombardment, as with radioactive particles or a combination of medications
dauernarkose	prolonged sleep
dauerschlaf	prolonged sleep
ersatz	synthetic or artificial
gegenhalten	involuntary resistance to passive movement, as in disorders of the cerebral cortex
grubelsucht	an obsessive/compulsive tendency to worry over trifles
leistungskern	functional part of a cell
mittelschmerz	pain between menstrual periods
schnauskrampf	a facial grimace resembling pouting
sitz (bath)	immersion of the hips and buttocks for relief of rectal, urethral, vaginal, or pelvic discomfort
steinstrasse	literally, "stone street"—residual stone fragments following extracorporeal shock wave lithotripsy

Reference: The entire section is being reprinted with permission from the author: Suzanne Gallivan, CMT.

REVIEW EXERCISES

I. For each of the singular forms below, provide the plural form.

1. criterion
2. arthritis
3. phenomenon
4. meniscus
5. urethra
6. nucleus pulposus
7. uterus
8. placenta previa
9. diagnosis
10. foramen

II. For each of the plural forms below, provide the singular form.

11. diverticula
12. epididymides
13. stamina
14. adnexa
15. biceps
16. conjunctivae
17. cerebra
18. verrucae vulgares
19. musculi trapezii
20. ganglia

ANSWER KEY

REVIEW EXERCISES

1. criteria
2. arthritides
3. phenomena
4. menisci
5. urethrae
6. nuclei polposi
7. uteri
8. placentae previae
9. diagnoses
10. foramina
11. diverticulum
12. epididymis
13. stamen
14. adnexa
15. biceps
16. conjunctiva
17. cerebrum
18. verruca vulgaris
19. musculus trapezius
20. ganglion

CHAPTER 3

Abbreviations and Acronyms

OBJECTIVES CHECKLIST

A prepared exam candidate will know the:

- ❏ Definitions and terminology related to abbreviations.
- ❏ Rules and exceptions governing use of abbreviations in the medical record.
- ❏ Rules and exceptions governing the use of acronyms and brief forms in the medical record.
- ❏ Rules for capitalizing and punctuating abbreviations, acronyms, and brief forms.

OVERVIEW

The use of abbreviations in health encounter documentation is widely prevalent. There are many factors and considerations that have to be taken into account when establishing practices and policies governing their use in transcription. The primary consideration for the expansion or retention of a dictated abbreviation should be the promotion of clarity. Attention must be paid to the potential for misinterpretation when encountering abbreviations in dictation. However, it is important to note there are other potential considerations that an MT will ultimately encounter in the workplace.

Facility Policy

As with other points of style and standards, provider/client preference will often be the final word on this issue. A healthcare provider or facility that is concerned about transcription costs, particularly in a per-unit billing environment, may restrict the expansion of many abbreviations despite the standards outlined here. Other providers and facilities may be more risk-management-minded and require the expansion of all abbreviations. It is important for the MT student to be aware that variability in the application of these standards may exist in the job setting.

Productivity

It is important to note that the decision to expand an abbreviation should never be made on the basis of its impact on productivity or potential wages, even in the absence of a company policy or provider preference. Transcribing a dictated abbreviation in abbreviated or expanded form should be based on the rules and exceptions outlined in this text with consideration for facility policies. The utilization of word expansion software to increase productivity often facilitates the quick and easy expansion of any and all abbreviations encountered in dictation; however, their expansion or retention should be judiciously considered based on these principles and *not* on productivity goals.

DEFINITIONS

Abbreviation A shortened form of a word or phrase used chiefly in writing, such as *USMC* for *United States Marine Corps*. Types: *Acronyms, Initialisms, & Brief Forms*

Acronym An abbreviation formed from the initial letters of each of the successive words or major parts of a compound term or of selected letters of a word or phrase **that is pronounced as a word** (*AIDS, GERD, LASIK*).

Initialism An abbreviation formed from the initial letters of each of the successive words or major parts of a compound term or of selected letters of a word or phrase **that is not pronounced as a word but by each letter** (*ALS, CPK, HIV*).

Brief Forms An abbreviation that results in a shortened form of a single word rather than the initial letters of a series of words (*phone, exam, Pap smear, labs*).

RULES AND EXCEPTIONS

I. When and Why

Transcribe abbreviations if they are commonly used and widely recognized. Again, clarity is the goal in making these transcription decisions. Keep in mind the following rules and exceptions:

A. **Terms dictated in full.** Do not use an abbreviation when a term is dictated in full.

Exception: units of measure (*milligrams, centimeters, etc.*) (see below)

B. **Diagnosis and operative titles.** Write out an abbreviation in full if it is used in the admission, discharge, preoperative, or postoperative diagnosis; consultative conclusion; or operative title. These are critical points of information, and their meanings must be clear to ensure accurate communication for patient care, reimbursement, statistical purposes, and medicolegal documentation.

DICTATED
DIAGNOSIS: AML.

TRANSCRIBED
DIAGNOSIS: AML.

Flag report for verification.

C. **Units of measure.**

1. Abbreviate most *metric* units of measure that accompany numerals and include virgule constructions. Use the same abbreviation for singular and plural forms. Do not use periods with abbreviated units of measure. Use these abbreviations only when a numeric quantity precedes the unit of measure.

   Examples:
   She was put on 2 L of oxygen.
   An approximately 2.5 cm incision was made.

   BUT

   The wound measured several centimeters.

2. Spell out common *nonmetric* units of measure to express weight, depth, distance, height, length, and width, except in tables. Do not abbreviate most nonmetric units of measure, except in tables.

   Examples:
   The baby weighed 8 pounds 9 ounces.
   She gave the child 2 tablespoons of Motrin.

D. **Dangerous and obscure abbreviations.** Do not use abbreviations found on the "Dangerous Abbreviations" list from the Institute for Safe Medication Practices (See Appendix 4). In addition to those found on the list, avoid any abbreviation that is obscure (like *a.c.b* for *before breakfast*) or any others that are potentially dangerous. For example, *b.i.w.* is both obscure *and* dangerous. It is intended to mean *twice weekly* but it could be mistaken for *twice daily*, resulting in a dosage frequency seven times that intended.

E. **Business names.** Some businesses are readily recognized by their abbreviations or acronyms and may be referred to by same if dictated and if there is reasonable assurance the business will be accurately identified by the reader. Most abbreviated forms use all capitals and do not use periods, but be guided by the entity's designated abbreviated form.

Examples:
IBM equipment
He is an ACLU attorney.
She found the item on eBay.

F. **Geographic names.** Abbreviate state and territory names when they are preceded by city, state, or territory name. Do not abbreviate names of states, territories, countries, or similar units within reports when they stand alone. Use abbreviations in state names in an address (such as in a letter or on an envelope).

Examples:
She was seen in an ER in Orlando, FL, a month ago.
The patient moved here 3 years ago from Canada.

G. **Units of time.** Do not abbreviate English units of time except in virgule constructions. Do not use periods with such abbreviations.

Examples:
The patient is 5 days old.
He will return in 1 week for followup.
Her IV was set to run at 10 mcg/min while in the ER.

II. Grammar & Punctuation

A. **Placement.**

1. A sentence may begin with a dictated abbreviation, or such abbreviated forms may be extended.

DICTATED
WBC was 9200.

TRANSCRIBED
WBC was 9200. *OR*
White blood count was 9200.

2. Avoid separating a numeral from its associated unit of measure or accompanying abbreviation; that is, keep the numeral and unit of measure together at line breaks.

..The specimen measured
4 cm in diameter.
OR
..The specimen measured 4 cm
in diameter.

NOT
..The specimen measured 4
cm in diameter.

B. **Capitalization.**

1. Capitalize all letters of most acronyms, but when they are extended, do not capitalize the words from which they are formed unless they are proper names.

Examples:
AIDS (*acquired immunodeficiency syndrome*)
BiPAP (*bilateral positive airway pressure*)
TURP (*transurethral resection of prostate*)

2. Do not capitalize abbreviations derived from Latin terms. The use of periods within or at the end of these Latin abbreviations remains the preferred style, although it is also acceptable to drop the periods for general Latin terms.

Use lowercase abbreviations with periods for Latin abbreviations that are related to doses and dosages. Avoid using all capitals because they emphasize the abbreviation rather than the drug name. Avoid lowercase abbreviations without periods because some may be misread as words.

Examples:

e.g.	exempli gratia	*for example*
et al.	et alii	*and others*
etc.	et cetera	*and so forth*
a.c.	ante cibum	*before food*
b.i.d.	bis in die	*twice a day*

3. Do not capitalize a brief form unless the extended form is routinely capitalized.

Examples:

segmented neutrophils	*segs*
examination	*exam*
Papanicolaou smear	*Pap smear*
Kirschner wire	*K-wire*

4. Do not capitalize most units of measure or their abbreviations. Learn the obvious exceptions, and consult appropriate references for guidance.

Examples:

meter	*m*	*kilogram*	*kg*
mole	*mol*	*centimeter*	*cm*

Exceptions:

liter	*L*	*kelvin*	*K*
milliliter	*mL*	*ampere*	*A*
decibel	*dB*	*hertz*	*Hz*
joule	*J*	*milliequivalent*	*mEq*

5. Always capitalize genus name abbreviations when they are accompanied by the species name.

Examples:
H influenzae
E coli
C difficile

C. **Punctuation.**

1. Do not use periods within or at the end of most abbreviations, including acronyms, abbreviated units of measure, and brief forms. Use a period at the end of abbreviated English units of measure if they may be misread without the period (only in virgule and table construction).

Examples:

wbc	*WBC*	*mg*	*cm*
exam	*prep*	*mEq*	*mL*

inch preferred to *in.*
(Do not use *in* for *inch* without a period.)

2. Do not use periods with abbreviated academic degrees and professional credentials.

Examples:
John Smith, MD
Mary Jones, CMT
Robert Williams, PhD

3. Use periods in lowercase drug-related abbreviations derived from Latin terms.

   Examples:
   b.i.d. *t.i.d.* *a.c.*
   p.r.n. *p.o.* *q.4 h.*

   NOTE: AAMT continues to discourage dropping periods in lowercase abbreviations that might be misread as words (*bid* and *tid*). If you must drop the periods, use all capitals, but keep in mind that the overuse of capitals, particularly in relation to drug doses and dosages, would draw more attention to the capitalized abbreviations than to the drug names themselves.

4. Periods may be used with courtesy title abbreviations (e.g., *Mr., Mrs.*) and following *Jr.* and *Sr.*, although there is a trend toward dropping them. Either remains acceptable, but be consistent.

5. Use a lowercase *s* without an apostrophe to form the plural of a capitalized abbreviation, acronym, or brief form.

   Examples:
   EKGs *PVCs* *exams*
   labs *monos* *CABGs*

6. Use 's to form the plural of lowercase abbreviations.

   Examples:
   rbc's *wbc's*

7. Use 's to form the plural of single-letter abbreviations.

   Examples:
   X's *K's* *flipped T's*

8. Add 's to most abbreviations or acronyms to show possession.

   Examples:
   The AMA's address is. . .
   AAMT's position paper on full disclosure states. . .

Ultimately, the application of these standards comes down to some fundamental, common sense principles. The objective, as stated initially, is to promote clarity in the healthcare record. An abbreviated form, when used, should meet this objective, and the application of capitalization or the use of punctuation to indicate plurality or possession should likewise promote clarity and be utilized consistently throughout the healthcare record. Of course, the overall goal of these standards is to encourage their consistent use across the entire healthcare delivery system.

REVIEW QUESTIONS

The goal of these questions is to test your knowledge of abbreviations and acronyms. Directions: Select the correct answer for the multiple-choice questions provided below. *Answers are provided at the end of this chapter.*

1. Which of the following is an example of an ACRONYM?
   A. COPD
   B. t.i.d.
   C. CABG
   D. lymphs
2. Which of the following is an example of a BRIEF FORM?
   A. cath
   B. mmHg
   C. BKA
   D. All of the above
3. Which is correctly transcribed?
   A. TITLE OF OPERATION: ORIF, left radius.
   B. DIAGNOSIS: Pyelonephritis with elevated blood urea nitrogen (BUN).
   C. TITLE OF OPERATION: Transurethral resection of the prostate (TURP).
   D. DIAGNOSIS: IDDM.
4. A measurement would be correctly indicated by which of the following?
   A. 2 cm
   B. 3 inches
   C. a few centimeters
   D. All of the above
5. Which would represent the incorrect transcription of a measurement?
   A. 4.5 cm
   B. 3 in
   C. 4 feet
   D. All of the above.
6. The Latin abbreviation referring to "twice per day" would be correctly transcribed as:
   A. bid
   B. B.I.D.
   C. b.i.d.
   D. BID
7. Which represents the incorrect capitalization of an abbreviation?
   A. Differential showed 58 SEGs.
   B. WBC was 48.2.
   C. Urinalysis revealed 8–10 wbc's.
   D. None of the above.
8. Which of the following is correctly pluralized?
   A. serial K's
   B. EKG's
   C. lymph's
   D. rbcs
9. Which of the following genus/species reference is correctly transcribed?
   A. staphylococcus aureus
   B. s. aureus
   C. S Aureus
   D. S aureus
10. Which of the following is correctly transcribed?
    A. The baby weighed 8 lbs 12 oz.
    B. She was instructed to return on a prn basis.
    C. We injected 10 mL of lidocaine.
    D. CBC showed WBC's of 9.2.

ANSWER KEY

REVIEW QUESTIONS ANSWER KEY

1. C
2. A
3. C
4. D
5. B
6. C
7. A
8. A
9. D
10. C

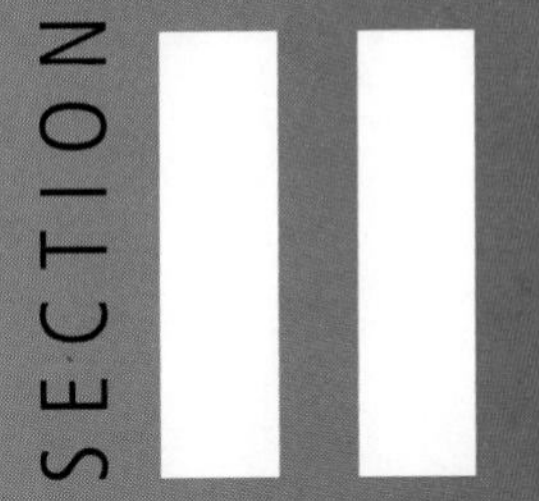

System Chapters

CHAPTER 4

Alternative Medicine

OBJECTIVES CHECKLIST

A prepared exam candidate will know the:

- ❑ Various types of treatment classified as alternative medicine.
- ❑ Basic philosophy of the major alternative therapies.
- ❑ Differences between Eastern and Western philosophy of health and treatment of disease.
- ❑ Most common herbs used in the various forms of alternative therapies.
- ❑ Most common nutritional supplements employed by the various forms of alternative therapies.
- ❑ Role that proper nutrition, exercise, and body mechanics play in the holistic model.

RESOURCES FOR STUDY

1. *Alternative Medicine: The Definitive Guide*
2. *The Professional's Handbook of Complementary and Alternative Medicines*
3. *Encyclopedia of Natural Medicine*

SAMPLE REPORTS

The following five reports are examples of reports you might encounter while transcribing alternative medicine.

ACUPUNCTURE REPORT

HISTORY OF PRESENT ILLNESS
The patient, a 40-year-old male, states that he has had pain in his knees with an intermittent clicking sound since his mid-teens. The discomfort occurs in the evenings and will often awaken him from sleep. It was first diagnosed as simply growing pains, but it continued to bother him and was next thought to be gout. Treatment for gout, however, did not help. Consultation with a sports medicine specialist and an orthopaedic physician led to several tests, including an arthritis panel, which was not remarkable. Radiology studies revealed questionable narrowing of the joints. MRI of the knees revealed a possible meniscal tear on the right.

The patient underwent bilateral arthroscopies, which revealed degenerative tears of the posterior horns of the medial menisci. Joint surfaces were normal, and there was no synovitis. Partial medial meniscectomy with resection of plica was performed bilaterally. The clicking improved, but there was no decrease in pain. He was then referred for acupuncture.

During our interview, the patient mentioned that over the past 5 years or so he has had increasing bouts of insomnia that he believes are caused by increased stress in his workplace and by the unrelenting discomfort in his knees that occurs during the night.

CLINICAL EVALUATION
Manipulation of the knee joints does not appear to cause pain, nor is there evidence of synovitis, effusion, or tenderness. There was, however, tenderness over the superior aspects of the bicipital grooves of both shoulders.

ACUPUNCTURE DIAGNOSES
1. Excess fire in jue yin-shao yang axis.
2. Emotional trauma related to increased workplace stress; external dragon, and perpetuation of the problem secondary to internal dragon.

TREATMENT RATIONALE
1. Disperse excess fire.
2. Tone the controlling element.
3. Release internal and external dragons.

TREATMENT PLAN
He will receive 6 acupuncture treatments, 1 each week. The 1st week will be N, N+1 in the jue yin-shao yang axis; LR3, LR5, MH6, TH5, and GB3, GB4, in dispersion.

HOLISTIC MEDICINE/ASSESSMENT AND PLAN

1. Weight loss. Plan to implement the recommendations based on food sensitivities. By eliminating foods that provoke the immune response, you will be able to shift metabolism and calories in the same direction. By following this diet on a regular basis, you should be able to lose 10 to 15 pounds the first month.
2. Reduce anxiety. Carry sublingual 5-HTP and use it in uneasy circumstances before the sweat begins. Learn breathing exercises and visualization to gain control of your autonomic nervous system. You have direct access to this system based on your integrated mental function. You should be able to learn and use these strategies very effectively.
3. Increase alertness. I believe this is all related to insomnia and poor sleep. Plan to have a dental re-positioner made as soon as possible to alleviate your snoring.
4. Muscle stiffness. Please take high-quality, pharmaceutical-grade mineral supplements, including calcium, zinc, magnesium, and vitamin D to address the problem of your chronic muscle spasm and bone mineral density. Take omega-3 oils to complement these mineral supplements and further reduce muscle spasm. Have deep tissue fascial-release-type massage once or twice a month. Learn and practice a regular stretching regime and use the breathing exercises learned for uneasy circumstances to help control the flow of energy through the body and prevent it from getting congested into the muscles and fascia as is happening now.
5. Irritable bowel symptoms. Plan to take natural aloe to reduce oxidative stress and ease bowel cramping. The mineral supplements and omega-3 oils will also help in this regard. Continue taking fiber on a regular basis and maintain a fluid intake of 100 ounces or more each day.
6. Spirituality. Keep looking and listening. Be as aware as you can. I believe that you can get connected to a much higher level of interconnectedness and from that gain wisdom, insight, and advantage. There is a lot more going on than we are sensually aware, but you have what it takes to know what that is.
7. Cardiovascular assessment. Your total cholesterol of 174 is within the normal range of 150–199. Your HDL, or helpful cholesterol, is barely adequate at 40 (40–70) and should be increased to provide cardioprotection. LDL, or harmful cholesterol, is too high at 113 (50–99) and poses a risk to your future coronary and cerebrovascular health. The noncholesterol-related risk factors homocysteine, fibrinogen, and hsCRP are within normal limits, but the independent risk factor for coronary artery disease and premature coronary dysfunction, called LP(a), is elevated at 66 with a normal of less than 48 and an optimal of less than 30. Please take the nutritional supplements known to lower LDL cholesterol and LP(a), consisting of pharmaceutical-grade flush-free niacin 2 g daily, vitamin C 2 g daily, omega-3 oils 2 g, and nattokinase twice a day. This combination of nutritional supplements should lower these risk factors and help improve your health future.
8. Mineral assessment. All trace, macro, and toxic minerals are within normal limits except for the trace mineral manganese. Manganese is important for protection against oxidative stress and inflammation. Please take a manganese supplement daily for the next 6 months to restore the level of this important trace mineral.
9. Carbohydrate metabolism. Your fasting insulin of 7 (2–18) and blood sugar of 90 (70–110) were within normal limits. Your 2-hour post-challenge insulin was elevated at 20 (2–18) indicating a state of excess insulin secretion and insulin resistance. This condition is called dysinsulinemia. Your 2-hour blood sugar was low at 86 (90–140) indicating a state of reactive hypoglycemia. Reactive hypoglycemia and dysinsulinemia are often seen together. They can

(continued)

be corrected and diabetes and other metabolic problems such as insulin resistance syndrome avoided by taking the natural substance CLA (conjugated linoleic acid) and by adapting the dietary recommendations listed in the addendum based on food sensitivities. This combined program will result in powerful changes in this important system.

10. Adrenal hormone. The adrenal gland makes 2 hormones from the same zone that enables you to respond to stress and recover from stress. The stress recovery hormone, DHEA, is normal at 183 (80–560), but your cortisol, that is the hormone that your gland releases in response to stress, is low at 8.5 (8.7 to 22.4). Frankly, I'm surprised it is not lower given the degree of exhaustion and stress you have endured over the past year. However, this needs to be restored via adequate adrenal support. By taking the antioxidants summarized in the prescription at the conclusion of this report along with the adaptogenic herbs licorice root, Panax ginseng, and ashwaganda, you should be able to recover from this state of insufficiency. Exercise is a vitally important part of that recovery program, as is adequate fluid intake. Please exercise regularly, drink plenty of fluids, and take the supplements described in this report in order to recover normal adrenal function. Let's recheck DHEA and cortisol in 6 weeks to be sure that this has been restored.
11. Bone status. You are beginning to show signs of early demineralization of the bone. Although you do not have osteoporosis at this time, that disease can evolve from this early stage if it is untreated. I suggest that we provide you with pharmaceutical-grade mineral replacement, omega-3 oils to reduce inflammation, and growth hormone to stimulate bone densification. Let's recheck your bone density in 6–12 months to see if healthy bone density has been restored.
12. Brain protection. All of these agents have been proven to improve one aspect or another of brain physiology. The key to brain health is to do most things right and not rely upon a supplement or group of supplements. Once you are doing most things right, try one or a combination of these agents to see if you think, remember, or feel better: ginkgo 240 mg, selegiline 2 mg, lipoic acid 100 mg, AL-carnitine 1 g, SAMe 200 mg twice a day, Enada (NADH 10 mg sublingual), and various amino acid combinations.

TRADITIONAL CHINESE MEDICINE TREATMENT FOR CHRONIC FATIGUE SYNDROME

HISTORY OF PRESENT ILLNESS

The patient is a 42-year-old female who has experienced the symptoms of chronic fatigue syndrome for approximately 5 years. She has been treated by a variety of practitioners, including medical doctors (one of whom diagnosed her as having yuppie flu), chiropractors, an herbalist, and most recently an acupuncturist. Although some drugs and treatments offered temporary relief, she has always relapsed into episodes of debilitating fatigue and loss of energy with chronic achiness and some problem with memory.

EXAMINATION

Keeping in mind that in traditional Chinese medicine deficiency can occur of yin, yang, qi, or blood, I felt the patient's pulse and examined her tongue and abdominal region, which revealed an obvious depletion of body substances and vital energy. Her liver was not adequately manufacturing proteins, hormones, or immune substances, and certain waste products were not efficiently eliminated.

TREATMENT

We discussed the need to eliminate simple sugars from her diet. It was recommended that, because her liver was the organ most affected, her diet include foods that lend support to it. She was advised to eat aduki beans several times each week. Other foods to include in her diet were cooked yams, fish, burdock, parsnips, and turnips.

She was advised that bitter herbs would improve assimilation. She was to take 2 to 4 capsules of gentian root twice daily before meals. She was to take ginger if she experienced gas or pain after eating or loose stools. I also recommended a capsule of an herbal formula of Ligustrum, American ginseng, and lychee berries. She was to take this 3 times daily.

FOLLOWUP

The patient understands that in order to attain optimal results, she must be faithful to the program that was outlined for her. Her history of having chronic fatigue syndrome for a significant time will surely require an investment of effort on her part before she enjoys a lasting benefit from treatment.

REIKI THERAPY NOTE

HISTORY OF PRESENT ILLNESS
The patient is a pleasant 37-year-old female who is currently undergoing chemotherapy for treatment of breast cancer. She was referred to me by her oncologist for Reiki therapy.

The patient understands that Reiki therapy is noninvasive and is used as a healing and stress-reducing technique in combination with her conventional cancer treatment. I also explained that we will repeat this therapy each week, more often if necessary.

TREATMENT
With the patient fully clothed, she reclined on a Reiki table with pillows beneath her head. Hands were placed over the usual 12 energy centers of the body.

The patient remained quiet throughout the session, and I believe she will receive benefit as therapy continues. She will return next week.

AROMATHERAPY CONSULTATION

HISTORY OF PRESENT ILLNESS

The patient has been experiencing considerable stress after the dissolution of a long-time relationship. This has led to frequent bouts of nausea, bloating, and diarrhea that have been diagnosed by her physician as indigestion and irritable bowel syndrome. Traditional medical treatment has been minimally successful, and she comes now for aromatherapy as recommended by a friend.

TREATMENT

I combined the essential oils of chamomile, peppermint, and fennel with a sweet almond carrier oil and massaged the abdomen.

RECOMMENDATIONS

I have recommended that she add 10 drops of chamomile essential oil to her bath water and soak for 15 minutes each night. She will return to see me in 1 week. I also recommended that she meditate in a quiet environment each morning and each evening for at least 15 minutes per session.

REVIEW QUESTIONS

The goal of these questions is to test your knowledge in the area of alternative medicine.

Directions: Select the correct answer for each of the multiple-choice questions provided below. *Answers are provided at the end of this chapter.*

1. An approach to medical care that emphasizes the study of all aspects of a person's health, including psychological as well as social and economic influences on health status, is called:
   A. Complementary
   B. Holistic medicine
   C. Eastern medicine
   D. Acupuncture
2. Chelation therapy is used to treat:
   A. Calcium deposits contributing to cardiovascular disease
   B. Iron overload
   C. Heavy metal toxicity
   D. All of the above
3. Biofeedback therapy has had widespread success in treating:
   A. Cancer in lieu of chemotherapy
   B. Migraine headaches
   C. Asthma attacks
   D. B and C
4. Reiki therapy involves the transfer of energy from the provider to the patient without:
   A. Being in the same room
   B. Touching the patient
   C. Any prior knowledge
   D. The use of mediating oils
5. According to traditional Chinese medicine, the universe is composed of five elements. They are:
   A. Earth, water, air, heaven, & hell
   B. Fire, wind, water, wood, & stars
   C. Fire, earth, metal, water, & wood
   D. Earth, wind, fire, heaven, & earth
6. Which of the following is sometimes used by acupuncturists in lieu of needles?
   A. Moxa
   B. Bamboo cup (cupping)
   C. Dong quai
   D. A and B
7. Some benefits of Shiatsu massage are said to include:
   A. Reversal of osteoporosis
   B. Improvement in CD-4 cell counts of AIDS patients
   C. Mobility improvement of frail, elderly patients
   D. Reduction of pain and muscle stiffness
8. In traditional Chinese medicine, the concept of opposing forces throughout the universe is called:
   A. Chi
   B. Yin and yang
   C. Meridians
   D. Ying and yan
9. In traditional Chinese medicine, meridians are energy pathways for:
   A. Chi
   B. Yin
   C. Yang
   D. Ki
10. The Oriental concept of turning architecture and lifestyle into an art form is called:
    A. Doshas
    B. Chi
    C. Feng shui
    D. Ayurveda

11. Rotating foods is a method of treating patients with:
    A. Finicky tastes
    B. Food allergies
    C. Gastritis
    D. Dysphagia

12. Feelings such as anger, depression, and sadness affect the body's physiologic processes in many ways and make an individual more susceptible to:
    A. Trauma
    B. Disease
    C. Malnutrition
    D. Arrested growth

13. A female massage therapist is called a:
    A. Masseur
    B. Massa
    C. Massini
    D. Masseuse

14. Steam, saunas, mineral soaks, and compresses are examples of:
    A. Hydrotherapy
    B. Body therapy
    C. Massage therapy
    D. Orthomolecular therapy

15. Combining acupressure with Western concepts of medicine to create improved healing is characteristic of:
    A. Orthomolecular medicine
    B. Soma
    C. Shiatsu
    D. Reflexology

16. Promoting mental images through verbal guidance or meditation is sometimes called "mind journeys" but is most often called:
    A. Biofeedback therapy
    B. Visualization therapy
    C. Qigong
    D. Herbal therapy

17. The recommended dosage of vitamin E is 400:
    A. mg
    B. IU (international units)
    C. mcg
    D. SI (standardized units)

18. The recommended dose of folic acid, which may be prescribed as an adjunctive treatment for depression, would be 800:
    A. mg
    B. IU (international units)
    C. mcg
    D. SI (standardized units)

19. Various forms of alternative medicine endeavor to reverse disease and promote health by removing toxic compounds and heavy metals in a process called:
    A. Catabolism
    B. Supplementation
    C. Detoxification
    D. Purification

20. Practitioners of holistic, naturopathic, and environmental medicine view the root cause of chronic fatigue syndrome to be associated with the:
    A. Immune system
    B. Cardiovascular system
    C. Digestive system
    D. Neurological system

21. Ginger is commonly used to treat:
    A. Menstrual pain
    B. Fatigue
    C. Headache
    D. Nausea

22. Mild depression is commonly treated with which of the following natural remedies:
    A. St. John's wort
    B. SAMe
    C. 5-HTP
    D. All of the above

23. Vitamins, minerals, and amino acids are central to the treatment of disease in:
    A. Homeopathy
    B. Ayurvedic medicine
    C. Orthomolecular medicine
    D. Traditional Chinese medicine

24. In homeopathy, the prescribed treatment is called:
    A. A remedy
    B. Chakra
    C. An aggravation
    D. Tincture

25. In homeopathy, the most dilute remedies are:
    A. The most potent
    B. The weakest
    C. The least effective
    D. Used as placebos

26. Nutritional support to stabilize blood sugar in patients with reactive hypoglycemia or pre-diabetic states might include supplementation with:
    A. Calcium
    B. Vitamin D
    C. Chromium
    D. Potassium

27. Leaky gut syndrome, caused by damage to the intestinal mucosa, is believed to be a significant cause of:
    A. Gastritis
    B. Autoimmune disorders
    C. Liver disease
    D. Ulcers

28. Which of the following therapies uses EDTA (ethylenediaminetetraacetic acid)?
    A. Rolfing
    B. Cell therapy
    C. Homeopathy
    D. Chelation

29. Dust, mold, chemicals, and certain foods are evaluated as a cause for chronic disease by physicians practicing:
    A. Environmental medicine
    B. Cellular therapy
    C. Homeopathy
    D. Orthomolecular medicine

30. Ma-huang, echinacea, ginkgo, and valerian are examples of:
    A. Asanas
    B. Herbs
    C. Meridians
    D. Doshas

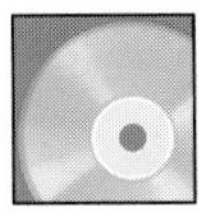

Please see the accompanying CD for additional review materials for this section.

PROOFREADING EXERCISES

These three proofreading exercises are provided to improve your skills in the area of editing and effective identification and correction of errors in the medical record.

Directions: Identify and correct the transcription errors found in the exercises below. *Answers are provided at the end of this chapter.*

PROOFREADING EXERCISE #1

ACUPUNCTURE REPORT

The patient returned for followup of her anxiety and depression associated with her younger brother's deaf. She is taking Ambien alternating with Xanax at night for sleep. In addition to the grief she is dealing with, she also is dealing with her parents-in-law.

Apparently, her in-laws are quite hostel towards the patient's husband. For reasons unclear to patient, the parents-in-law have decided not to come to the patient's daughter's wedding this summer. Her husband is under severe stress and, consequently, the patient finds herself playing the roll of the person who glues the extended family together. She is in the center of taking care of her 6 children, her husband, and her elderly mother. She has some anxiety and increasing dysphonia.

I am going to start her on Lexapro 5 mg at 6:00 p.m.

Otherwise, acupuncture was performed: GV-20, GV-22, GV-24.5, followed by Chong Mo stimulated with 2 Hz. Bilateral KI-3, HT-3, and four gaits were also piqured with KI-3 simulated for 30 minutes as well.

I will see her back again in 2 weeks for followup and support.

PROOFREADING EXERCISE #2

NATURAL REMEDIES FOR MULTIPLE SCLEROSIS

HISTORY OF PRESENT ILLNESS

The patient is a 50-year-old Caucasian female who has had the diagnosis of relapsing/remitting multiple sclerosis for approximately 5 years when plaques were discovered in the brainstem and spinal cord on MRI. The patient's primary complaint at that time was a la meet sign, which caused her significant discomfort. This was treated successfully with Tergal, and that treatment continues today.

The patient comes now to seek alternative care, hoping to avoid advancement of the disease and additional drug therapies. We discussed the disease process, and I advised her that there are no known cures. It is, however, believed that there are some natural remedies that appear to slow the progression and help alleviate certain symptoms such as fatigue.

PLAN

I have asked the patient to follow this regiment for 3 weeks and report her progress. I explained to her that it has been successful for many of the multiple sclerosis patients that I see. The plan is as follows:

1. Replace animal protein with plant protein.
2. Increase intake of fish fiber.
3. Eliminate milk and milk products and reduce other diary intake.
4. Increase originally grown fruits and vegetables in diet.
5. Use olive oil, peanut oil, or cannula oil as main sources of fat.
6. Brew fresh tea daily using ginger route.
7. Take a multi vitamin and an anti oxidant daily.
8. Walk 20 minutes each day during the cool time of day.
9. Mediate in a quiet environment for at least 30 minutes each day.
10. Check into the local multiple sclerosis support group.

PROOFREADING EXERCISE #3

The patient is a 49-year-old housewife who is referred for assessment of chronic back pain and consideration of acupuncture treatment.

The patient began to experience lower back pain in early 2004, at which time she had returned to school to be a personal trainer. She stated that once in class for a few hours, she started to have lower lumber and sacral pain. The pain is band-like, radiating across the back but not to the hip. Standing for a prolonged period of time will also bring on the pain. Sometimes when she bends, she will get some exacerbation. She has had neuromuscular message, which appeared to have helped some for short periods of time. She also found that using a tin unit was somewhat effective; however, once the lower back pain was relieved, the pain would travel up to the midback. She also has perisinus pain in her lower thoracic region. The patient has taken Vicoprofen, about 3 tablets a day, for the past 2 months.

The patient denies being depressed. She was able to sleep pretty well until about February of this year when her husband developed some neurologic problems. He sleeps fitfully, so the patient is unable to sleep through the night. For the past 2 months, she has been taking Zantac 1 mg at night, which has helped. Her appetite is good and her libido is intact.

SOCIAL AND DEVELOPMENTAL HISTORY
She was married at age 25 for 16 years with no children. Her husband was an alcoholic. She was married to her second husband for 6 months, as he was physically abusive. She has been married to her third husband for 1 year. She states that this marriage is good; however, her husband recently has become very ill.

EXAMINATION
Patient is 5-feet-6-inches tall and weighs 119 pounds. She is alert and oriented. She appears 2-BU thymic with a full range of aft. On examination, she has minimal palpable muscle tenderness in her lower back muscles as well as in her paraspinous muscles. When she bends down, she points to her PFIS region as being tender. Patient does not have any evidence of delusional beliefs or perceptual distortions. She denies any suicidal dilations.

(continued)

IMPRESSION
Chronic axil back pain with some myofascial tightness.

RECOMMENDATION
Acupuncture may be able to relieve some of the mild facial pain for this lady, and I am going to perform treatment on her today.

TREATMENT
The patient assumed a zone position. KI-BL, N, M+1 protocols were performed with low-frequency simulation followed by local points from T7 region down to her S1 foremen laterally to PSIS region. The needles were left in place for 20 minutes. After the needles had been removed, I asked patient to do some range of motion exercises. She did not verbalize any increase in pain.

ANSWER KEYS

REVIEW QUESTIONS ANSWER KEY

1. B
2. A
3. D
4. B
5. C
6. D
7. D
8. B
9. A
10. C
11. B
12. B
13. D
14. A
15. C
16. B
17. B
18. C
19. C
20. A
21. D
22. D
23. C
24. A
25. A
26. C
27. B
28. D
29. A
30. B

PROOFREADING EXERCISE #1 KEY

Incorrect word—death

Incorrect word—hostile

Incorrect spelling—role

Incorrect term—dysphoria

Incorrect word—stimulated

Incorrect spelling—gates

ACUPUNCTURE REPORT

The patient returned for followup of her anxiety and depression associated with her younger brother's deaf. She is taking Ambien alternating with Xanax at night for sleep. In addition to the grief she is dealing with, she also is dealing with her parents-in-law.

Apparently, her in-laws are quite hostel towards the patient's husband. For reasons unclear to patient, the parents-in-law have decided not to come to the patient's daughter's wedding this summer. Her husband is under severe stress and, consequently, the patient finds herself playing the roll of the person who glues the extended family together. She is in the center of taking care of her 6 children, her husband, and her elderly mother. She has some anxiety and increasing dysphonia.

I am going to start her on Lexapro 5 mg at 6:00 p.m.

Otherwise, acupuncture was performed: GV-20, GV-22, GV-24.5, followed by Chong Mo stimulated with 2 Hz. Bilateral KI-3, HT-3, and four gaits were also piqured with KI-3 simulated for 30 minutes as well.

I will see her back again in 2 weeks for followup and support.

PROOFREADING EXERCISE #2 KEY

NATURAL REMEDIES FOR MULTIPLE SCLEROSIS

HISTORY OF PRESENT ILLNESS

The patient is a 50-year-old Caucasian female who has had the diagnosis of relapsing/remitting multiple sclerosis for approximately 5 years when plaques were discovered in the brainstem and spinal cord on MRI. The patient's primary complaint at that time was a la meet sign, which caused her significant discomfort. This was treated successfully with Tergal, and that treatment continues today.

The patient comes now to seek alternative care, hoping to avoid advancement of the disease and additional drug therapies. We discussed the disease process, and I advised her that there are no known cures. It is, however, believed that there are some natural remedies that appear to slow the progression and help alleviate certain symptoms such as fatigue.

PLAN

I have asked the patient to follow this regiment for 3 weeks and report her progress. I explained to her that it has been successful for many of the multiple sclerosis patients that I see. The plan is as follows:

1. Replace animal protein with plant protein.
2. Increase intake of fish fiber.
3. Eliminate milk and milk products and reduce other diary intake.
4. Increase originally grown fruits and vegetables in diet.
5. Use olive oil, peanut oil, or cannula oil as main sources of fat.
6. Brew fresh tea daily using ginger route.
7. Take a multi vitamin and an anti oxidant daily.

Incorrect term—Lhermitte

Incorrect drug—Tegretol

Incorrect word—regimen

Missing word—fish and fiber

Incorrect word—dairy

Incorrect word—canola

Incorrect word—organically

Incorrect spelling—root

Use combined form—multivitamin

Use combined form—antioxidant

Incorrect term—meditate

8. Walk 20 minutes each day during the cool time of day.
9. Mediate in a quiet environment for at least 30 minutes each day.
10. Check into the local multiple sclerosis support group.

PROOFREADING EXERCISE #3 KEY

Incorrect term—lumbar

Incorrect term—massage

Incorrect term—paraspinous

Incorrect term—TENS

Incorrect drug—Xanax

The patient is a 49-year-old housewife who is referred for assessment of chronic back pain and consideration of acupuncture treatment.

The patient began to experience lower back pain in early 2004, at which time she had returned to school to be a personal trainer. She stated that once in class for a few hours, she started to have lower lumber and sacral pain. The pain is band-like, radiating across the back but not to the hip. Standing for a prolonged period of time will also bring on the pain. Sometimes when she bends, she will get some exacerbation. She has had neuromuscular message, which appeared to have helped some for short periods of time. She also found that using a tin ~~unit~~ was somewhat effective; however, once the lower back pain was relieved, the pain would travel up to the midback. She also has perisinus pain in her lower thoracic region. The patient has taken Vicoprofen, about 3 tablets a day, for the past 2 months.

The patient denies being depressed. She was able to sleep pretty well until about February of this year when her husband developed some neurologic problems. He sleeps fitfully, so the patient is unable to sleep through the night. For the past 2 months, she has been taking Zantac 1 mg at night, which has helped. Her appetite is good and her libido is intact.

SOCIAL AND DEVELOPMENTAL HISTORY

She was married at age 25 for 16 years with no children. Her husband was an alcoholic. She was married to her second husband for 6 months, as he was physically abusive. She has been married to her third husband for 1 year. She states that this

Incorrect format—no hyphens

Incorrect abbreviation—PSIS

Incorrect term—axial

Incorrect term—myofascial

Incorrect term—stimulation

Incorrect term—to be euthymic

Incorrect term—affect

Incorrect term—ideations

Incorrect term—prone

Incorrect term—foramen

marriage is good; however, her husband recently has become very ill.

EXAMINATION

Patient is 5-feet-6-inches tall and weighs 119 pounds. She is alert and oriented. She appears 2-BU thymic with a full range of aft. On examination, she has minimal palpable muscle tenderness in her lower back muscles as well as in her paraspinous muscles. When she bends down, she points to her PFIS region as being tender. Patient does not have any evidence of delusional beliefs or perceptual distortions. She denies any suicidal dilations.

IMPRESSION

Chronic axil back pain with some myofascial tightness.

RECOMMENDATION

Acupuncture may be able to relieve some of the mild facial pain for this lady, and I am going to perform treatment on her today.

TREATMENT

The patient assumed a zone position. KI-BL, N, M+1 protocols were performed with low-frequency simulation followed by local points from T7 region down to her S1 foremen laterally to PSIS region. The needles were left in place for 20 minutes. After the needles had been removed, I asked patient to do some range of motion exercises. She did not verbalize any increase in pain.

CHAPTER 5

Cardiology/Cardiac Surgery/ Thoracic Surgery

OBJECTIVES CHECKLIST

A prepared exam candidate will know the:

- ❑ Combining forms, prefixes, and suffixes related to the body system.
- ❑ Basic structures of the heart and how they function together.
- ❑ Major vessels of the circulatory system as well as the difference in vessel types and functions.
- ❑ Flow of blood along its full circulatory path and the correct order of coronary structures through which blood flows during the oxygenation process.
- ❑ Electrophysiology of the heartbeat, from the role of the sinoatrial node to ventricular contraction.
- ❑ Fundamentals of blood pressure and the indications of elevated and depressed diastolic and systolic levels.
- ❑ Common signs and symptoms associated with coronary and/or circulatory dysfunction or disease.
- ❑ Major disease processes associated with the heart and vessels and the general treatment course for each.
- ❑ Diagnostic imaging and nuclear medicine studies used in the assessment and treatment of heart/vessel disease.
- ❑ Terminology related to an electrocardiogram (EKG), including the accurate transcription of leads and trace findings.
- ❑ Laboratory tests used in the diagnosis and ongoing evaluation of heart/vessel disease.
- ❑ Commonly prescribed medications, by type, for diseases and symptoms related to the heart, vessels, and circulation.

RESOURCES FOR STUDY

1. *The Language of Medicine*
   Chapter 11: Cardiovascular System, pp. 383–439.
2. *H&P: A Nonphysician's Guide to the Medical History and Physical Examination*
   Chapter 8: Review of Systems: Cardiovascular, pp. 71–81.
   Chapter 23: Examination of the Heart, pp. 217–221.
3. *Human Diseases*
   Chapter 8: Diseases of the Cardiovascular System, pp. 105–126.
4. *Laboratory Tests & Diagnostic Procedures in Medicine*
   Chapter 4: Measurement of Temperature, Rates, Pressures and Volumes (Cardiovascular Measurements, Noninvasive Cardiac Measurements, and Invasive Cardiovascular Procedures), pp. 42–48.
   Chapter 6: Electrocardiography, pp. 75–92.
   Chapter 20: Blood Chemistry (Electrolytes and Acid-Base Balance, Arterial Blood Gases, and Enzymes), pp. 355–400.
5. *The AAMT Book of Style for Medical Transcription*
   Cardiology, pp. 57–63.
6. *Understanding Pharmacology for Health Professionals*
   Chapter 15: Cardiovascular Drugs, pp. 150–177.

SAMPLE REPORTS

The following four reports are examples of reports you might encounter while transcribing cardiology, cardiac surgery, or thoracic surgery.

OPERATIVE REPORT

DATE OF OPERATION
05/01/2004

ATTENDING SURGEON
John Smith, MD.

PREOPERATIVE DIAGNOSIS
End-stage cardiomyopathy.

POSTOPERATIVE DIAGNOSIS
End-stage cardiomyopathy.

PROCEDURE PERFORMED
Heart transplantation.

ANESTHESIA
General endotracheal.

JUSTIFICATION FOR PROCEDURE
The patient is a 65-year-old man with ischemic cardiomyopathy. He had been evaluated for heart transplantation at this facility and placed on the national computer waiting list.

PROCEDURE IN DETAIL
On the night of this surgery, a suitable donor was identified. The patient had previous laryngeal cancer with radiation to the neck, and he was brought to the operating room somewhat early because difficulty with his airway was anticipated. For this reason, he underwent fiberoptic awake intubation which was accomplished without difficulty. A left subclavian Swan-Ganz catheter was placed, as was a radial arterial line and a Foley catheter. With notification from the donor site that the heart was acceptable, the anterior chest, abdomen, groin, and legs were prepped with Betadine and draped as a sterile field.

With notification from the donor site that the heart had been harvested, we began the operation by making a skin incision over the sternum. The sternum was then split in the midline with a saw. A self-retaining retractor was placed, and the pericardium was opened to the right side of the midline. Heparin was administered, and cannulation pursestrings were placed in the ascending aorta, high right superior vena cava, and low lateral right atrium. Cannulation was accomplished and the connection was made to the heart/lung machine.

With notification that the heart had arrived in town, cardiopulmonary bypass was instituted, and a vent was placed through the right superior pulmonary vein through a pursestring. With the heart in the hospital, we cross-clamped the aorta, snugged down on tapes which had been placed around the inferior vena cava and superior vena cava, and divided the superior vena cava, the

(continued)

ascending aorta after cross-clamping it, the pulmonary artery, the inferior vena cava, and then the left atrium. The heart was then removed and hemostasis was obtained at the left atrial cuff.

The donor heart was then brought into the room and prepared for implantation. There was no patent foramen ovale. The pulmonary artery was shortened appropriately, as was the left atrial cuff. The anastomosis was begun on the left side. We placed a 3-0 Prolene suture in a running fashion to accomplish the left atrial anastomosis. Just prior to completion of this anastomosis, the left ventricular vent was placed across the mitral valve and continued on gentle suction. A 4-0 Prolene suture was then used, interrupted in two places, to anastomose the inferior vena cava of the donor and the recipient. A 5-0 Prolene suture was then used to anastomose the pulmonary artery of the donor and recipient, again using interrupted technique at three different points. The ascending aorta was then anastomosed using a running 4-0 Prolene suture in two layers reinforced by pledgets. After completion of the inner layer, the left ventricular vent was turned off, the aortic root was allowed to fill with left ventricular blood, a vent was placed in the ascending aorta and placed on gentle suction, and the cross-clamp was removed. The outer layer was then accomplished using a second layer of running Prolene. The superior vena cava was then anastomosed using a running 6-0 Prolene, which was interrupted in four spots to prevent pursestringing.

The heart began to beat spontaneously, first with an idioventricular rhythm and then subsequently with a nice, normal sinus rhythm. We checked for bleeding and found one spot on the left atrium; this was oversewn with 3-0 Prolene. Pacing wires were placed on the surface of the atrium and the ventricle. The superior vena cava cannula was clamped and removed, and the cannulation site was repaired in longitudinal fashion using a running 6-0 Prolene. The heart was then reperfused for a total of one-half the ischemic interval, or 92 minutes. We then weaned from cardiopulmonary bypass without a great deal of difficulty. There was a significant amount of bleeding from the posterior wall of the aortic anastomosis, and this required several sutures to control. Ultimately, however, we were able to get it under control.

The patient then remained quite hemodynamically labile over the next several minutes, with blood pressures as high as 200 and as low as 90. He gradually stabilized and we were able to administer Protamine and remove the cannulas after reinfusion of all shed blood.

The pursestring sutures were secured and all suture lines were inspected and found to be hemostatic. Two chest tubes were then brought in through separate stab wounds in the mediastinum and secured with silk sutures. After a final check for hemostasis, we went ahead and closed the sternum using interrupted figure-of-8 stainless steel wires. The skin and subcutaneous layers were then closed with absorbable sutures. A dry sterile dressing was applied. The chest tubes were placed for Pleur-evac suction. Sponge, laparotomy pad, instrument, and needle counts were reported as correct at the end of the case.

TOTAL BYPASS TIME
146 minutes.

TOTAL ISCHEMIC TIME
148 minutes.

ADDENDUM
The patient was cooled to 28°C on cardiopulmonary bypass.

OPERATIVE REPORT

DATE OF OPERATION
05/01/2004

ATTENDING SURGEON
John Smith, MD.

PREOPERATIVE DIAGNOSIS
Ventricular tachycardia.

POSTOPERATIVE DIAGNOSIS
Ventricular tachycardia.

PROCEDURE PERFORMED
Placement of automatic implantable cardioverter-defibrillator (AICD).

ANESTHESIA
General endotracheal.

JUSTIFICATION FOR PROCEDURE
The patient is a 75-year-old man with a history of ventricular fibrillation and tachycardia.

PROCEDURE IN DETAIL
At the time of surgery, the patient was brought to the operating room and placed in the supine position where he underwent general endotracheal anesthesia without any difficulty. The patient was prepped with Betadine scrub and Betadine paint and draped in the usual sterile fashion.

An incision was then made in the left deltopectoral fold, and a pocket was made underneath the pectoralis major muscle. A percutaneous stick was then made into the left subclavian vein and attached to the guide wire. It should be noted that, during this, some air was retrieved, and the patient had a small pneumothorax for which a left chest tube was placed at the end of the procedure without difficulty.

Once the guide wire was in, the AICD lead was implanted. This was a Corpus model #1234, serial #123456, with threshold measurements of 1.1 milliampere, 600 ohms resistance, 16 millivolt R-wave, and a 0.6 volt threshold. The patient then had inducible ventricular fibrillation with a 15-joule shock and returned to normal sinus rhythm. This was done a second time, and he returned to normal sinus rhythm once again.

After this, the patient did well, and the wound was irrigated with antibiotic solution and closed with a 3-0 Vicryl subcutaneous layer and a 4-0 Vicryl subcuticular layer. The patient was transferred to the recovery room in stable condition.

ECHOCARDIOGRAM

M-MODE ECHOCARDIOGRAM

AORTIC VALVE LEVEL
The aortic valve opening is normal. The aortic root motion is normal. The left atrial intracavitary dimensions are increased.

MITRAL VALVE LEVEL
The mitral valve opening is normal. The DE and EF slopes are reduced. The E-point septal separation is increased. There is no pericardial effusion.

LEFT VENTRICULAR LEVEL
The left ventricular and septal wall thickness is increased. The left ventricular intracavitary dimensions are increased.

IMPRESSION
1. Mild concentric left ventricular hypertrophy.
2. Dilated left ventricle.
3. Reduced left ventricular function by increased E-point septal separation.
4. Dilated left atrium.

2-D ECHOCARDIOGRAM, DOPPLER AND COLOR FLOW

The 2-dimensional echocardiographic study revealed increased left ventricular and septal thickness. The left ventricular and septal wall motion and contractility revealed generalized diffuse hypokinesia. The intracavitary dimensions of the left ventricle are increased during systole and diastole. The left atrial intracavitary dimensions are increased. The aortic root motion is reduced. The aortic root and mitral anulus are thickened. There is no evidence of intracavitary mass, thrombus or pericardial effusion.

The right ventricular wall motion and contractility are normal.

DOPPLER STUDIES
The Doppler studies reveal a regurgitant jet across the mitral valve with a jet velocity of 4.25 m/s with a gradient of 72 mmHg. The E and A velocities appeared to be fairly normal with decreased deceleration time and evidence of increased left ventricular relaxation time. However, the E and the A velocities could not be sampled. Pulmonary studies were not obtained.

Transtricuspid Doppler interrogation revealed a regurgitant jet with a jet velocity of 3.2 m/s with a calculated right ventricular systolic pressure of 50 mmHg. The transaortic and pulmonic valve Doppler studies are unremarkable, with normal velocities.

IMPRESSION
1. Left ventricular and systolic and diastolic dysfunction.
2. Mild concentric left ventricular hypertrophy.
3. Dilated left ventricle and left atrium.
4. Thickening of the aortic root and mitral anulus.

MYOCARDIAL PERFUSION IMAGING

MYOCARDIAL PERFUSION IMAGING AT REST AND WITH EXERCISE

HISTORY
A 63-year-old female with known coronary artery disease and recurrent chest pain.

INDICATION
Chest pain.

PROCEDURE
The patient exercised on a treadmill for a total of 9 minutes, reaching stage IV of the Bruce protocol, achieving an estimated workload of 7 METs. The heart rate was 80 bpm at baseline and increased to 171 bpm at peak exercise, representing 109% of age-predicted maximal heart rate. The blood pressure response was normal.

The patient did not have chest pain during the procedure. The electrocardiogram showed ST changes which were inconclusive.

The patient's heart was tomographically imaged with 10 mCi of Myoview (^{99m}Tc-tetrofosmin) at rest and 29 mCi of Myoview before gated acquisition was performed.

FINDINGS
There was no evidence of significant motion artifact or extracardiac uptake. Left ventricular hypertrophy was noted with diastolic dysfunction. Anteroseptal wall motion abnormalities were noted. LVEF was calculated at 40%. There were anteroapical and anteroseptal perfusion defects on stress images that were partially reversible on the rest images.

IMPRESSION
1. Left ventricular hypertrophy.
2. Diastolic dysfunction.
3. Anteroapical and anteroseptal perfusion defects with stress.
4. Technically difficult test.

REVIEW QUESTIONS

The goal of these questions is to test your knowledge in the areas of cardiology, cardiac surgery, and thoracic surgery.

Directions: Select the correct answer for each of the multiple-choice questions provided below. *Answers are provided at the end of this chapter.*

1. A heartbeat less than 60 is termed:
   - A. Tachycardia
   - B. Bradycardia
   - C. Thrombosis
   - D. Fibrillation
2. A heartbeat greater than 100 is termed:
   - A. Fibrillation
   - B. Tachycardia
   - C. Bradycardia
   - D. Ischemia
3. Another term for defibrillation is:
   - A. Cardioversion
   - B. Angiography
   - C. Pacemaker implantation
   - D. Doppler technique
4. The heart's internal pacemaker is called the:
   - A. SA node
   - B. AV node
   - C. Bundle of His
   - D. Circle of Willis
5. Cardiac standstill is also called:
   - A. Myocardial infarction
   - B. Ventricular fibrillation
   - C. Asystole
   - D. Atrial fibrillation
6. The largest artery in the human body is the:
   - A. Femoral
   - B. Tricuspid
   - C. Carotid
   - D. Aorta
7. Inflammation of the internal cardiac sac is called:
   - A. Myocarditis
   - B. Aortic insufficiency
   - C. Endocarditis
   - D. Myocardial infarction
8. In a CABG procedure, the following incision is made:
   - A. Mid-sternal
   - B. Mid-axillary
   - C. Pfannenstiel
   - D. McBurney
9. An aortic dissection can result in:
   - A. Heart transplant
   - B. Death
   - C. Supraventricular tachycardia
   - D. Stent placement
10. The ejection fraction is an indication of:
    - A. Intracardiac blood pressure
    - B. The efficiency of the pumping action
    - C. Peripheral blood pressure
    - D. The level of cardiac ischemia present
11. A patient with a history of rheumatic fever is at increased risk for:
    - A. Wolff-Parkinson-White syndrome
    - B. Tachybradycardia syndrome
    - C. Subacute bacterial endocarditis [SBE]
    - D. Thromboangiitis obliterans

12. A patient with new-onset atrial fibrillation is started on heparin and Coumadin. Which lab tests will be used to monitor the patient's response to these medications?
    A. CBC with differential and SMA-7
    B. PT, PTT, and INR
    C. IgA, IgG, and Monospot test
    D. Platelet count, D-dimer, and fibrin split products

13. Which of these tests would be ordered for a patient experiencing retrosternal chest pain?
    A. AST, ALT, and GGTP
    B. Amylase, lipase, and serum protease level
    C. MI factor, PPD, and catecholamine level
    D. EKG, CK-MB, and troponin-I

14. A doctor is dictating on her cell phone from the beach. You hear her say that the patient is being discharged on Lasix once a day, but the sound quality is unclear so you cannot tell whether the dose is 14 or 40. Which is the correct dose of Lasix?
    A. 14 mg q.d.
    B. 40 mg q.d.
    C. 14 mEq q.d.
    D. 40 mEq q.d.

15. Which catheter would be used to monitor the hemodynamic status in a patient with septic shock?
    A. Groshong
    B. Coude
    C. Foley
    D. Swan-Ganz

16. A patient with coronary artery disease amenable to intervention by stenting might undergo a:
    A. CABG
    B. PTCA
    C. BACTEC
    D. CASS

17. Which of these might be visualized on a cardiac catheterization?
    A. Celiac artery
    B. Brachial artery
    C. Azygous vein
    D. Circumflex artery

18. Purkinje fibers are:
    A. Striated muscle fibers
    B. Specialized lung fibers
    C. Specialized conductive myocardial fibers
    D. Part of the bundle of His

19. Which medication is routinely given for at least 30 days following stent placement?
    A. An ACE inhibitor
    B. Plavix
    C. A beta blocker
    D. Coumadin

20. Transposition of the great vessels only occurs in:
    A. Neonates
    B. The elderly
    C. Premature infants
    D. Heart attack survivors

21. An irregular heart rate may require:
    A. Ventricular fibrillation
    B. Coronary artery bypass grafting
    C. Pacemaker implantation
    D. Heart transplant

22. Which of the following is not a predisposing factor for myocardial infarction?
    A. Elevated HDL
    B. Elevated LDL
    C. Diabetes
    D. Hypertension

23. A patient with atrial fibrillation might have this finding on physical examination:
    A. A regular heartbeat
    B. An irregularly irregular heartbeat
    C. Bradycardia
    D. Rubs

24. To help prevent endocarditis, an individual might take the following medication prior to dental surgery:
    A. An antihistamine
    B. An anticoagulant
    C. An antibiotic
    D. An antiplatelet agent

25. With a blood pressure of 125/80, which is the systolic reading?
    A. 125
    B. 80
    C. 45 (the difference between 125 and 80)
    D. 250 (the total of 125 and 80)

26. What drug is given as the antidote to digoxin toxicity?
    A. Dilacor
    B. Digitek
    C. Didronel
    D. Digibind

27. The carotid artery is located in the:
    A. Arm
    B. Neck
    C. Wrist
    D. Leg

28. Hypertrophy and failure of the right heart ventricle is called:
    A. Pulmonary embolism
    B. ASD
    C. Tetralogy of Fallot
    D. Cor pulmonale

29. Idiopathic persistently elevated blood pressure is called:
    A. Hypertension
    B. Hypotension
    C. Essential hypertension
    D. Nonessential hypertension

30. Chest pain resulting from myocardial ischemia is called:
    A. Coronary artery disease
    B. Aortic insufficiency
    C. Angina pectoris
    D. Congestive heart failure

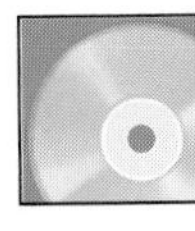

Please see the accompanying CD for additional review materials for this section.

PROOFREADING EXERCISES

These four proofreading exercises are provided to improve your skills in the area of editing and effective identification and correction of errors in the medical record.

Directions: Identify and correct the transcription errors found in the exercises below. *Answers are provided at the end of this chapter.*

PROOFREADING EXERCISE #1

INDICATIONS FOR PROCEDURE
Stroke. The patient had a central retinal artery occlusion and a right carotid bruits.

PROCEDURE
Real-time ultrasound duplex imaging of the parotids was performed, including color-flow Doppler.

INTERPRETATION
The right column carotid artery has mild intimate thickening but no significant stenosis. The right internal carotid artery has evidence of 30% plaque at its origin but no significant flow acceleration or hemodynamically significant narrowing. The right external carotid artery has mild irregularities.

The left column carotid artery has minimal intimate thickening. The left internal carotid artery has mild plaque at its origin but no significant stenosis or flow acceleration. The left external carotid artery has minimal irregularities.

The vertebral flow is plantigrade bilaterally.

CONCLUSION
Mild bilateral carotid plaques with no significant stenosis.

PROOFREADING EXERCISE #2

TECHNICAL
This is a fairly good quality study.

2-DIMENSIONAL ECHOCARDIOGRAM (2-D ECHO)
Ventricle looks to be of normal size with fare wall motion, although the septal motion appears slightly diminished. Dejection fraction is better than 70%. Chamber size looks normal. Left atria appears slightly enlarged. There is closure of the mitral and aortic leaflets. The mitral leaflet separation appears diminished, possibly indicating some amount of mitral stenosis. No intramural thrombus; no perichordal fluid.

DOPPLER/COLOR-FLOW IMAGING
There is some turbulence to mitral inflow; however, the peak velocity recorded is only 2 meters, which gives a mean gradient of about 16 mmHg. There is mild aortic regurgitation and miner tricuspid regurgitation. The tricuspid velocity is 37, giving a pressure gradient of about 65, indicating moderate pulmonary hypertension.

FINAL IMPRESSION
1. Normal study.
2. No intraneural thrombus or mass.
3. No valvular vegetations seen.
4. There is mild mitral stenosis with noncalcified valve.
5. There is moderate pulmonary hypertension.
6. Mild chaotic regurgitation.
7. Left atrium is slightly enlarged.
8. No pericardial fluid.

PROOFREADING EXERCISE #3

INDICATIONS
The patient is a 69-year-old female presenting for cardiac catherization, coronary angiography, and possible intervention. The patient presented with unstable angina culminating in a non-que-wave infarction with persistent pain.

The risks and benefits of the procedure were explained to the patient and family. I believe they understood and they agreed to proceed.

PROCEDURE
An intravenous line was established. The right groin was shaved. The patient was given prednisone 60 mg PO and Benadryl 50 mg orally, as well as Plavix 300 mg, aspirin 325 mg, a heparin bullous followed by infusion, which was stopped on transfer to the cath lab, and an Integrilin bullous and infusion following standard protocol. She was brought to the cath lab where the right groin was prepped and draped in the usual manner. Xylocaine 2% was infused in this area.

Using the Seldinger technique, a 6-french sheath was introduced into the right femoral artery. Additional Heparin was not given. Cineangiography of the left coronary artery was then performed in the LAO, RAO, and hemiaxial projections, and this catheter was then changed for a 6-French #4 right Judkins catheter. The right coronary artery could not be engaged; this catheter was used to engage a graph to the left circumflex and a graph to the RCA. Pictures were taken in multiple views. The same catheter was used to engage the left internal mammary artery. Cineangiography of this vessel was performed in the AP projection.

Left ventriculography was not performed.

HEMODYNAMICS
Systolic pressures were normal to mildly elevated. The LB was not entered; LVEDP was not measured.

(continued)

ANGIOGRAPHY

1. Left ventriculogram was not performed.
2. Right coronary artery: The right coronary artery was not selectively engaged. Hand injection of the aortic route revealed no patent native RCA.
3. Reverse sanguinous graft to the RCA: This graft was patient; inserted into the RCA just proximal to the PDA. The proximal RCA filled with contrast with injection of this graft. The PDA itself was small, as well as the distal RCA beyond the PDA. This was extremely and diffusely diseased.
4. Reverse sanguinous graft to the circumflex: This was 100% obstructed proximally.
5. The third graft was not found, and was reportedly closed upon review of her previous catheterizations.
6. Left internal mammary artery: This was patent and had no obstruction. However, it did not insert into the corollary arteries and looked to be a good vessel for bypass purposes if needed.
7. Left main coronary artery: This gave rise to the left exterior descending coronary artery and the left circumflex coronary artery.

PROOFREADING EXERCISE #4

REASON FOR CONSULTATION
Palpitations and hypertension.

The patient is a 53-year-old female with a 1-year history of labial hypertension and palpitations. She was started on pharmacological intervention for hypertension 1 year ago. Most recently she developed nonexertional chest pain and palpitations described as a rapid and forceful beating of the heart. With some adjustments in her pharmacological regimen, her blood pressure has improved and her palpitations improved somewhat but they persist. Outpatient clear study was done, which was normal, with an ejection fraction of 96%. An echocardiogram was done which demonstrated a suggestion of hypertensive heart disease with diastolic dysfunction but no significant left ventricular hypotonia. Thyroid function tests were normal as was a chest x-ray.

The patient has tried to limit her caffeine intake. She is not using alcohol to excess. She is avoiding stimulants and over-the-counter decongestants.

CURRENT MEDICATIONS
She is on Benicar AZT 40/25 mg a day, Cardizem LA 360 mg a day.

PAST MEDICAL HISTORY
Remarkable for hypertension of 1 year's duration. She has had a previous hysterectomy, tonsillectomy, and some type of hip surgery.

ALLERGIES
She states she is allergic to sulfa drugs.

SOCIAL HISTORY
She is married. She works in management. She is a reformed smoker of approximately 15 years. Rare intake of ethenol.

FAMILY HISTORY
Father died of "old age" at age 90. Mother died of some type of oropharyngeal carcinoma at the age of 65. Siblings are hypertensive.

(continued)

REVIEW OF SYSTEMS
She does note some easy fatigability. No recent change in weight. No recent fever or chills. Denies chronic headaches, history of glaucoma or cataracts. She has some mild dyspnea on exertion and pendent edema. Nonexertional chest pain. No history of asthma, chronic cough. No hemoptysis, hematemesis, melena, or hematochezia. Denies dysuria, urgency, or frequency. Denies myalgias or arthralgias. No history of seizure or stroke. Denies easy bruising or bleeding diaphysis. No history of thyroid disorder.

PHYSICAL EXAMINATION
GENERAL: This is a pleasant, somewhat anxious-appearing white female in no distress.
VITAL SIGNS: Weight is 154 pounds, blood pressure is 152/76, heart rate is 170 and regular.
HEENT: Pupils are equal, round, and reactive to light. Sclerae are not icteric. Mucous membranes are moist.
NECK: Good carotid upstrokes. No carotid bruits heard. Jugulovenous distention is not appreciated. Thyromegaly is not detected.
LUNGS: Clear to auscultation and percussion.
HEART: Regular rate and rhythm. PMI is not displaced. S1 and S2 are normal. I do not hear a significant murmur, dollop, rub, or click.
ABDOMEN: Soft. No masses, tenderness, or organomegaly.
EXTREMITIES: Good distal pulses without peripheral edema.

ELECTROCARDIOGRAM
EKG is that of sinus arrhythmia but is otherwise normal.

IMPRESSION
1. Palpations–cause undetermined.
2. Label hypertension.

RECOMMENDATION
To further evaluate her palpitations, an agent recorder will be sent home with the patient to document whether or not there is any significant brady- or tachydysrhythmia present. We will see her back once representative rhythm strips have been submitted. In the meantime, I have instructed her on a low-chromium diet and a good exercise program to see if we can augment her antihypertensive treatment with nonpharmacological means.

ANSWER KEYS

REVIEW QUESTIONS ANSWER KEY

1. B
2. B
3. A
4. A
5. C
6. D
7. C
8. A
9. B
10. B
11. C
12. B
13. D
14. B
15. D
16. B
17. D
18. C
19. B
20. A
21. C
22. A
23. B
24. C
25. A
26. D
27. B
28. D
29. C
30. C

PROOFREADING EXERCISE #1 KEY

INDICATIONS FOR PROCEDURE
Stroke. The patient had a central retinal artery occlusion and a right carotid bruits.

Use singular form—bruit

PROCEDURE
Real-time ultrasound duplex imaging of the parotids was performed, including color-flow Doppler.

Incorrect term—carotids

INTERPRETATION
The right column carotid artery has mild intimate thickening but no significant stenosis. The right internal carotid artery has evidence of 30% plaque at its origin but no significant flow acceleration or hemodynamically significant narrowing. The right external carotid artery has mild irregularities.

Incorrect term—common

Incorrect term—intimal

The left column carotid artery has minimal intimate thickening. The left internal carotid artery has mild plaque at its origin but no significant stenosis or flow acceleration. The left external carotid artery has minimal irregularities.

Incorrect term—common

Incorrect term—intimal

The vertebral flow is plantigrade bilaterally.

Incorrect term—antegrade

CONCLUSION
Mild bilateral carotid plaques with no significant stenosis.

PROOFREADING EXERCISE #2 KEY

TECHNICAL
This is a fairly good quality study.

2-DIMENSIONAL ECHOCARDIOGRAM (2-D ECHO)
Ventricle looks to be of normal size with fare wall motion, although the septal motion appears slightly diminished. Dejection fraction is better than 70%. Chamber size looks normal. Left atria appears slightly enlarged. There is closure of the mitral and aortic leaflets. The mitral leaflet separation appears diminished, possibly indicating some amount of mitral stenosis. No intramural thrombus; no perichordal fluid.

DOPPLER/COLOR-FLOW IMAGING
There is some turbulence to mitral inflow; however, the peak velocity recorded is only 2 meters, which gives a mean gradient of about 16 mmHg. There is mild aortic regurgitation and miner tricuspid regurgitation. The tricuspid velocity is 37, giving a pressure gradient of about 65, indicating moderate pulmonary hypertension.

FINAL IMPRESSION
1. Normal study.
2. No intraneural thrombus or mass.
3. No valvular vegetations seen.
4. There is mild mitral stenosis with noncalcified valve.
5. There is moderate pulmonary hypertension.
6. Mild chaotic regurgitation.
7. Left atrium is slightly enlarged.
8. No pericardial fluid.

Incorrect spelling—fair

Incorrect word—ejection

Incorrect form—singular atrium

Incorrect term—pericardial

Incorrect spelling—minor

Should be abnormal

Incorrect term—intramural

Incorrect term—aortic

PROOFREADING EXERCISE #3 KEY

Incorrect spelling—catheterization

Incorrect term—Q-wave

INDICATIONS
The patient is a 69-year-old female presenting for cardiac catherization, coronary angiography, and possible intervention. The patient presented with unstable angina culminating in a non-que-wave infarction with persistent pain.

The risks and benefits of the procedure were explained to the patient and family. I believe they understood and they agreed to proceed.

PROCEDURE
An intravenous line was established. The right groin was shaved. The patient was given prednisone 60 mg PO and Benadryl 50 mg orally, as well as Plavix 300 mg, aspirin 325 mg, a heparin bullous followed by infusion, which was stopped on transfer to the cath lab, and an Integrilin bullous and infusion following standard protocol. She was brought to the cath lab where the right groin was prepped and draped in the usual manner. Xylocaine 2% was infused in this area.

Incorrect term—bolus

Using the Seldinger technique, a 6-french sheath was introduced into the right humoral artery. Additional Heparin was not given. Cineangiography of the left coronary artery was then performed in the LAO, RAO, and hemiaxial projections, and this catheter was then changed for a 6-French #4 right Judkins catheter. The right coronary artery could not be engaged; this catheter was used to engage a graph to the left circumflex and a graph to the RCA. Pictures were taken in multiple views. The same catheter was used to engage the left internal mammary artery. Cineangiography of this vessel was performed in the AP projection.

Incorrect term—femoral

Capitalize proper nouns—French

Incorrect word—graft

Left ventriculography was not performed.

Incorrect abbreviation—LV

HEMODYNAMICS

Systolic pressures were normal to mildly elevated. The LB was not entered; LVEDP was not measured.

ANGIOGRAPHY

1. Left ventriculogram was not performed.
2. Right coronary artery: The right coronary artery was not selectively engaged. Hand injection of the aortic route revealed no patent native RCA.
3. Reverse sanguinous graft to the RCA: This graft was patient; inserted into the RCA just proximal to the PDA. The proximal RCA filled with contrast with injection of this graft. The PDA itself was small, as well as the distal RCA beyond the PDA. This was extremely and diffusely diseased.
4. Reverse sanguinous graft to the circumflex: This was 100% obstructed proximally.
5. The third graft was not found, and was reportedly closed upon review of her previous catheterizations.
6. Left internal mammary artery: This was patent and had no obstruction. However, it did not insert into the corollary arteries and looked to be a good vessel for bypass purposes if needed.
7. Left main coronary artery: This gave rise to the left exterior descending coronary artery and the left circumflex coronary artery.

Incorrect word—root

Incorrect term—saphenous

Incorrect word—patent

Incorrect term—coronary

Incorrect term—anterior

PROOFREADING EXERCISE #4 KEY

Incorrect term—labile

Flag—this is not a normal value for ejection fraction

Incorrect term—nuclear

Incorrect term—hypertrophy

Incorrect abbreviation—HCT

Incorrect spelling—ethanol

REASON FOR CONSULTATION
Palpitations and hypertension.

The patient is a 53-year-old female with a 1-year history of labial hypertension and palpitations. She was started on pharmacological intervention for hypertension 1 year ago. Most recently she developed nonexertional chest pain and palpitations described as a rapid and forceful beating of the heart. With some adjustments in her pharmacological regimen, her blood pressure has improved and her palpitations improved somewhat but they persist. Outpatient clear study was done, which was normal, with an ejection fraction of 96%. An echocardiogram was done which demonstrated a suggestion of hypertensive heart disease with diastolic dysfunction but no significant left ventricular hypotonia. Thyroid function tests were normal as was a chest x-ray.

The patient has tried to limit her caffeine intake. She is not using alcohol to excess. She is avoiding stimulants and over-the-counter decongestants.

CURRENT MEDICATIONS
She is on Benicar AZT 40/25 mg a day, Cardizem LA 360 mg a day.

PAST MEDICAL HISTORY
Remarkable for hypertension of one year's duration. She has had a previous hysterectomy, tonsillectomy, and some type of hip surgery.

ALLERGIES
She states she is allergic to sulfa drugs.

SOCIAL HISTORY
She is married. She works in management. She is a reformed smoker of approximately 15 years. Rare intake of ethenol.

Incorrect term—dependent

FAMILY HISTORY

Father died of "old age" at age 90. Mother died of some type of oropharyngeal carcinoma at the age of 65. Siblings are hypertensive.

REVIEW OF SYSTEMS

She does note some and easy fatigability. No recent change in weight. No recent fever or chills. Denies chronic headaches, history of glaucoma or cataracts. She has some mild dyspnea on exertion and pendent edema. Nonexertional chest pain. No history of asthma, chronic cough. No hemoptysis, hematemesis, melena, or hematochezia. Denies dysuria, urgency, or frequency. Denies myalgias or arthralgias. No history of seizure or stroke. Denies easy bruising or bleeding diaphysis. No history of thyroid disorder.

Incorrect term—diathesis

PHYSICAL EXAMINATION

GENERAL: This is a pleasant, somewhat anxious-appearing white female in no distress.

VITAL SIGNS: Weight is 154 pounds, blood pressure is 152/76, heart rate is 170 and regular.

Flag—probably incorrect value

HEENT: Pupils are equal, round, and reactive to light. Sclerae are not icteric. Mucous membranes are moist.

NECK: Good carotid upstrokes. No carotid bruits heard. Jugulovenous distention is not appreciated. Thyromegaly is not detected.

Incorrect spelling—jugular venous

LUNGS: Clear to auscultation and percussion.

HEART: Regular rate and rhythm. PMI is not displaced. S1 and S2 are normal. I do not hear a significant murmur, dollop, rub, or click.

Incorrect term—gallop

ABDOMEN: Soft. No masses, tenderness, or organomegaly.

EXTREMITIES: Good distal pulses without peripheral edema.

ELECTROCARDIOGRAM
EKG is that of sinus arrhythmia but is otherwise normal.

IMPRESSION
1. Palpations–cause undetermined.
2. Label hypertension.

RECOMMENDATION
To further evaluate her palpitations, an agent recorder will be sent home with the patient to document whether or not there is any significant brady- or tachydysrhythmia present. We will see her back once representative rhythm strips have been submitted. In the meantime, I have instructed her on a low-chromium diet and a good exercise program to see if we can augment her antihypertensive treatment with nonpharmacological means.

Incorrect term—palpitations

Incorrect word—labile

Incorrect word—event

Incorrect word—sodium

CHAPTER 6

Emergency Medicine

OBJECTIVES CHECKLIST

A prepared exam candidate will know the:

- ☐ Basics of emergency medicine including assessment, triage, diagnostic intervention, and stabilization.
- ☐ Role of Advanced Cardiac Life Support (ACLS) protocol in resuscitation and critical cardiac intervention.
- ☐ ABCs (airway, breathing & circulation) of trauma evaluation as used on scene and in the emergency room.
- ☐ Fundamentals of the mental status exam as well as terminology unique to psychiatric assessment in the emergency setting.
- ☐ Typical first-line treatment course for most common presenting complaints in the emergency setting.
- ☐ Diagnostic imaging and laboratory studies related to emergency medicine.
- ☐ Interventional medications administered in critical treatment, particularly resuscitation, drug overdose, poisoning, envenomization, and acute trauma.
- ☐ Medications administered routinely for common presenting complaints.

RESOURCES FOR STUDY

1. *H&P: A Nonphysician's Guide to the Medical History and Physical Examination*
   Chapter 1: General Remarks on the History, pp. 13–24.
   Chapter 2: Chief Complaint and History of Present Illness, pp. 25–34.
   Chapter 28: The Formal Mental Status Examination, pp. 273–280.

2. *Human Diseases*
   Chapter 6: Trauma and Poisoning, pp. 73–86.
   Chapter 20: Mental Disorders, pp. 315–332.

3. *Laboratory Tests and Diagnostic Procedures in Medicine*
   Chapter 4: Measurement of Temperature, Rates, Pressures and Volumes, pp. 39–60.
   Section VI (Chapters 19–24). *Note: Information in all of these chapters is pertinent to Emergency Medicine but will also be well covered in other chapters of this text.*

4. *Understanding Pharmacology for Health Professionals*
   Chapter 16: Emergency Drugs, pp. 178–191.
   Chapter 17: Anticoagulant and Thrombolytic Drugs, pp. 185–191.
   Chapter 26: Analgesic Drugs, pp. 296–310.
   Chapter 32: Intravenous Fluids and Blood Products, pp. 373–385.

SAMPLE REPORTS

The following four reports are examples of reports you might encounter while transcribing emergency medicine.

OPERATIVE NOTE

DATE OF OPERATION
02/21/2004

SURGEON OF RECORD
John Smith, MD.

PREOPERATIVE DIAGNOSIS
Left index finger cellulitis.

POSTOPERATIVE DIAGNOSIS
Left index finger cellulitis.

PROCEDURE PERFORMED
Hickman catheter placement.

ANESTHESIA
Monitored anesthesia care.

COMPLICATIONS
None noted.

ESTIMATED BLOOD LOSS
Minimal.

INTRAVENOUS FLUIDS
200 mL of Crystalloid.

INDICATIONS FOR PROCEDURE
The patient is a 33-year-old Haitian male who had a gunshot wound to his left index finger and subsequently underwent surgery by the orthopedic hand service. This included having a piece of hardware placed. The patient presented to the surgical emergency room today with purulent drainage from his finger and underwent incision and drainage of his left index finger. The patient will require long-term antibiotics and, for this reason, a Hickman catheter was requested by the orthopedic team.

PROCEDURE IN DETAIL
The patient was given intravenous sedation and then prepped and draped in the usual sterile fashion, still in the surgical emergency room. We then proceeded to cannulate the left subclavian vein and passed a guide wire through the needle.

Then we made a tunnel under the skin with an exit approximately 4 cm below our initial cannulation site. After that, we measured the Hickman catheter, making sure the cuff would be at the level of the skin of the lower incision and the tip would be at the level of the superior vena

(continued)

cava. After that, we proceeded, using the Seldinger technique, to introduce the dilator and introducer into the left subclavian vein. After removal of the dilator, good blood return was seen and we proceeded to introduce the Hickman catheter through the sheath, which was then removed. Good blood flow was obtained from the Hickman catheter.

At that time, an x-ray was obtained, noting the presence of no pneumothorax and the tip of the catheter at the level of the superior vena cava.

We then approximated the skin edges using 4-0 Vicryl in an inverted fashion, following which we applied a dry dressing.

OPERATIVE REPORT

DATE OF OPERATION
01/06/2004

SURGEON OF RECORD
John Jones, MD.

PREOPERATIVE DIAGNOSIS
Gunshot wound to the abdomen.

POSTOPERATIVE DIAGNOSES
1. Gunshot wound to the abdomen.
2. Laceration of the duodenum.
3. Injury to the head of the pancreas.
4. Injury to the inferior vena cava.
5. Injury to the right renal artery.

PROCEDURES PERFORMED
1. Closure of stomach laceration.
2. Closure of duodenal laceration.
3. Drainage of pancreas.
4. Repair of renal artery.
5. Repair of inferior vena cava.

ANESTHESIA
General endotracheal anesthesia.

JUSTIFICATION FOR PROCEDURE
This is an 18-year-old known gang member who presented to the trauma center with a gunshot wound to the abdomen.

PROCEDURE IN DETAIL
The patient was brought to the operating room in the trauma center, placed in the supine position, and prepped and draped in the usual sterile fashion. The abdomen was entered through a long midline incision. Upon entering the abdomen, the abdomen was packed to control bleeding.

Examination of the abdomen revealed the following injuries: There was a long laceration of the greater curvature of the stomach. There was a hole through-and-through on the head of the pancreas and a small laceration of the duodenum. The bullet projectile also caused a large right retroperitoneal hematoma. The right side of the colon was mobilized and the duodenum was kocherized. Kocherization of the duodenum revealed the through-and-through injury to the head of the pancreas and also revealed the small hole through the duodenum mentioned previously.

After the right side of the colon was mobilized, it was evident that the bullet had gone through the hilum of the right kidney, and exploration of that area revealed that the renal artery had been lacerated and there was also a small hole in the inferior vena cava. The small hole in the inferior vena cava was closed with figure-of-8 sutures of 5-0 Prolene. The renal artery was controlled proximally and distally and was completely divided and débrided. Following this, a primary anastomosis was performed with 6-0 Prolene interrupted stitches.

(continued)

The examination of the rest of the abdomen was normal, and the abdomen was thoroughly irrigated with normal saline, following which a Jackson-Pratt drain was placed over the head of the pancreas and the duodenum.

The patient tolerated the procedure well and was transferred to the postanesthesia recovery unit in good general condition.

EMERGENCY ROOM REPORT

CHIEF COMPLAINT/HISTORY OF PRESENT ILLNESS

The patient is a 40-year-old black male who was, unfortunately, shot by his brother this evening. The patient was shot in both legs. The patient then dove down the stairs. The patient was brought to the emergency room by EMS with stable vital signs complaining of pain in both legs. The patient denies injuries elsewhere. The patient admits to abusing cocaine and alcohol today as well.

ALLERGIES

The patient is ALLERGIC to HALDOL, PROLIXIN, and THORAZINE.

MEDICATIONS

Valium and Tylenol #3.

PAST MEDICAL HISTORY

His medical problems include a history of schizophrenia.

SOCIAL HISTORY

The patient admits to polysubstance abuse as well as alcohol abuse. The patient also smokes cigarettes.

PAST SURGICAL HISTORY

Positive for a gunshot wound to the abdomen in the past with intraoperative repair.

PHYSICAL EXAMINATION

GENERAL: The patient is well-developed, well-nourished black male in moderate, nonrespiratory distress, presenting on a backboard with C-collar immobilization.
VITAL SIGNS: The patient's initial vital signs include an oral temperature of 97, pulse 70, respiratory rate 20 with a blood pressure of 91/50. At the time of transfer, his blood pressure was 115/61 (sitting) and his saturation was 100% on 100% oxygen via face mask.
SKIN: Revealed gunshot wounds to the right mid-thigh and to the left mid-shin with no exit wounds.
HEENT: Extraocular movements are intact and pupils are equally round and reactive to light. ENT examination was negative.
NECK: Supple.
CHEST: Lungs are clear anteriorly.
HEART: Regular rate and rhythm.
ABDOMEN: Reveals good bowel sounds, soft, nontender, nondistended, and otherwise negative.
GENITALIA: Normal.
EXTREMITIES: He has a gunshot wound to the right midthigh with no exit wound and a gunshot wound to the left midtibia and fibula with no exit wound. There are good femoral pulses, dorsalis pedis, and 2+ posterior tibialis pulses bilaterally and full range of motion at the toes except for decreased sensation to the left 5th toe. Otherwise, there is normal sensation.
NEUROLOGICAL: The patient is somewhat lethargic but he has a Glasgow coma scale of 15, and he is oriented x3 and otherwise nonfocal.

(continued)

DIAGNOSTIC STUDIES

His labs reveal a pH of 7.3, pCO_2 of 38, a pO_2 of 202, a HCO_3 of 18, and this is on 100% oxygen by mask. Coagulation studies reveal a PT of 12, an INR of 1.2, and a PTT of 26.4. The patient's urine is essentially negative but it does reveal a small amount of hematuria, and the patient's ABO/Rh type is O positive. The patient's urine drug screen revealed benzodiazepines and cocaine metabolites. A CBC revealed a white count of 9.8, hemoglobin and hematocrit of 12 and 35.1, respectively, with platelets of 305 and an MCV of 80. The patient's Chem-12 revealed a BUN of 23, a creatinine of 1.3, sodium 138, and bicarbonate 17.8. Alcohol level is 210. EKG revealed normal sinus rhythm with left ventricular hypertrophy.

EMERGENCY DEPARTMENT COURSE

The patient was given a tetanus toxoid booster and 2 g of Ancef as well as 1 unit of blood secondary to the initial low blood pressure reading. The patient had a Foley catheter placed and a hard cervical collar placed with towels to bolster the head, and this was secured at the forehead and the chin. The patient's left lower extremity was splinted with a short-leg splint and the right with a long-leg splint. The patient was given morphine 4 mg IV for pain and also received 1 L of normal saline and 2 L of lactated Ringers with a resultant output of 350 mL of urine.

I did speak with Dr. Smith, who is the trauma surgeon at Johnson Hospital, and their emergency room physician has accepted the patient for transfer. The patient's x-rays have been copied, as were all records and lab studies. These records will accompany the patient on transfer to the other hospital.

FINAL DIAGNOSES

1. Status post gunshot wounds to lower extremities; right femur fracture and left tibia fracture.
2. Polysubstance illicit drug ingestion.

EMERGENCY ROOM REPORT

CHIEF COMPLAINT/HISTORY OF PRESENT ILLNESS

The patient is a 30-year-old female who does not have a doctor at this hospital. She was brought to the emergency room by the paramedics. It seems that she was found "down" in the street, unconscious, with labored breathing.

ALLERGIES

No information is available at this time.

CURRENT MEDICATIONS

Her tetanus immunization status is unknown.

PHYSICAL EXAMINATION

VITAL SIGNS: Blood pressure 90/50, pulse 120, respirations 10, temperature 99.
GENERAL: The patient is unconscious, not responding, and incoherent. She smells of alcohol.
HEENT: Pupils are equal, round and sluggishly reactive to light. The patient has multiple abrasions of the face with swelling of her upper lip. The patient also has multiple superficial avulsive lacerations particularly involving the left periorbital area.
NECK: A C-collar is in place, and she is in full spinal precautions.
CHEST: Auscultation reveals rales and rhonchi.
HEART: Tachycardia is present.
ABDOMEN: No distention, feels soft, bowel sounds are difficult to hear.
EXTREMITIES: Upper extremities have no swelling, no deformities, and she moves all joints normally. Lower extremities have no swelling, no deformities, and she moves all joints normally.
NEUROLOGICAL: Cranial nerves intact. No motor or sensory deficits.

DIAGNOSTIC STUDIES

The patient had a CT of the head done which was negative. A CT of the C-spine was also negative as were the chest and pelvic CTs. Among the laboratory work, the alcohol level is 409, glucose 85, BUN 9, creatinine 0.6, sodium 143, potassium 3.8, chloride 111. The WBC count is 4.4, hemoglobin is 13.7 with a hematocrit of 40, neutrophils of 31, lymphocytes of 43, and monocytes of 8.4.

EMERGENCY DEPARTMENT COURSE

The patient was started on normal saline wide open followed by D5 normal saline at 125 mL/hour. She received thiamine 100 mg IV and also Ancef 2 grams IV piggyback and a tetanus shot. The laceration of the left orbital area was sutured with 5-0 nylon. We notified the trauma surgeon on-call, and the patient is being admitted to his service for further evaluation and management.

FINAL DIAGNOSES

1. Head and facial trauma.
2. Alcohol abuse/alcohol intoxication.

REVIEW QUESTIONS

The goal of these questions is to test your knowledge in the area of emergency medicine.

Directions: Select the correct answer for each of the multiple-choice questions provided below. *Answers are provided at the end of this chapter.*

1. A common type of fracture seen in young children:
   - A. Epicondylar
   - B. Greenstick
   - C. LeFort
   - D. Bimalleolar
2. A "both bone" fracture is a common term for which of these?
   - A. Atlas and axis
   - B. Tibia and femur
   - C. Radius and ulna
   - D. Mandible and maxilla
3. A toddler who accidentally inhaled a small bead comes to the ER making strange, harsh noises while breathing. These noises are called:
   - A. Rales
   - B. Rhonchi
   - C. Stridor
   - D. Croup
4. A patient is brought to the ER with chest pain. An MI is suspected. Which of these tests is most likely to be ordered?
   - A. CK-MB
   - B. BNP
   - C. ANA
   - D. TURP
5. A patient having a hypertensive emergency might have which of these findings on exam?
   - A. Papillary edema
   - B. Papillary rupture
   - C. Papilledema
   - D. Pupillary edema
6. What score is used to assess a trauma patient's condition and chances of survival?
   - A. Gleason score
   - B. SCSI score
   - C. TIMI-3 score
   - D. Glasgow Coma Score
7. Hemothorax can cause:
   - A. Opacification of the costophrenic angle
   - B. The "bends"
   - C. Ecchymosis of the breasts
   - D. Generalized pruritus
8. Which of these findings is associated with a CVA?
   - A. Loss of nasolabial fold
   - B. Ketosis
   - C. Cholesteatoma
   - D. Positive Tinel sign
9. A common reason for someone with BPH to present to the ER:
   - A. Headache
   - B. Diplopia
   - C. Intractable vomiting
   - D. Urinary retention
10. A person with decreased sensorium is said to be:
    - A. Depressed
    - B. Obtunded
    - C. Uninhibited
    - D. Manic-depressive
11. A patient who has been seizing for more than 30 minutes is said to have:
    - A. Status asthmaticus
    - B. Petit mal seizures
    - C. Status epilepticus
    - D. Grand mal seizures

12. A patient comes into the ER and blood tests reveal a subtherapeutic phenytoin level. What disorder does this patient have?
    A. Cystic fibrosis
    B. Schizophrenia
    C. Epilepsy
    D. Diabetes

13. Which of these conditions might cause nuchal rigidity?
    A. Fracture of the distal radius
    B. Preterm labor with placental abruption
    C. Migraine headache
    D. Meningitis

14. A patient with COPD comes to the ER with dyspnea. To assess oxygenation, the doctor would order a/an:
    A. TIA
    B. ABG
    C. DOE
    D. IABP

15. A stat VQ scan would be ordered for a patient suspected of having:
    A. Pulmonary embolism
    B. Appendicitis
    C. Ruptured abdominal aortic aneurysm
    D. Placenta previa

16. Upon presentation to the ER, the patient has hematemesis, which is:
    A. A blood infection
    B. A blood dyscrasia
    C. Vomiting blood
    D. Blood clots

17. Upon presentation to the ER, the patient is diaphoretic. This means she is:
    A. Breathing rapidly
    B. Profusely sweating
    C. Extremely nauseated
    D. Spiking a temperature

18. An x-ray of the kidneys, ureters, and bladder is abbreviated as:
    A. IVP
    B. VCUG
    C. KUB
    D. ROM

19. A patient who is described as being "A&O x 4" is found to be alert and oriented to:
    A. Person, place, time, and family members
    B. Person, time, event, and president
    C. Person, place, time, and event
    D. Person, place, event, and president

20. A cerebral concussion is usually caused by:
    A. Blunt trauma
    B. Loss of consciousness
    C. Cerebral aneurysm
    D. Headache

21. Damage to the right side of the brain may cause:
    A. Right-sided paralysis
    B. Quadriplegia
    C. Left-sided paralysis
    D. Paraplegia

22. Paralysis of the trunk and lower extremities is called:
    A. Hemiplegia
    B. Quadriplegia
    C. Paraplegia
    D. Cardioplegia

23. A patient with life-threatening ventricular fibrillation would be given:
    A. Lidocaine HCl
    B. Benzocaine
    C. Marcaine
    D. Xylocaine

24. A presenting complaint of "chest pain" that is reproduced upon palpation of the sternum would most likely be indicative of:
    A. Peptic ulcer disease
    B. Myocardial infarction
    C. Angina pectoris
    D. Costochondritis

25. The Heimlich maneuver is sometimes used to:
    A. Ease delivery of twins
    B. Expel an object obstructing the airway
    C. Test for meningitis
    D. Check vision in a cataract patient

26. Which condition is correctly matched with its indicator?
    A. Gout–tophi
    B. Hypercholesterolemia–Heberden node
    C. Rheumatoid arthritis–xanthelasma
    D. Parkinson disease–uremia

27. Why would a physician order a DAU?
    A. For suspected pregnancy
    B. For suspected CVA
    C. For suspected drug abuse
    D. For suspected MI

28. If an ER physician dictates, "The patient's ABCs were addressed." What does he/she mean by this?
    A. Airway, Blood Flow, and Consciousness
    B. Airway, Breathing, and Consciousness
    C. Airway, Breathing, and Circulation
    D. Airway, Blood, and Consciousness

29. ACLS protocols address which of the following:
    A. Defibrillation, airway management, and use of drugs and medications
    B. Methodology used to determine nursing home placement
    C. Implementation of a DNR request by a family
    D. Management of palliative care given to terminal patients

30. A woman presents to the ER with complaints of bleeding and cramping and passage of some mucoid-like material per vagina. She may have a/an:
    A. Infection with Chlamydia
    B. Ectopic pregnancy
    C. Threatened or incomplete abortion
    D. Birth control device in place

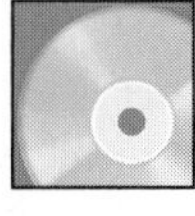

Please see the accompanying CD for additional review materials for this section.

PROOFREADING EXERCISES

These four proofreading exercises are provided to improve your skills in the areas of editing and effective identification and correction of errors in the medical record.

Directions: Identify and correct the transcription errors found in the exercises below. *Answers are provided at the end of this chapter.*

PROOFREADING EXERCISE #1

CHIEF COMPLAINT/HISTORY OF PRESENT ILLNESS
The patient is a 66-year-old female who does not have a doctor at this hospital. She was therefore referred to Dr. Jones, the OB/GYN physician on-call today. Her chief complaint is that of alleged sexual assault which happened 2 days ago. The patient said that she is 4-6 weeks pregnant. She denied any abdominal pain or any vaginal bleeding. She did not seek medical attention until today.

PHYSICAL EXAMINATION
VITAL SIGNS: Blood pressure 111/61, pulse 82, respirations 20, temperature 98.
GENERAL: The patient is unconscious, responsive, and coherent.
HEENT: Pupils are equal, round, and reactive to light. No hematoma of the scalp.
NECK: Subtle.
CHEST: Clear.
HEART: Heart sounds are normal.
ABDOMEN: No distention, feels soft, bowel sounds present. Her uterus is palpated just below the cubic margin.
PELVIC EXAMINATION: No lacerations, no bleeding; the uterus is about 4 to 6 weeks and no annexal masses are felt.

(continued)

DIAGNOSTIC STUDIES
The patient had a CBC, SMA-7 and a beta aCG test done. Her pregnancy test was positive. We also did a serum quantitative pregnancy test. Electrolytes are normal. Alcohol level is zero. Her drug screen, however, is positive for both marijuana and cocaine. We also obtained gonorrhea and chlamydia cultures. A cervical culture was also prepared. Her urinalysis was negative.

EMERGENCY DEPARTMENT COURSE
We contacted social services and the police department. The patient received Rocephin 250 mg IM for prophylactic. She will be followed by her private medical doctor.

FINAL DIAGNOSES
1. Alleged sexual assault.
2. Enterouterine pregnancy.

PROOFREADING EXERCISE #2

CHIEF COMPLAINT
The patient is a 20-year-old female who was brought by EMS following ingestion of an overdose of aspirin in a suicidal gesture. This ingestion occurred following an argument with his family about 15 minutes prior to presentation.

CURRENT MEDICATIONS
None.

PHYSICAL EXAMINATION
VITAL SIGNS: Temperature 96, pulse 120, respirations 24, blood pressure 146/68.
GENERAL: She is morbidly obese at over 300 pounds on her 5′6″ frame. She appears unkept.
HEENT: Normal cephalic and atraumatic. Eyes are normal. ENT normal.
NECK: Supple. No jugular venous distension or carotid bruit.
CHEST: Clear to auscultation and percussion.
HEART: Auscultation revealed regular sinus rhythm with a 2/6 systolic ejection murmur best heard over the left sternal border.
ABDOMEN: Soft and nontender but dentulous. Bowel sounds are normoactive.
GENITALIA: Deferred.
RECTAL EXAMINATION: Differed.
EXTREMITIES: She moves all 4 extremities to command.
NERVOUS SYSTEM: No sign of focal deficit. No sign of meningismus.

DIAGNOSTIC STUDIES
Her salicylate level was 6 mg/dL, acetaminophen level was less then 10.

EMERGENCY DEPARTMENT COURSE
The patient was given 50 grams of charcoal in sorbitol and normal saline to run at 125 mL per hour. She also received Xanax 300 mg and Maalox 1 ounce. Dr. Smith was consulted, and the patient will be admitted for an aspirin overdose in a suicide attempt. A psychiatric consultation has also been requested.

FINAL DIAGNOSES
1. Acetaminophen overdose.
2. Suicide attempt.

PROOFREADING EXERCISE #3

HISTORY OF PRESENT ILLNESS
The history is that of a pink left eye and ear pain. The patient is a 3-year-old child who has had a pink-tinged left eye for 1 day and has complained of ear pain primarily on the left side. She also has a cough and congestion. She saw her primary doctor yesterday, was reportedly diagnosed with bronchitis, and was placed on amoxicillin, and her mother was given a prescription for that as well as albuterol to be used on an as-needed basis. She has had no fever for the past severe days. Her mother reports that she has not yet filled the prescription for the amoxicillin but she has given her the atenolol at home.

PAST MEDICAL HISTORY
She has no prior episodes of wheezing. She has essentially been healthy.

CURRENT MEDICATIONS
Albuterol, as noted above.

ALLERGIES
She has no known medication allergies.

IMMUNIZATIONS
Up to date.

PHYSICAL EXAMINATION
VITAL SIGNS: Temperature was 99.7, pulse 86, respiratory rate 16 and her weight is 17.6 kg.
GENERAL: She is alert, well developed, well nourished and in no acute distress.
HEENT: Normocephalic and atraumatic. Pupils were equal, round and reactive to light. Her left conjunctivae was slightly pink without discharge. Her right conjunctivae was clear. She did have rhinorrhea. Her mucous membranes are moist. Her oropharynx is clear. Her right tympanic membrane had erythema peripherally with good hand marks. Her left tympanic membrane was bright red with diminished hand marks.
NECK: Supple. She had shoddy cervical lymphadenopathy bilaterally. There were no masses.

(continued)

CHEST: Lungs were clear to auscultation bilaterally.
HEART: Regular rate and rhythm, normal S1 and S2 with no murmur, rub, click or gallop.
ABDOMEN: Soft, nontender, nondistended, with good bowel sounds, no masses, and no hepatosplenomegaly.
NEUROLOGICALLY: She was alert, with normal gate, moving all 4 extremities, and was grossly nonfocal.

FINAL DIAGNOSES

1. Acute osteitis media bilaterally but primarily on the left side.
2. Mild conjunctivitis on the left.

DISCHARGE INSTRUCTIONS

She was instructed not to fill the prescription for amoxicillin but rather was given a prescription for Augmentin, which should help with both her eye and ears. Her prescription was for 40 mg/mL, and she is to take 1 teaspoon p.o. b.i.d. for the next 10 days. In addition, mother should encourage plenty of fluids, and the child should return to the emergency room or see her pediatrician if there is no improvement in her condition in 3 days.

PROOFREADING EXERCISE #4

HISTORY OF PRESENT ILLNESS

The patient is an 80-year-old African-American male with a history of diabetes mellitus and severe vascular accident who was brought into the emergency room by his daughter after he was found unresponsive in bed. The patient reportedly had become more lethargic in the past 2 days prior to his presentation, and the patient's daughter was reportedly unable to awaken him on the day of presentation. The patient was noted to have a blood sugar of 332 in the emergency room.

The patient was found to be comatose, and a detailed history was unobtainable other than that provided by the patient's daughter.

PAST MEDICAL HISTORY

Significant for diabetes mellitus and a history of severe vascular accident with a residual right paresis.

ALLERGIES

No known drug allergies.

MEDICATIONS

Glucophage and aspirin.

PHYSICAL EXAMINATION

GENERAL: Revealed an elderly African-American male who is unresponsive and comatose except to painful stimuli. He was in no acute respiratory distress.
VITAL SIGNS: His blood pressure was 100/51, pulse 81, respiratory rate 20 and temperature was 93.8.
HEENT: Normocephalic and atraumatic, with exophthalmos.
NECK: Supple with no jugular venous distension.
CHEST: Bilateral rhoncal.
CARDIOVASCULAR SYSTEM: S1 and S2 with no S3.
ABDOMEN: Soft and nondistended.
EXTREMITIES: No pitting edema.
CENTRAL NERVOUS SYSTEM: The patient was comatose.

(continued)

LABORATORY FINDINGS

Blood glucose was 732, BUN 76, creatinine 3.5, chloride 117, bicarbonate 13. There were positive ketones and sodium was 154, potassium 60. White blood cells were 17.7, hemoglobin 7.8, hematocrit 84 and platelets 372. A CT scan of the head revealed a right occipital farse. An arterial blood gas showed a Ph of 7.34, pCO_2 of 20, a pO_2 of 46, and oxygen saturation of 100% on 1 L of oxygen. Urinalysis showed moderate blood, too numerous to count white blood cells, 3+ bacteria, and 2+ trichomonas.

HOSPITAL COURSE

The patient was admitted to the intensive care unit and a "do not resuscitate (DNR)" order was signed by the patient's daughter. The patient was placed on a 100% nonrebreather mask. The patient was given IV fluids of normal saline. The patient was started on an insulin drip, and he had arterial blood gases, a Chemistry-7, and Accu-Cheks monitored very closely.

The patient was pancultured and started on imperfect antibiotics for possible sepsis. The patient was started on cereal CPKs and CK-MBs, and a nephrology consultation was obtained. The patient was also started on warming blankets, and a dopamine strip was continued to keep his systolic blood pressure above 90.

Subsequently, the patient was found unresponsive without pulse or respirations, and his pupils were fixed and dilated. He was pronounced expired at 16:30 on 04/15/2004.

EXPIRATION DIAGNOSES

1. Septic anemia due to urosepsis.
2. Cerebrovascular accident.
3. Diabetic ketosis.
4. Dehydration.
5. Acute renal failure.
6. Hyperthermia.
7. Anemia.
8. Electrolyte imbalance with hyponatremia.

ANSWER KEYS

REVIEW QUESTIONS ANSWER KEY

1. B
2. C
3. C
4. A
5. C
6. D
7. A
8. A
9. D
10. B
11. C
12. C
13. D
14. B
15. A
16. C
17. B
18. C
19. C
20. A
21. C
22. C
23. A
24. D
25. B
26. A
27. C
28. C
29. A
30. C

PROOFREADING EXERCISE #1 KEY

Flag patient age (patient is pregnant)

CHIEF COMPLAINT/HISTORY OF PRESENT ILLNESS
The patient is a 66-year-old female who does not have a doctor at this hospital. She was therefore referred to Dr. Jones, the OB/GYN physician on-call today. Her chief complaint is that of alleged sexual assault which happened 2 days ago. The patient said that she is 4-6 weeks pregnant. She denied any abdominal pain or any vaginal bleeding. She did not seek medical attention until today.

PHYSICAL EXAMINATION
VITAL SIGNS: Blood pressure 111/61, pulse 82, respirations 20, temperature 98.
GENERAL: The patient is unconscious, responsive, and coherent.
HEENT: Pupils are equal, round, and reactive to light. No hematoma of the scalp.
NECK: Subtle.
CHEST: Clear.
HEART: Heart sounds are normal.
ABDOMEN: No distention, feels soft, bowel sounds present. Her uterus is palpated just below the cubic margin.
PELVIC EXAMINATION: No lacerations, no bleeding; the uterus is about 4 to 6 weeks and no annexal masses are felt.

Incorrect word—conscious

Incorrect word—supple

Incorrect word—pubic

Incorrect term—adnexal

DIAGNOSTIC STUDIES
The patient had a CBC, SMA-7 and a beta aCG test done. Her pregnancy test was positive. We also did a serum quantitative pregnancy test. Electrolytes are normal. Alcohol level is zero. Her drug screen, however, is positive for both marijuana and cocaine. We also obtained gonorrhea and chlamydia cultures. A cervical culture was also prepared. Her urinalysis was negative.

Incorrect abbreviation—hCG

Incorrect spelling—prophylaxis

Wrong term—Intrauterine

EMERGENCY DEPARTMENT COURSE

We contacted social services and the police department. The patient received Rocephin 250 mg IM for prophylactic. She will be followed by her private medical doctor.

FINAL DIAGNOSES

1. Alleged sexual assault.
2. Enterouterine pregnancy.

PROOFREADING EXERCISE #2 KEY

CHIEF COMPLAINT
The patient is a 20-year-old female who was brought by EMS following ingestion of an overdose of aspirin in a suicidal gesture. This ingestion occurred following an argument with his family about 15 minutes prior to presentation.

Gender reversal—her

CURRENT MEDICATIONS
None.

PHYSICAL EXAMINATION
VITAL SIGNS: Temperature 96, pulse 120, respirations 24, blood pressure 146/68.

GENERAL: She is morbidly obese at over 300 pounds on her 5′6″ frame. She appears unkept.

Incorrect word—unkempt

HEENT: Normal cephalic and atraumatic. Eyes are normal. ENT normal.

Incorrect spelling—normocephalic

NECK: Supple. No jugular venous distension or carotid bruit.

CHEST: Clear to auscultation and percussion.

HEART: Auscultation revealed regular sinus rhythm with a 2/6 systolic ejection murmur best heard over the left sternal border.

ABDOMEN: Soft and nontender but dentulous. Bowel sounds are normoactive.

Incorrect term—pendulous

GENITALIA: Deferred.

RECTAL EXAMINATION: Differed.

Incorrect word—Deferred

EXTREMITIES: She moves all 4 extremities to command.

NERVOUS SYSTEM: No sign of focal deficit. No sign of meningismus.

DIAGNOSTIC STUDIES
Her salicylate level was 6 mg/dL, acetaminophen level was less then 10.

Incorrect word—than

Incorrect drug—Zantac

Contradicts diagnostic studies and previous statements—should be aspirin.

EMERGENCY DEPARTMENT COURSE

The patient was given 50 grams of charcoal in sorbitol and normal saline to run at 125 mL per hour. She also received Xanax 300 mg and Maalox 1 ounce. Dr. Smith was consulted, and the patient will be admitted for an aspirin overdose in a suicide attempt. A psychiatric consultation has also been requested.

FINAL DIAGNOSES

1. Acetaminophen overdose.
2. Suicide attempt.

PROOFREADING EXERCISE #3 KEY

HISTORY OF PRESENT ILLNESS
The history is that of a pink left eye and ear pain. The patient is a 3-year-old child who has had a pink-tinged left eye for 1 day and has complained of ear pain primarily on the left side. She also has a cough and congestion. She saw her primary doctor yesterday, was reportedly diagnosed with bronchitis, and was placed on amoxicillin, and her mother was given a prescription for that as well as albuterol to be used on an as-needed basis. She has had no fever for the past severe ~~days~~. Her mother reports that she has not yet filled the prescription for the amoxicillin but she has given her ~~the~~ atenolol at home.

Incorrect word—several

Incorrect drug—albuterol

PAST MEDICAL HISTORY
She has no prior episodes of wheezing. She has essentially been healthy.

CURRENT MEDICATIONS
Albuterol, as noted above.

ALLERGIES
She has no known medication allergies.

IMMUNIZATIONS
Up to date.

PHYSICAL EXAMINATION
VITAL SIGNS: Temperature was 99.7, pulse 86, respiratory rate 16 and her weight is 17.6 kg.

GENERAL: She is alert, well developed, well nourished and in no acute distress.

HEENT: Normocephalic and atraumatic. Pupils were equal, round and reactive to light. Her left conjunctivae was slightly pink without discharge. Her ~~right~~ conjunctivae was clear. She did have rhinorrhea. Her mucous membranes are moist. Her oropharynx is clear. Her right tympanic membrane

Incorrect spelling—singular conjunctiva

had erythema peripherally with good hand marks. Her left tympanic membrane was bright red with diminished hand marks.
NECK: Supple. She had shoddy cervical lymphadenopathy bilaterally. There were no masses.
CHEST: Lungs were clear to auscultation bilaterally.
HEART: Regular rate and rhythm, normal S1 and S2 with no murmur, rub, click or gallop.
ABDOMEN: Soft, nontender, nondistended, with good bowel sounds, no masses, and no hepatosplenomegaly.
NEUROLOGICALLY: She was alert, with normal gate, moving all 4 extremities, and was grossly nonfocal.

FINAL DIAGNOSES

1. Acute osteitis media bilaterally but primarily on the left side.
2. Mild conjunctivitis on the left.

DISCHARGE INSTRUCTIONS

She was instructed not to fill the prescription for amoxicillin but rather was given a prescription for Augmentin, which should help with both her eye and ears. Her prescription was for 40 mg/mL, and she is to take 1 teaspoon p.o. b.i.d. for the next 10 days. In addition, mother should encourage plenty of fluids, and the child should return to the emergency room or see her pediatrician if there is no improvement in her condition in 3 days.

Incorrect word—landmarks

Incorrect word—shotty

Incorrect spelling—gait

Incorrect term—otitis

Flag—conflicts with physical exam

Incorrect dose—Augmentin dispensed as 400 mg/mL

PROOFREADING EXERCISE #4 KEY

HISTORY OF PRESENT ILLNESS
The patient is an 80-year-old African-American male with a history of diabetes mellitus and severe vascular accident who was brought into the emergency room by his daughter after he was found unresponsive in bed. The patient reportedly had become more lethargic in the past 2 days prior to his presentation, and the patient's daughter was reportedly unable to awaken him on the day of presentation. The patient was noted to have a blood sugar of 332 in the emergency room. The patient was found to be comatose, and a detailed history was unobtainable other than that provided by the patient's daughter.

Wrong words—cerebrovascular

PAST MEDICAL HISTORY
Significant for diabetes mellitus and a history of severe vascular accident with a residual right paresis.

Incomplete term—hemiparesis

ALLERGIES
No known drug allergies.

MEDICATIONS
Glucophage and aspirin.

PHYSICAL EXAMINATION
GENERAL: Revealed an elderly African-American male who is unresponsive and comatose except to painful stimuli. He was in no acute respiratory distress.
VITAL SIGNS: His blood pressure was 100/51, pulse 81, respiratory rate 20 and temperature was 93.8.
HEENT: Normocephalic and atraumatic, with exophthalmos.
NECK: Supple with no jugular venous distension.
CHEST: Bilateral rhoncal.
CARDIOVASCULAR SYSTEM: S1 and S2 with no S3.
ABDOMEN: Soft and nondistended.

Incorrect term—rhonchi

EXTREMITIES: No pitting edema.
CENTRAL NERVOUS SYSTEM: The patient was comatose.

LABORATORY FINDINGS
Blood glucose was 732, BUN 76, creatinine 3.5, chloride 117, bicarbonate 13. There were positive ketones and sodium was 154, potassium 60. White blood cells were 17.7, hemoglobin 7.8, hematocrit 84 and platelets 372. A CT scan of the head revealed a right occipital farse. An arterial blood gas showed a Ph of 7.34, pCO_2 of 20, a pO_2 of 46, and oxygen saturation of 100% on 1 L of oxygen. Urinalysis showed moderate blood, too numerous to count white blood cells, 3+ bacteria, and 2+ trichomonas.

Flag—improbable value for potassium

Flag—improbable value for hematocrit

Incorrect term—infarct

Incorrect format—pH

HOSPITAL COURSE
The patient was admitted to the intensive care unit and a "do not resuscitate (DNR)" order was signed by the patient's daughter. The patient was placed on a 100% nonrebreather mask. The patient was given IV fluids of normal saline. The patient was started on an insulin drip, and he had arterial blood gases, a Chemistry-7, and Accu-Cheks monitored very closely.

Incorrect term—Chem-7

The patient was pancultured and started on imperfect antibiotics for possible sepsis. The patient was started on cereal CPKs and CK-MBs, and a nephrology consultation was obtained. The patient was also started on warming blankets, and a dopamine strip was continued to keep his systolic blood pressure above 90.

Incorrect word—empiric

Incorrect spelling—serial

Incorrect word—drip

Subsequently, the patient was found unresponsive without pulse or respirations, and his pupils were fixed and dilated. He was pronounced expired at 16:30 on 04/15/2004.

Incorrect word—septicemia

Should be hypothermia based on temperature reported above

EXPIRATION DIAGNOSES

1. Septic anemia due to urosepsis.
2. Cerebrovascular accident.
3. Diabetic ketosis.
4. Dehydration.
5. Acute renal failure.
6. Hyperthermia.
7. Anemia.
8. Electrolyte imbalance with hyponatremia.

Should be hypernatremia based on sodium value reported above

CHAPTER 7

Hematology/Oncology

OBJECTIVES CHECKLIST

A prepared exam candidate will know:

- ❑ All combining forms, prefixes, and suffixes related to the blood system and to oncology.
- ❑ Composition and formation of the blood.
- ❑ Stages of blood cell development from stem cell to full differentiation.
- ❑ Role and function of each blood component, including the breakdown of each leukocyte type and its percentage in the blood.
- ❑ Physiology of clot formation.
- ❑ Different blood groups that identify human blood and the role of antigens and antibodies in determining blood type and preventing agglutination.
- ❑ Characteristics of tumors and the differences between benign and malignant neoplasms.
- ❑ Physiology of carcinogenesis and the role of DNA/RNA in cellular malignancy.
- ❑ Different environmental agents and hereditary factors that contribute to the development of cancer.
- ❑ Differences among carcinomas, sarcomas, and mixed-tissue tumors, as well as the tissues from which they derive.
- ❑ Diseases and disorders of each type of blood cell, of clotting, and of the bone marrow.
- ❑ Laboratory studies used in the identification and treatment of hematologic disorders and diseases.
- ❑ Gross and microscopic pathological descriptions used to indicate the appearance of tumors on examination.
- ❑ Grading and staging systems used to classify neoplasms.
- ❑ Four major approaches to cancer treatment (surgery, radiation therapy, chemotherapy, and biological therapy) and the terminology related to each.
- ❑ Common medications prescribed for blood disorders and diseases and for the side effects and symptoms associated with radiation and chemotherapy.

RESOURCES FOR STUDY

1. *The Language of Medicine*
   Chapter 13: Blood System, pp. 488–528.
   Chapter 19: Cancer Medicine (Oncology), pp. 770–816.
2. *Human Diseases*
   Chapter 5: Neoplasia, pp. 57–72.
   Chapter 16: Disorders of Blood cells, Blood-Forming Tissues, and Blood Coagulation, pp. 241–258.
3. *Laboratory Tests & Diagnostic Procedures in Medicine*
   Section V: Anatomic Pathology, pp. 223–314.
   Chapter 19: Hematology, Coagulation and Blood Typing, pp. 323–354.
4. *Understanding Pharmacology for Health Professionals*
   Chapter 17: Anticoagulant and Thrombolytic Drugs, pp. 139–142.
   Chapter 30: Chemotherapy Drugs, pp. 337–364.
   Chapter 32: Intravenous Fluids and Blood Products, Blood and Blood Cellular Products, pp. 378–382.
5. *The AAMT Book of Style*
   Blood counts and Blood groups, pp. 39–40.
   Blood types, p. 41.
   Cancer classifications, pp. 50–56.
   Laboratory data and values: hemoglobin and hematocrit, p. 232.
   Laboratory data and values: tumor cell markers, p. 233.

SAMPLE REPORTS

The following four reports are examples of reports you might encounter while transcribing hematology and oncology.

FOLLOWUP

HISTORY
The patient is a 25-year-old woman, G3 P2 A0, who is being followed for idiopathic thrombocytopenic purpura developed during her third pregnancy. She was started on prednisone at 1 mg/kg per day when she came in with a platelet count of 40,000, easy bruising, and marked petechiae. Her platelet count responded to prednisone. Although she has not come in as scheduled because she was too busy, her platelet count had increased to 161,000 on March 22. At that time, I decreased the dose to 60 mg per day. The patient comes in today for reevaluation.

REVIEW OF SYSTEMS
She has had no fever. She has had the normal weight change expected from her pregnancy. No malaise, no dizziness. SKIN: No ulcers, spots, bleeding, changes in color or texture. HEENT: No headaches, sinus problems, hoarseness, visual or hearing problems. CARDIORESPIRATORY: No cough, sputum production, hemoptysis, dyspnea, paroxysmal nocturnal dyspnea, orthopnea, chest pain, palpitations, or cyanosis. GASTROINTESTINAL: Mild heartburn. No dysphagia, odynophagia, abdominal pain, tenesmus, bleeding, or change in bowel habits. GENITOURINARY: Negative. MUSCULOSKELETAL: Basically negative. NERVOUS: Negative. LYMPHATIC: Negative.

PHYSICAL EXAMINATION
HEENT: Intact external ocular movements, no nystagmus, oropharynx clear. NECK: Supple. No JVD, no lymph nodes. HEART: Regular rhythm, no murmurs. LUNGS: Clear. ABDOMEN: Soft, bowel sounds positive. Gravid uterus, normal size.

LABORATORY
CBC done today shows a platelet count of 139,000.

IMPRESSION
1. Pregnancy.
2. Idiopathic thrombocytopenic purpura.

PLAN
1. Will decrease prednisone to 40 mg p.o. daily.
2. CBC and differential in 2 weeks.
3. Office visit in 4 weeks.

FOLLOWUP

The patient is a 75-year-old gentleman with stage IIIB non-small-cell lung cancer who received his first cycle of chemotherapy with carboplatin and Taxol on 4/27. The dosage is 225 mg/m^2 of Taxol and carboplatin to an AUC of 6. However, the patient's BSA was capped at 2 m^2 and the initial dose was reduced by 20%. The patient comes in today for reevaluation. He is feeling very well and has had no major complaints. He is breathing better than he has in a long time.

REVIEW OF SYSTEMS
The rest of the review of systems is per questionnaire.

PHYSICAL EXAMINATION
On physical examination, his height is 6 feet, weight is 200 pounds, BSA 2.08 m^2, blood pressure 150/70, pulse 80, temperature 97.9. HEENT: Intact external ocular movements, no nystagmus, oropharynx clear. NECK: Supple. No JVD, no lymph nodes. His face is not as swollen as on prior evaluations. HEART: Regular rhythm. LUNGS: Clear. ABDOMEN: Soft, bowel sounds positive. No liver or spleen enlargement. EXTREMITIES: No edema or cyanosis. NEUROLOGICAL: Nonfocal.

IMPRESSION
1. Non-small-cell lung cancer stage IIIB (T4 N2 M0).
2. Superior vena cava syndrome, much improved.
3. Syndrome of inappropriate antidiuretic hormone secretion, so far not evaluated.

PLAN
1. Will do CBC and differential today.
2. Office visit on May 19 with chest x-ray, PA and lateral, and CBC and differential for possible chemotherapy.

CONSULTATION

The patient is a 76-year-old lady with no prior history of systemic disease who is referred by Dr. Smith for evaluation of lymphoma. She presented approximately 1 year ago with a mass in the right side of her neck which has increased in size. She has also developed other nodules in the opposite side of the neck. I am told the lymph nodes showed low-grade lymphoma with gene-rearrangement status and negative flow cytometry. Final pathology is still pending. I am consulted for recommendations for further treatment.

PAST MEDICAL HISTORY
Gastroesophageal reflux and occasional wheezing. Osteoarthritis.

PAST SURGICAL HISTORY
Cholecystectomy, appendectomy, and bladder resection.

MEDICATIONS
Prevacid and Vioxx.

ALLERGIES
None.

FAMILY HISTORY
Positive for COPD in most of her 10 siblings and in her father. There is also a history of lung cancer in a few of her siblings who were smokers.

SOCIAL HISTORY
She is married with 2 children. She does not work. She has never used alcohol, drugs, or cigarettes.

REVIEW OF SYSTEMS
Occasional shortness of breath, usually in the morning and related to postnasal drip, none on exercise. Otherwise, negative as per questionnaire.

PHYSICAL EXAMINATION
On physical examination, her weight is 203 pounds, height 5 feet 3 1/2 inches, BSA 1.95 m^2, blood pressure 110/70, pulse 80. She is conscious, oriented and alert. HEENT: Intact external ocular movements, no nystagmus, oropharynx clear. Patient is edentulous. NECK: Supple. No thyromegaly. Trachea is midline. There are lymph nodes palpable measuring about 3 × 3 cm in the submandibular area as well as smaller lymph nodes along the cervical areas on both sides. Also, there are lymph nodes in the supraclavicular region. They are non-matted. Cranial nerves are intact. No JVD. HEART: Regular rhythm, no murmurs. LUNGS: Clear. ABDOMEN: Soft, bowel sounds positive. No liver or spleen enlargement. NEUROLOGICAL: Nonfocal. SKIN: No petechiae or eruptions.

I performed a bone marrow aspirate and biopsy on the right iliac crest. Patient was prepped with Betadine and infiltrated with 1% lidocaine. The procedure was indicated for staging of her lymphoma. She did not have any complications.

(continued)

IMPRESSION

Non-Hodgkin lymphoma, currently being staged, but at least stage II. By preliminary report, it looks like a low-grade lymphoma. I discussed with the patient, her daughter, and husband for more than 90 minutes the characteristics of low-grade lymphomas and her expected prognosis. In general, low-grade lymphomas are characterized by indolent clinical behavior and comparatively long survival with a median survival between 6 and 10 years. Most patients have advanced stage disease at diagnosis and only about 10–20% have stage I or II. There is a very low potential for cure when the disease presents in the more advanced stages and the treatment is usually palliative. Since the patient is having some discomfort, she would be a candidate for treatment.

ADDENDUM

Basically, her CT scan of the chest was negative as well as her bone marrow biopsy. The CT scan of the abdomen shows mild retroperitoneal adenopathy in the infrarenal region as well as near the obturator muscle. She also has lymphadenopathy around the right common femoral vein and inguinal adenopathy, most measuring between 1 and 2 cm. This would definitely convert her from stage II to stage III. This has further implications for her prognosis. In general, for localized, low-grade non-Hodgkin lymphoma of the head and neck, the treatment of choice is involved-field radiation therapy with or without adjuvant chemotherapy. This results in 5-year survival of over 50%. However, if she has stage III disease, she is not a candidate for radiation at all and would have to have chemotherapy. After explaining this, we have decided to do a PET scan as well as MUGA scan, since the patient would be receiving CHOP chemotherapy which has Adriamycin. We will see again after the PET scan to evaluate whether she needs chemotherapy only or chemotherapy with radiation.

EVALUATION

The patient is a 46-year-old woman with no prior history of systemic illness who about 6 years ago was evaluated for enlarged submandibular lymph nodes. The patient is quite apprehensive, but after several questions, she tells me it was diagnosed as hypertrophic adenopathy. She was told to follow with them regularly because it might change. She was scared and did not want to get a bone marrow biopsy which was offered at that time. One to 2 years ago, she started to develop axillary lymph nodes and finally she went to see Dr. Smith who did a biopsy of a cervical lymph node which showed lymphocytic lymphoma/CLL. She is referred for recommendations on further management.

PAST MEDICAL HISTORY
As above.

PAST SURGICAL HISTORY
Laparoscopic cholecystectomy due to gallstones in February of 2000.

FAMILY HISTORY
Father is alive with diabetes. Her mother died but she does not know the cause of her death. She has 2 brothers in good health and a sister in good health.

TOXIC HABITS
She quit smoking cigarettes several years ago.

SOCIAL HISTORY
She has been married for 27 years and has 2 children, ages 15 and 25.

REVIEW OF SYSTEMS
Remarkably negative. She does not have fever, chills, or weight loss. She only notices the lymph nodes when she looks in the mirror. She gets shortness of breath with exercise, but she has no chest pain. She occasionally has nausea and heartburn. The rest of the review of systems is per questionnaire.

PHYSICAL EXAMINATION
On physical examination, her weight is 150 pounds, height 5 feet 4 inches, blood pressure 158/89, pulse 98. She is conscious, oriented, and alert. HEENT: Intact external ocular movements, no nystagmus, oropharynx clear. NECK: Supple. No JVD. No thyromegaly. She has extensive shotty adenopathy bilaterally in the submandibular, cervical, and supraclavicular regions, some of them as large as 4 cm. HEART: Regular rhythm, no murmurs. LUNGS: Clear. ABDOMEN: Soft, bowel sounds positive. No liver or spleen enlargement. EXTREMITIES: She does have bilateral axillary lymphadenopathy, large and shotty. No inguinal lymphadenopathy.

LABORATORY DATA
Biopsy of the lymph nodes as described. CBC drawn on 3/29 shows a WBC of 10,200 with 25% lymphocytes, hemoglobin of 10.4 with hematocrit of 31.8, MCV of 74, and RDW of 18, which is quite suggestive of iron deficiency anemia.

CT scan of the chest shows evidence of supraclavicular and axillary lymph nodes, and CT scan of the abdomen shows several intraabdominal mesenteric nodes and periaortic nodes.

(continued)

IMPRESSION

Small lymphocytic lymphoma/CLL, currently asymptomatic except for shotty adenopathy. I would like to try a low-dose regimen with low toxicity such as CVP. Another option would be Fludara, but the schedule would be daily for 5 days and she cannot work under those conditions. Patient will not even consider a bone marrow biopsy at this time. Actually, except for bulky disease, she does not have other known bad prognostic features, although I have not done a bone marrow biopsy. My plan for now is to start chemotherapy with Cytoxan, vincristine, and prednisone and watch closely to see if we can induce remission. Side effects were explained to the patient and she was given written information about chemotherapy.

PLAN

1. Cytoxan 400 mg/m^2 plus vincristine 2 mg/m^2 plus prednisone 60 mg IV on day 1 for 3 weeks.
2. Bone marrow aspirate and biopsy. Patient is quite reluctant to have this done.
3. Iron sulfate 300 mg p.o. t.i.d.
4. CBC and differential today and then in 10 days for nadir counts.
5. Metabolic panel, LDH, beta-2-microglobulin, SPEP and immunofixation, iron, TIBC, and ferritin.
6. Office visit next week.

REVIEW QUESTIONS

The goal of these questions is to test your knowledge in the areas of hematology and oncology.

Directions: Select the correct answer for each of the multiple-choice questions provided below. *Answers are provided at the end of this chapter.*

1. Hypoechoic nodules are detected in breast tissue using:
   A. Blood tests
   B. Ultrasound
   C. Mammogram
   D. Breast physical examination

2. The scale used to record functional capacity (ability to perform activities of daily living) for cancer patients is called:
   A. Wechsler
   B. Glasgow
   C. Karnofsky
   D. Apgar

3. BRCA-1 and BRCA-2 are:
   A. Genes associated with a higher incidence of leukemia
   B. Genes associated with a higher incidence of breast cancer
   C. Cells associated with breast cancer
   D. Estrogen receptors

4. A fibroadenoma is:
   A. A metastatic breast cancer
   B. An early form of breast cancer
   C. A benign breast tumor
   D. A breast lump with early invasion of cancer

5. What is ductal carcinoma in situ (DCIS)?
   A. A metastatic breast cancer
   B. Benign tumor in the breast tissue
   C. Breast cancer which has not metastasized
   D. An invasive breast cancer

6. Arimidex, Femara, and Nolvadex are hormonal drugs used to treat:
   A. Breast cancer
   B. Prostate cancer
   C. Anemia
   D. CML

7. A partial, arrested, or non-apparent form of disease is called:
   A. Benign
   B. Metastatic
   C. Forme fruste
   D. HER2/neu

8. Which of the following is a naturally occurring protein produced by recombinant DNA technology, used to treat cancers and viral infections?
   A. Interferon alfa-2a
   B. Interferon alpha
   C. Taxotere
   D. Casodex

9. The PET scan has become a valuable tool in staging breast cancer because:
   A. The type of breast cancer can be determined without biopsy
   B. Metastatic disease to lymph nodes can usually be seen even when nodes cannot be felt
   C. The aggressiveness of the tumor can be determined
   D. Hormonal therapy can be decided on prior to surgery

10. What does T/N/M stand for when describing cancer?
    A. Tumor/Nonoperative/Mastopexy
    B. Tumor/Negativity/Malignancy
    C. Throat/Nose/Mouth
    D. Tumor/Nodes/Metastasis

11. Surgery done to sustain a cancer patient or alleviate pain is called:
    A. Adjuvant
    B. Preventive surgery
    C. Palliative surgery
    D. Brachytherapy

12. Which of the following is a monoclonal antibody therapy for lymphoma?
    A. Rituxan
    B. Adriamycin
    C. Xeloda
    D. Zinecard

13. A type of neoplasm that affects bone marrow is called:
    A. Sarcoma
    B. Osteosarcoma
    C. Adenoma
    D. Leukemia

14. Epogen and Procrit (epoetin alfa) are used to treat which of the following common side effects of chemotherapy?
    A. Nausea
    B. Anemia
    C. Hair loss
    D. Loss of appetite

15. One type of malignant tumor of the kidney is called:
    A. Retinoblastoma
    B. Burkitt lymphoma
    C. Wilms tumor
    D. Astrocytoma

16. A patient with severe leukopenia might require:
    A. Transfusion with 10 units of FFP (fresh frozen plasma)
    B. Reverse isolation to prevent infection
    C. Acetaminophen 650 mg p.o. q.4 h. around-the-clock
    D. Emergency endotracheal intubation

17. A patient has had these blood tests ordered: Ferritin level, B-12 level, folate level, and total iron binding capacity. A differential diagnosis might include:
    A. Jaundice
    B. Iron-deficiency anemia
    C. Malabsorption syndrome
    D. Chronic fatigue syndrome

18. Casodex, Eulexin, Zoladex, and Lupron are treatments used for:
    A. Breast cancer
    B. Leukemia
    C. Lymphoma
    D. Prostate cancer

19. Which of the following is not a routine part of a complete blood count (CBC)?
    A. Red cell indices
    B. Hemoglobin
    C. Platelet count
    D. Reticulocyte count

20. The complex process by which platelets, plasma, and fibrin interact to control bleeding is called:
    A. Phagocytosis
    B. Hematopoiesis
    C. Coagulation
    D. Plasmapheresis

21. Macrocytosis, anisocytosis, and poikilocytosis are terms used to describe:
    A. Red cells
    B. White cells
    C. Platelets
    D. Tumor cells

22. The major categories of formed elements in the blood include:
    A. Phagocytes, histiocytes, and erythrocytes
    B. Erythrocytes, leukocytes, and platelets
    C. Platelets, metamyelocytes, and prolymphocytes
    D. Neutrophils, eosinophils, and basophils

23. Factor VIII is a clotting factor most often prescribed for:
    A. Eye surgery
    B. Hemophiliacs
    C. Cancer patients
    D. Platelet aggregation

24. A patient has the following lab values: Electrophoresis positive for hemoglobin S, elevated reticulocyte count, and nucleated RBC and target cells seen on peripheral smear. A likely diagnosis would be:
    A. Pernicious anemia
    B. Aplastic anemia
    C. Sickle cell anemia
    D. Leukemia

25. ITP is the abbreviation for:
    A. Idiopathic thrombocytopenic purpura
    B. Immune thrombocytic purpura
    C. Idiopathic T-cell proliferation
    D. Both A & B

26. Cancers which develop from plasma cells are called:
    A. Myelomas
    B. Leukemia
    C. Lymphomas
    D. Gliomas

27. A type of cancer that causes painless, progressive enlargement of lymph nodes, spleen, and other lymphoid tissue and is associated with Reed-Sternberg cells is called:
    A. Leukemia
    B. Lymphoid hyperplasia
    C. Hodgkin disease
    D. Non-Hodgkin lymphoma

28. The Philadelphia chromosome is pathognomonic for:
    A. CML
    B. Lymphoma
    C. Breast cancer
    D. Prostate cancer

29. Which of the following is a list of lung cancer types?
    A. Adenocarcinoma, oat cell, and anaplastic
    B. Epidermoid, anaplastic, and oat cell
    C. Small cell, adenocarcinoma, and lymphocytic
    D. Oat cell, squamous cell, large cell

30. A WBC count of 100,000 would indicate:
    A. A normal white cell count
    B. A slightly elevated white cell count
    C. A decreased WBC
    D. A markedly elevated count typical of leukemia

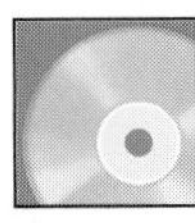

Please see the accompanying CD for additional review materials for this section.

PROOFREADING EXERCISES

These three proofreading exercises are provided to improve your skills in the areas of editing and effective identification and correction of errors in the medical record.

Directions: Identify and correct the transcription errors found in the exercises below. *Answers are provided at the end of this chapter.*

PROOFREADING EXERCISE #1

Mr. Smith is a 63-year-old gentleman with hormone-secretory prostate cancer who is currently on withdrawal from coronal therapy. He comes in today for reevaluation. He had been sent to the vascular surgeon for intermittent claudication mostly on the left lower extremity distally from the knee. On his last visit on April 11, he was feeling much better and his pain was markedly improved. Now, he is having much more pain again which now radiates from the lip all the way down the leg. He has decreased strength in that leg.

REVIEW OF SYSTEMS
The rest of the review of systems is unchanged since last visit. He has had radiotherapy to the hip and cervical area.

PHYSICAL EXAMINATION
He is conscious, oriented and alert. HEENT: Intact external ocular movements, no nystagmus, oropharynx clear. NECK: Supple. No JVD, no lymph nodes. HEART: Regular rhythm, no murmurs. LUNGS: Clear. ABDOMEN: Soft, bowel sounds positive. No liver or spleen enlargement. EXTREMITIES: No edema or cyanosis. NEUROLOGICAL: Nonfocal except as noted with decreased strength in the left leg, mostly distally.

LABORATORY DATA
Last PFA was 162. MRI ordered by Dr. Jones shows a retro peroneal mass extending into the lower vertebral bodies and the spinal canal with primary involvement of L3, L4 and L5 vertebral bodies and partial relapse of each.

(continued)

IMPRESSION
Hormone-refractory prostate cancer now with painful involvement of L3-L5 region. The pane seems more like nerve impingement than actual spinal cord repression. The patient has had multiple irradiations, so I am concerned that giving him mediation at this point will be too suppressive. I will watch him closely over the next couple of days and start him on dexamethasone and Vexol. If there is not an improvement or if his condition deteriorates, I will send him for radiation.

PLAN
1. Chemotherapy tomorrow.
2. Start dexamethasone 8 mg p.o. b.i.d. today.

PROOFREADING EXERCISE #2

The patient is a 62-year-old woman with focally-advanced breast cancer who had quite significant residual disease after fore cycles of neon adjuvant chemotherapy with AC. She underwent right modified radicle mastectomy with axiliary dissection and 4 additional cycles of Paxil. She then received radiotherapy to her chest wall and axilla which she finished in January. In late April of this year, she was admitted to Memorial Hospital with shortness of breath and a DVT on the left side. The shortness of breath was secondary to a right-sided pleural effusion which was tapped. This showed malignant sails. A bone scan was also positive for multiple metastatic disease. She was treated with pan iduronate 90 mg IV on 4/25 and she was discharged on Femara 2.5 mg daily. She comes in today for reevaluation. She is feeling much better. Her shortness of breath is stable and she tolerates exercise better. She continues with occasional pain in the scapular region of the left shoulder and she is having hot flashes. She is currently on Coumadin 7.5 mg q.d.

REVIEW OF SYSTEMS
GENERAL: She denies fever, weight change, malacia, or dizziness. SKIN: No ulcers, spots, bleeding, or changes in color or texture. HEENT: No headaches, sinus problems, hoarseness, visual or hearing problems. CARDIORESPIRATORY: No cough. Shortness of breath as described. No chest pain. GASTROINTESTINAL: Denies dysphasia, odynophagia, heartburn. GENITOURINARY: Negative. MUSCULOSKELETAL: Left-sided pain which is better than it was when she had a full-blown DVT.

PHYSICAL EXAMINATION
On physical examination, her weight is 226 pounds, which is 2 pounds less than prior visit, blood pressure 140/80, pulse 80. She is conscious, oriented, and alert. HEENT: Intact external ocular movements, no nystagmus, oropharynx clear. NECK: Supple. No JVD, no lymph nodes. HEART: Regular rhythm, no murmurs. LUNGS: Left lung clear. Right lung has a pleural fusion covering practically two-thirds of the lung. ABDOMEN: Soft, bowel sounds positive. No liver or spleen enlargement. EXTREMITIES: No edema or cyanosis. NEUROLOGICAL: Nonfocal.

(continued)

IMPRESSION

1. Metastatic breast cancer, currently on neuronal therapy.
2. Status post BVT with implantation of an interior vena cava filter. Patient is currently on Coumadin.

PLAN

1. PT/IMR and CBC drawn today. Not available at the time of dictation.
2. Abreva 90 mg IV over 3 hours on May 23.
3. Continue Femara.
4. Will see again on May 23.

PROOFREADING EXERCISE #3

The patient is a 30-year-old gentleman who comes in today to discuss the results of his bone marrow biopsy for asymptomatic neutropenia. His biopsy basically shows a cellular furrow with good evidence of trilineage granulopoiesis but profound neutropenia. There is no evidence of malignancy or myeloic dysplasia. Since he has normal granulopoiesis with relative monocytosis, this would indicate either a drug affect or chronic B-9 neutropenia. The patient however denies the use of any medications prescribed or over-the-counter. He did use some herbal supplements with ma huang and ginseng for about 6 months last year but stopped in October. If that had a drug effect, it should have gotten better by now. He is not having any symptoms, and except for a couple of upper respiratory tract infections earlier this year, he has been feeling well. His ANC is 500.

LABORATORY DATA
CBC done today shows a WBC of 1.8 with an AMC of 500. Neutral fills on parenteral smear appear normal. There are no blacks on peripheral smear.

IMPRESSION
Neutropenia, etiology unknown. Given that the patient is asymptomatic and that he has mild mono cytosis, this might be chronic benign neutropenia or even cyclic neutropenia which is an even rarer disease. However, with his normal peripheral smear, I doubt he has leukemia. Other differential diagnoses would include a drug-induced reaction verses early myelomalacia and even aplasia. Since he is asymptomatic, we will also have to rule-out other infections such as HIV or thyroid dysfunction as well as B-12 deficiency.

PLAN
1. CBC and deferential today.
2. HIV, TSH, T_3, T_4 and B-12, methyl malonic acid, serum homocysteine.

ANSWER KEYS

REVIEW QUESTIONS ANSWER KEY

1. B
2. C
3. B
4. C
5. C
6. A
7. C
8. A
9. B
10. D
11. C
12. A
13. D
14. B
15. C
16. B
17. B
18. D
19. D
20. C
21. A
22. B
23. B
24. C
25. D
26. A
27. C
28. A
29. D
30. D

PROOFREADING EXERCISE #1 KEY

Incorrect term—refractory

Incorrect word—hip

Incorrect term—hormonal

Mr. Smith is a 63-year-old gentleman with hormone-secretory prostate cancer who is currently on withdrawal from coronal therapy. He comes in today for reevaluation. He had been sent to the vascular surgeon for intermittent claudication mostly on the left lower extremity distally from the knee. On his last visit on April 11, he was feeling much better and his pain was markedly improved. Now, he is having much more pain again which now radiates from the lip all the way down the leg. He has decreased strength in that leg.

REVIEW OF SYSTEMS
The rest of the review of systems is unchanged since last visit. He has had radiotherapy to the hip and cervical area.

PHYSICAL EXAMINATION
He is conscious, oriented, and alert. HEENT: Intact external ocular movements, no nystagmus, oropharynx clear. NECK: Supple. No JVD, no lymph nodes. HEART: Regular rhythm, no murmurs. LUNGS: Clear. ABDOMEN: Soft, bowel sounds positive. No liver or spleen enlargement. EXTREMITIES: No edema or cyanosis. NEUROLOGICAL: Nonfocal except as noted with decreased strength in the left leg, mostly distally.

Incorrect abbreviation—PSA

Incorrect term—collapse

Incorrect term—retroperitoneal

LABORATORY DATA
Last PFA was 162. MRI ordered by Dr. Jones shows a retro peroneal mass extending into the lower vertebral bodies and the spinal canal with primary involvement of L3, L4 and L5 vertebral bodies and partial relapse of each.

Incorrect spelling—pain

Incorrect term—compression

Incorrect term—Taxol

Incorrect term—radiation

IMPRESSION
Hormone-refractory prostate cancer now with painful involvement of L3-L5 region. The pane seems more like nerve impingement than actual spinal cord repression. The patient has had multiple irradiations, so I am concerned that giving him mediation at this point will be too suppressive. I will watch him closely over the next couple of days and start him on dexamethasone and Vexol. If there is not an improvement or if his condition deteriorates, I will send him for radiation.

PLAN

1. Chemotherapy tomorrow.
2. Start dexamethasone 8 mg p.o. b.i.d. today.

PROOFREADING EXERCISE #2 KEY

The patient is a 62-year-old woman with focally-advanced breast cancer who had quite significant residual disease after fore cycles of non adjuvant chemotherapy with AC. She underwent right modified radicle mastectomy with axiliary dissection and 4 additional cycles of Paxil. She then received radiotherapy to her chest wall and axilla which she finished in January. In late April of this year, she was admitted to Charleton Hospital with shortness of breath and a DVT on the left side. The shortness of breath was secondary to a right-sided pleural effusion which was tapped. This showed malignant sails. A bone scan was also positive for multiple metastatic disease. She was treated with pan iduronate 90 mg IV on 4/25 and she was discharged on Femara 2.5 mg daily. She comes in today for reevaluation. She is feeling much better. Her shortness of breath is stable and she tolerates exercise better. She continues with occasional pain in the scapular region of the left shoulder and she is having hot flashes. She is currently on Coumadin 7.5 mg q.d.

REVIEW OF SYSTEMS

GENERAL: She denies fever, weight change, malacia, or dizziness. SKIN: No ulcers, spots, bleeding, or changes in color or texture. HEENT: No headaches, sinus problems, hoarseness, visual or hearing problems. CARDIORESPIRATORY: No cough. Shortness of breath as described. No chest pain. GASTROINTESTINAL: Denies dysphasia, odynophagia, heartburn. GENITOURINARY: Negative. MUSCULOSKELETAL: Left-sided pain which is better than it was when she had a full-blown DVT.

Incorrect term—locally

Incorrect word—4

Incorrect term—neoadjuvant

Incorrect spelling—radical

Incorrect word—axillary

Incorrect drug—Taxol

Incorrect word—cells

Incorrect drug—pamidronate

Incorrect term—malaise

Incorrect spelling—dysphagia

PHYSICAL EXAMINATION

On physical examination, her weight is 226 pounds, which is 2 pounds less than prior visit, blood pressure 140/80, pulse 80. She is conscious, oriented, and alert. HEENT: Intact external ocular movements, no nystagmus, oropharynx clear. NECK: Supple. No JVD, no lymph nodes. HEART: Regular rhythm, no murmurs. LUNGS: Left lung clear. Right lung has a pleural fusion covering practically two-thirds of the lung. ABDOMEN: Soft, bowel sounds positive. No liver or spleen enlargement. EXTREMITIES: No edema or cyanosis.

NEUROLOGICAL: Nonfocal.

IMPRESSION

1. Metastatic breast cancer, currently on neuronal therapy.
2. Status post BVT with implantation of an interior vena cava filter. Patient is currently on Coumadin.

PLAN

1. PT/IMR and CBC drawn today. Not available at the time of dictation.
2. Abreva 90 mg IV over 3 hours on May 23.
3. Continue Femara.
4. Will see again on May 23.

Incorrect term—effusion

Incorrect term—hormonal

Incorrect term—inferior

Incorrect abbreviation—DVT—spell out deep vein thrombosis

Incorrect abbreviation—INR

Incorrect drug—Aredia

PROOFREADING EXERCISE #3 KEY

The patient is a 30-year-old gentleman who comes in today to discuss the results of his bone marrow biopsy for asymptomatic neutropenia. His biopsy basically shows a cellular furrow with good evidence of trilineage granulopoiesis but profound neutropenia. There is no evidence of malignancy or myeloic dysplasia. Since he has normal granulopoiesis with relative monocytosis, this would indicate either a drug affect or chronic B-9 neutropenia. The patient however denies the use of any medications prescribed or over-the-counter. He did use some herbal supplements with ma huang and ginseng for about 6 months last year but stopped in October If that had a drug effect, it should have gotten better by now. He is not having any symptoms, and except for a couple of upper respiratory tract infections earlier this year, he has been feeling well. His ANC is 500.

LABORATORY DATA

CBC done today shows a WBC of 1.8 with an AMC of 500. Neutral fills on parenteral smear appear normal. There are no blacks on peripheral smear.

IMPRESSION

Neutropenia, etiology unknown. Given that the patient is asymptomatic and that he has mild mono cytosis, this might be chronic benign neutropenia or even cyclic neutropenia which is an even rarer disease. However, with his normal peripheral smear, I doubt he has leukemia. Other differential diagnoses would include a drug-induced reaction verses early myelomalacia and even aplasia. Since he is asymptomatic, we will also have to rule-out other infections such as HIV or thyroid dysfunction as well as B-12 deficiency.

PLAN

1. CBC and deferential today.
2. HIV, TSH, T_3, T_4 and B-12, methyl malonic acid, serum homocysteine.

Incorrect term—marrow

Use combined form—myelodysplasia

Incorrect term—benign

Incorrect spelling—effect

Incorrect abbreviation—ANC

Incorrect term—neutrophils

Incorrect term—peripheral

Incorrect term—blasts

Use combined form—monocytosis

Incorrect spelling—versus

Incorrect term—myelodysplasia

Incorrect term—differential

Use combined form—methylmalonic

CHAPTER 8

Allergy/Immunology/ Rheumatology

OBJECTIVES CHECKLIST

A prepared exam candidate will know:

- ❑ All combining forms, prefixes, and suffixes related to the immune system.
- ❑ Anatomy of the lymphatic system, including the role of lymph, lymph vessels, and lymph nodes.
- ❑ Anatomy and function of the spleen and thymus gland.
- ❑ Physiology of the immune response as well as the difference between natural and acquired immunity.
- ❑ Role and relationship of antigens and antibodies.
- ❑ Signs, symptoms, and diseases related to the lymphatic and immune systems.
- ❑ Allergic and immunologic triggering factors for disease.
- ❑ Imaging and diagnostic studies used in the identification and treatment planning of lymphatic and immunologic disorders.
- ❑ Laboratory studies related to the diagnosis and treatment of lymphatic and immunologic disorders.
- ❑ Common medications prescribed for lymphatic and immunologic disorders.
- ❑ Transcription standards pertaining to allergies and lymphocytes.
- ❑ Fundamentals of rheumatic disease and the common disorders associated with rheumatology.
- ❑ Common laboratory tests ordered for rheumatic conditions.
- ❑ Medications commonly prescribed for rheumatic disorders, symptoms, and diseases.

RESOURCES FOR STUDY

1. *The Language of Medicine*
   Chapter 14: Lymphatic and Immune Systems, pp. 529–558.
   Chapter 15: Musculoskeletal System, Pathological Conditions, pp. 587–591.
2. *H&P: A Nonphysician's Guide to the Medical History and Physical Examination*
   Chapter 14: Review of Systems: Skin, pp. 125–130.
3. *Human Diseases*
   Chapter 4: The Immune System, pp. 43–56.
4. *Laboratory Tests & Diagnostic Procedures in Medicine*
   Chapter 16: Normal Anatomy and Histology, pp. 225–250.
   Chapter 17: Procedures and Practice in Anatomic Pathology, pp. 251–278.
   Chapter 18: Pathologic Change and Pathologic Diagnosis (Inflammation, Allergy, and Infection), pp. 283–288.
5. *Understanding Pharmacology for Health Professionals*
   Chapter 19: Ear, Nose and Throat, pp. 205–216.
   *Note: Chapter 18 (Pulmonary Drugs) also contains medications given for allergy and should be reviewed in this section.
6. *The AAMT Book of Style for Medical Transcription*
   Allergies, p. 19.
   Lymphocytes, pp. 245–246.

SAMPLE REPORTS

The following five reports are examples of reports you might encounter while transcribing allergy, immunology, and rheumatology.

HISTORY & PHYSICAL

HISTORY
The patient presents for followup of a cough. She did see the allergist and was found to be allergic to grass, dust mites, and molds. She is currently taking Claritin-D daily; Flovent 110 mcg/dose, 2 puffs b.i.d.; Serevent 2 puffs b.i.d.; and Rhinocort 2 sprays each nostril b.i.d.; as well as albuterol p.r.n. She does not have any shortness of breath. Her cough is much improved. She is taking some measures around the house to help with her allergies; however, she has not been very aggressive about this. Her only remaining complaint is hoarseness, which occurs toward the end of the day.

PHYSICAL EXAMINATION
GENERAL: On exam, she is alert and in no acute distress.
VITAL SIGNS: Respirations were 20, blood pressure 130/90, and saturation 96%.
LUNGS: The lungs are clear with good air movement bilaterally.
HEENT: The throat is clear; there may be a slight amount of mucus.
NECK: Supple.
CHEST: Respirations are clear with good air movement.
CARDIOVASCULAR: Regular.
ABDOMEN: Soft and nontender.
EXTREMITIES: No edema.

IMPRESSION
Mild asthma with ongoing cough secondary to allergies and postnasal drip. She seems fairly well controlled on the current regimen. I am not sure that she is not having some ongoing, low-grade postnasal drip that accounts for her hoarseness; however, it may also be secondary to the Flovent.

PLAN
The plan at this time is to switch the Flovent to 44 mcg so she can get the same antiinflammatory effect with less hoarseness. I advised the patient once again to gargle well after use, which she states she is doing. I have advised her that after a couple of months she can come off the Flovent and see if just controlling her sinuses will be enough to stop the cough from recurring, and I did talk to her in more detail about trying to control her environment for the allergies.

HISTORY & PHYSICAL

HISTORY

I had the pleasure of seeing this woman, who is self referred for an evaluation of dyspnea. She has had a diagnosis of asthma since 1986 when she acquired 2 cats. Subsequent evaluation demonstrated significant extrinsic asthma with allergies to cats, feathers, and cottonwood. When she avoids these triggers, she very rarely has asthma symptoms and equally rarely has to use her albuterol metered-dose inhaler. She subsequently remodeled her house and has hardwood and tile flooring.

She was well until the last month when she noticed an increase in her dyspnea. She walks for exercise and noticed more dyspnea when walking at the moderate pace of 3 miles per hour. This occurs when she walks indoors and outdoors, although it seems to be worse inside. Parenthetically, her dyspnea seems better when breathing cold air. She has also noticed a significant amount of coughing in the last month, especially nocturnally. This has caused her husband to sleep in an adjacent room. She also noticed worsening of these symptoms over the Thanksgiving weekend when exposed to burning leaves and last summer when she was in Santa Fe and exposed to particulate matter from a nearby forest fire. Her typical asthma symptoms are chest tightness, shortness of breath, wheezing, and coughing.

PAST MEDICAL HISTORY

1. Gastroesophageal reflux symptoms. She has a chronic H. pylori infection and has received 3 treatment regimens of antibiotics without success. As long as she avoids tomatoes, citrus, caffeine, and chocolate and sleeps on 4 pillows, she has reflux symptoms only 1–2 times a month.
2. Hysterectomy for fibroids.
3. Benign cystic disease of her breasts with lumps removed in 1988 and 2001.
4. Right oophorectomy in 1998.

ALLERGIES

Sulfa, latex, and Ceclor, which all cause blotchiness and predominantly skin manifestations. Also allergic to iodine dye, which causes shortness of breath and an increase in blood pressure, and bee stings.

MEDICATIONS

1. Tums as needed for GERD symptoms.
2. Albuterol metered-dose inhaler.
3. Multivitamins.
4. Vitamin E.
5. EpiPen.

FAMILY HISTORY

Notable for her mother having breast cancer, bladder cancer, and metastatic colon cancer, although she is still alive at age 78. Her maternal grandmother had breast cancer and colon cancer.

SOCIAL HISTORY

Notable for 1/2-pack-a-day habit for 12 years, which she quit when she became pregnant at age 30. She is currently a housewife, having sold her business 2 years ago, and has been successfully participating in a Weight Watchers program, with weight loss from 177 to 150 pounds.

(continued)

REVIEW OF SYSTEMS
Notable for the absence of constitutional symptoms, fevers, chills, night sweats, myalgias, arthralgias, nasal congestion, painful or watery eyes, nausea, vomiting, constipation, diarrhea, or paresthesias. The remainder of her systems review is negative.

PHYSICAL EXAMINATION
VITAL SIGNS: Her heart rate is 108, blood pressure 136/78, weight is 58, and respiratory rate is 18.
HEENT: Notable for nasal mucosal erythema with mild congestion. Pharynx is normal. Mouth shows normal dentition.
NECK: Supple without thyromegaly or lymphadenopathy.
LUNGS: Clear to auscultation and percussion bilaterally.
CARDIOVASCULAR: Exam demonstrates a normal S1 and S2 without an S3, S4, murmurs, rubs, or clicks.
ABDOMEN: Exam demonstrates normal bowel sounds without tenderness, masses, or palpable organomegaly.
EXTREMITIES: Without clubbing, cyanosis, or edema.
NEUROLOGIC: Exam is nonfocal, and her affect is rather anxious.

IMPRESSION
She is a woman with a 16-year history of asthma who presents with progressive dyspnea on exertion and worsening cough of 1 month's duration. First on the differential diagnosis is a worsening of her asthma. Gastroesophageal reflux disease or other respiratory diseases are other considerations, although are less likely at this time.

PLAN
In conjunction with the patient, we have decided on an empiric trial of an inhaled corticosteroid. I have given her a sample of Advair 250/50 and asked her to use 1 puff b.i.d. I have also refilled her albuterol metered-dose inhaler and given her a prescription for a peak flow meter at her request. I will obtain baseline spirometry and, at the patient's request, obtain a PA and lateral chest x-ray to exclude other potential etiologies for her dyspnea.

She will call me in a couple of weeks to let me know of any progress with the treatment of these symptoms. Otherwise, I will plan to see her again in followup after the new year.

FOLLOWUP REPORT

The patient was seen on July 1, 2004. The patient comes in today after being off methotrexate since I saw her in the office back in May. She has been off methotrexate since that time and has noticed increasing swelling and tenderness in her joints. She has had a marked increase in pain and swelling in her MCPs, PIPs, feet, and ankles. We had to hold the methotrexate because of elevated liver function tests. I did repeat the LFTs on November 5, 2002, and she had an elevated gamma GT of 218, an elevated alkaline phosphatase of 194, and the isoenzymes revealed predominantly hepatobiliary fraction. Her other liver function tests were normal.

The patient's physical exam revealed marked synovitis in MCPs, PIPs, wrists, elbows, ankles, and MTPs. Her chest was clear to percussion and auscultation.

The patient is having an active flare of rheumatoid arthritis. We needed to stop the methotrexate because of her elevated liver function tests. I am also having her hold the Celebrex at the present time so that we can evaluate the etiology of her liver function elevation. I did suggest that she be evaluated, and an appointment has been made. We will repeat the liver function tests off the Celebrex in 2 weeks, however.

I am concerned about the patient's heavy workload. She is doing a great deal of heavy lifting at work, which is of great concern. Her x-rays revealed an erosion in her right hand at the radial base of the proximal phalanx, and the patient is going to need more therapy for remission. I did discuss Enbrel with the patient and her daughter and gave them one of the pamphlets about biologic therapy. In the meantime I did have her increase her prednisone, with warnings, to 10 mg a day for a week and then tapering to 7.5 mg a day.

I did express concern over the fact that her swelling may inhibit her ability to get off her left fourth finger wedding ring. I told them to try to soap it off after the swelling goes down with the prednisone, but to call me if they are not able to do so.

In this patient with active rheumatoid arthritis, we will need to increase her therapy, probably with Enbrel, but we will need to keep her off methotrexate while evaluating her liver function tests.

FOLLOWUP REPORT

HISTORY
It was my pleasure to see this delightful woman in rheumatologic followup. I saw her at my new office and have not yet received the copy of her records. The patient has been taking Mobic 15 mg a day, along with nortriptyline, Femhrt, Synthroid, Combivent, and Pulmicort.

As you know, the patient has had a history of a positive ANA that was felt to be possibly drug-induced. She has, over the last several months, experienced much less knee pain and has had no rash. In general, she is doing well on the Mobic with good relief.

With respect to the patient's previous history of fibromyalgia, she states that she has had some increased stiffness and diffuse pain but that it "comes and goes."

The patient has noted some increased bilateral hand pain and stiffness, as well as some slight increase in her heel pain.

The patient is followed by you for her hypothyroidism and states that she has a followup planned next month with you for her thyroid.

The patient states that she recently saw you for her increasing exercise intolerance. She was prescribed Pulmicort, which seems to be helping. She does state, however, that her pulmonary function tests revealed a worsening in her diffusion capacity. The patient has had followup for an abnormality in her chest CT and has a planned followup in the near future.

The patient is postmenopausal and has been taking Femhrt. She will be discussing with you the issue of hormone replacement at her followup appointment.

PHYSICAL EXAM
The patient's physical exam was remarkable for a mild, erythematous, maculopapular rash on her anterior chest. Her blood pressure was 150/80. She had patellofemoral crepitus in her knees and hallux valgus in her feet, without any active synovitis in her other joints. Her chest was clear to percussion and auscultation.

PLAN
I did ask the patient to obtain labs, including anti-DNA, C3, C4, and sedimentation rate, as well as her other connective tissue blood workup.

Certainly, if her diffusion capacity is decreasing and there is any consideration of interstitial lung disease, we may have to pursue a high resolution CT scan to evaluate her, with possible further workup if there is concern about connective tissue disease involving her lungs. I will forward a copy of this letter, and we will discuss this after her labs are back. I did tell the patient about her slightly elevated blood pressure, which she will be following up with you as well. I will be discussing the patient's results with her next week, but I told her to call if she has any questions or concerns. We did plan a followup appointment in 3 months, but I told her to call me if she has any exacerbation of her symptomatology before that time.

It is my pleasure to provide rheumatologic followup on this delightful woman.

HISTORY & PHYSICAL

HISTORY

The patient is a 53-year-old female with a past medical history of systemic lupus erythematosus that was complicated with vasculitis of her temporal arteries, in which she had a stroke and also had a partial loss of her vision. She comes in today for a followup visit and stated that, in general, she is doing better, but she is very concerned that, since she has been on a high dose of prednisone, she is having significant weight gain. Occasionally, she has some headaches, but she doesn't have any other complaints.

CURRENT MEDICATIONS

CellCept 1 g p.o. b.i.d., prednisone 60 mg a day, calcium with vitamin D, and antihypertensive medications.

PHYSICAL EXAMINATION

Weight 228 pounds, height is 6-3/4 inches, blood pressure 150/92, pulse 90, and respiratory rate 20. Her temperature is 97.8 degrees. She is well developed and not in acute distress. She does not have any oral ulcers. Her neck is supple. The lungs are clear to auscultation bilaterally. The heart was regular without murmurs. The musculoskeletal exam is negative for synovitis. There is no edema.

IMPRESSION

This is a patient with systemic lupus erythematosus complicated with vasculitis of the temporal arteries.

RECOMMENDATIONS

Because she is having significant side effects with the prednisone, I am going to increase the CellCept to 1.5 g p.o. b.i.d., and I am going to start a slow tapering of the prednisone by 5 mg every other day. To evaluate activity of her lupus, I ordered complement levels, CBC, double-stranded DNA, and urinalysis. I will follow up with the patient in 6 weeks.

REVIEW QUESTIONS

The goal of these questions is to test your knowledge in the areas of allergy, immunology, and rheumatology.

Directions: Select the correct answer for each of the multiple-choice questions provided below. *Answers are provided at the end of this chapter.*

1. Which condition below is an autoimmune disorder characterized by the formation of blisters with extensive erosion of healthy skin and mucous membranes? This disease is chronic, relapsing, and potentially fatal.
   A. Systemic lupus erythematosus
   B. Scleroderma
   C. Pemphigus vulgaris
   D. Mycosis fungoides
2. The medical term for hives is:
   A. Psoriasis
   B. Eczema
   C. Urticaria
   D. Scabies
3. The cause of scleroderma is a disorder of the:
   A. Immune system
   B. Endocrine system
   C. Musculoskeletal system
   D. Cardiovascular system
4. Systemic scleroderma usually results in death from:
   A. Renal failure
   B. Stroke
   C. Sepsis
   D. Malnutrition
5. A butterfly rash on the facial cheeks is a classic sign of:
   A. Rheumatoid arthritis
   B. Systemic lupus erythematosus
   C. Ankylosing spondylitis
   D. Vasculitis
6. Another common term for asthma is:
   A. Chronic obstructive pulmonary disease
   B. Reactive airway disease
   C. Allergic rhinitis
   D. Acute bronchitis
7. A neoplastic malignancy of the lymphatic system is called:
   A. Epstein-Barr
   B. Fibroadenoma
   C. Hodgkin disease
   D. Lymphadenitis
8. The Raji cell assay is helpful in evaluating:
   A. Autoimmune diseases
   B. Cold agglutinins
   C. Rheumatoid factors
   D. Antinuclear antibodies
9. HLA-DW3 is associated with several autoimmune diseases. HLA is the abbreviation for:
   A. Human lymphocyte antibody
   B. Human leukocyte antigen
   C. Humoral leukocyte autoantibody
   D. Histocompatible leukocyte antigen
10. ANA are almost always detected in patients with:
    A. SLE
    B. Rheumatic fever
    C. Allergies
    D. Immunosuppression
11. Autoantibodies are:
    A. Made against the patient's own tissues
    B. Injected to fight infection such as hepatitis
    C. Created even if the patient isn't exposed to an antigen
    D. Used in vaccines

12. ANA, which is often positive in autoimmune diseases, is the abbreviation for:
    A. Anaphylactic shock
    B. Autonomic antibodies
    C. Antinuclear antigens
    D. Antinuclear antibodies

13. A patient complaining of painful joints, especially in the hands and feet, with warmth and swelling would likely be tested for:
    A. Systemic lupus erythematosus
    B. Rheumatoid factor
    C. A & B
    D. Uric acid

14. Rheumatoid arthritis is often treated with which class of drugs:
    A. COX-2 inhibitors
    B. NSAIDS
    C. Salicylates
    D. All of the above

15. The inability to form antibodies is called:
    A. Agammaglobulinemia
    B. Hypogammaglobulinemia
    C. Hypergammaglobulinemia
    D. Hypoalbuminemia

16. Which of the following tests is used to identify specific antibodies in the serum in order to diagnose and identify allergies?
    A. ELISA
    B. LE
    C. RF
    D. RAST

17. Which of the following is a nonspecific laboratory test used to assess inflammation?
    A. UA
    B. ESR
    C. RIA
    D. ANA

18. Patients who are immunosuppressed are susceptible to:
    A. Non-Hodgkin lymphoma
    B. Multiple myeloma
    C. Anaphylaxis
    D. Opportunistic infections

19. A laboratory test used to separate and quantify immunoglobulins using electrical currents is called:
    A. Agglutination
    B. Immunofluorescence
    C. Immunoelectrophoresis
    D. ELISA

20. Which of these is not an autoimmune disease?
    A. Lupus erythematosus
    B. Rheumatoid arthritis
    C. Osteoarthritis
    D. Sjögren disease

21. The quantity of antibodies measured in serum is often expressed as a:
    A. Nadir
    B. Titer
    C. Trough value
    D. Peak value

22. Which of the following is not an area of lymph node concentration?
    A. Inguinal
    B. Cervical
    C. Brachial
    D. Axillary

23. Which of the following correctly lists the various classes of immunoglobins?
    A. IgA, IgE, IgM, IgG
    B. IgC, IgH, IgM, IgD
    C. IgO, IgA, IgN, IgG
    D. IgB, IgD, IgM, IgF

24. Treating disease with techniques such as vaccines and monoclonal antibodies is called:
    A. Chemotherapy
    B. Immunotherapy
    C. Cryotherapy
    D. Antibiotic therapy

25. A protein produced by the body in response to bacteria, viruses, or foreign tissue is called a/an:
   A. Complement
   B. Albumin
   C. Antigen
   D. Antibody

26. Which of the following is not used to treat rheumatoid arthritis?
   A. Methotrexate
   B. Sulfasalazine
   C. COX-2 inhibitors
   D. Soma

27. Zyrtec, Claritin, and brompheniramine are examples of what class of drugs?
   A. Antihistamines
   B. Decongestants
   C. Antibiotics
   D. Mast cell inhibitors

28. Corticosteroids are used to treat disorders of the immune system by:
   A. Blocking histamine
   B. Inhibiting the inflammatory response
   C. Killing infectious agents
   D. Blocking pain receptors

29. A side effect of long-term corticosteroid use is:
   A. Delayed hypersensitivity
   B. Paget disease
   C. Osteoporosis
   D. Gout

30. Which of the following is not a congenital immunodeficiency syndrome?
   A. Agammaglobulinemia
   B. Lupus erythematosus
   C. SCID
   D. Wiskott-Aldrich syndrome

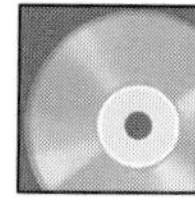

Please see the accompanying CD for additional review materials for this section.

PROOFREADING EXERCISES

These four proofreading exercises are provided to improve your skills in the areas of editing and effective identification and correction of errors in the medical record.

Directions: Identify and correct the transcription errors found in the exercises below. *Answers are provided at the end of this chapter.*

PROOFREADING EXERCISE #1

CHIEF COMPLAINT
The patient is a 7-year-old male who presents to the emergency department today with his mother complaining of bilateral swollen thighs with drainage beginning this morning.

HISTORY OF PRESENT ILLNESS
The patient states that he was playing outside in a field all day yesterday. He began having mild symptoms of nasal congestion, diarrhea, and watery eyes. The patient states he woke up this morning with puffiness around the eyes and scant drainage or discharge from both eyes. The patient states that the puffiness has improved and he no longer has pleuritis or drainage from the eyes but he still has mild nasal congestion, which has continuously improved throughout the morning. The patient denies fevers, sweats or chills, nausea, vomiting, diarrhea, constipation, or any trauma to the face or eye area. He denies any change in vision, and he denies difficulty breathing or shortness of breath. Finally, he denies wheezing.

PAST MEDICAL/SURGICAL HISTORY
The patient has no significant past medical history.

ALLERGIES
No known drug allergies.

CURRENT MEDICATIONS
He is not currently taking any medication.

IMMUNIZATIONS
Up-to-date.

(continued)

PHYSICAL EXAMINATION

VITAL SIGNS: Temperature is 98.6, pulse 72, respirations 20, blood pressure 110/57.

GENERAL: The patient is a well-developed, well-nourished 77-year-old male in no acute distress.

SKIN: Warm and dry with normal fervor and normal pigmentation. No rashes or lesions are noted. He appears well hydrated.

HEENT: Head is normocephalic, atraumatic and nontender. Eyes: There is mild puffiness in the paraorbital area and mild pruritus. There is no dejection and the conjunctiva are anicteric. There is no drainage or discharge. Pupils were equal, round, regular, and reactive to light. Extraocular movements are intact. Funduscopic examination is clear. Ears: Tympanic membranes are clear bilaterally. Nose: There is mild nasal congestion bilaterally. No drainage or discharge. Mares have a mild decrease in patency bilaterally. Throat: Oropharynx is clear.

NECK: No preauricular, cervical, or infundibular lymphadenopathy, and there is full range of motion.

CHEST: Lungs clear bilaterally. No wheezes, rales, or round eye.

HEART: Regular rate and rhythm, without murmurs, gallops, rubs, or clicks.

EXTREMITIES: The patient moves all extremities through full range of motion and is well coordinated.

NEUROLOGICAL: No focal deficits.

DIAGNOSIS

1. Allergic conjunctivitis.
2. Allergic initis.

DISCHARGE INSTRUCTIONS

Mother was given a prescription for Claritin 100 mg 1 p.o. q.d. The child was instructed to take all medication as prescribed and to follow up with his primary care physician in 3–4 days or return to the emergency department as needed.

PROOFREADING EXERCISE #2

The patient's rheumatoid arthritis remains nicely controlled on combined Endal 50 mg per week and methotrexate 15 mg per week on Monday plus folic acid 4 mg per day. No current side reactions to the medications.

The patient has not had complications so far in terms of infections, lymphoma, or other tumors, though the patient does understands risks associated with these treatments. On the other hand, the risks of uncontrolled RA are so severe that the patient wants to continue this current regimen anyway.

The patient does have stiffness and aching in the hands, neck, and back. The patient's first CNCs are prominent and subluxed. Grip is relatively poor and neck mobility is somewhat limited inspection, extension, and rotation, though there is no atopy, radiculopathy, or reflex change. Color, temperature, and pulses are good.

The patient still has dryness, better on Evoxac. Apparent Sjögren syndrome related to the RA but not severe.

The patient is tired, lethargic, and has poor stamina related to a degree of fibromyalgia remaining after an L-tryptophan reaction lead to hemophilia myalgia syndrome. Again, the blood elements have been normal, and there is no overt inflammatory feature. Overall, the patient functions in the home with activities of daily giving but cannot work because of the problems associated with RA, OA, and fiber myalgia.

Lab to be done today and every 2 months.

PROOFREADING EXERCISE #3

REASON FOR ADMISSION
A cute asthmatic attack.

HISTORY OF PRESENT ILLNESS
The patient is a 22-year-old male with a history of brachial asthma who presented to the emergency room complaining of wheezing, shortness of breath, and cough for a few days. The patient stated that the extreme heat caused him to have an asthmatic attack. Extreme temperatures, both cold and hot, usually exacerbate his asthma. He uses his red lighter at home but his symptoms got progressively worse. He was wheezing and was using excess muscles of respiration. He had difficulty catching his breadth and, therefore, he presented to the emergency room.

The patient denied any cynical episodes. He also reports a cough with some conductive sputum of whitish coloration. He denied any fevers or chills. The patient was seen in the emergency room where he was evaluated. He had several up graft treatments, but he was subsequently wheezing and was using accessory muscles for respiration. Therefore, he was admitted.

PAST MEDICAL/SURGICAL HISTORY
Positive for bronchial asthma. The patient has had several admissions in the past for management of his asthmatic attacks.

ALLERGIES
No known drug allergies.

MEDICATIONS
Multivitamins only.

SOCIAL HISTORY
The patient is unemployed. He denied any elicit drug or alcohol use.

FAMILY HISTORY
Noncontributory.

(continued)

REVIEW OF SYSTEMS

Significant for shortness of breath, associated wheezing, and the use of accessory muscles for respiration. He also reports a cough with some productive sputum but denied any fever or chills.

PHYSICAL EXAMINATION

GENERAL: This is a medium-built male who is wheezing; however, he is alert and responsive.

VITAL SIGNS: Temperature is 97, pulse is 128, respiratory rate 22, and blood pressure is 143/108.

HEENT: The head is atraumatic without any lesions. Pupils are equally round and reactive to light and accommodation, extraocular muscles are intact.

LUNGS: The lungs showed diffuse exploratory and inventory wheezing throughout his lungs with diffuse breathe sounds at the bases.

CARDIOVASCULAR: Normal sinus rhythm, without any gallops or murmurs.

ABDOMEN: Soft and bowel sounds are present.

EXTREMITIES: No edema. Pulses are equal and symmetrical.

NEUROLOGICAL: There are no focal deficits.

IMPRESSION

1. Acute asthmatic attack, likely secondary to extreme temperatures.
2. Asthmatic bronchitis.

PLAN

The plan is to admit the patient for management. The patient will be given atenolol updraft treatments and we will also start the patient on prednisone. We will follow his arterial blood gases, and further management will depend upon the patient's clinical course.

PROOFREADING EXERCISE #4

REASON FOR CONSULTATION
Evaluation and management of show grin as well as arthritis.

HISTORY OF PRESENT ILLNESS
The patient is a 76-year-old Caucasian female with a history of coronary artery disease, status post PTCH x3 and stinting, history of multiple pulmonary emboli, antiphospholipid syndrome, Sjögren syndrome, and osteoarthritis. She stated that she was diagnosed with Sjögren syndrome 7 years ago based on dry mouth and dry eye symptoms. She denied any blood tests or autopsy to confirm this diagnosis. She states that she has been using eyedrops as needed for her high eyes and drinking fluids, especially water, when her mouth becomes dry. With regard to her arthritis, she states that she has been having joint pains for a number of years, mainly effecting her ankles and her knees, and occasionally her hands. She states that sometimes her joints will swell. Morning stiffness lasts less than 5 minutes. Joint pain is worse with significant activity. She denied any nodules, molar rash or other rashes, photosensitivity, aural or vaginal ulcers, and Ray nod phenomenon, but she did report fatigue, some hair loss, and upper body myalgias. With regard to her antiphospholipid syndrome (AVS), she was diagnosed in 1996 after having suffered from a myocardial infraction as well as pulmonary embolus. She has been on chronic Coumadin therapy for several years now. There is no documentation of serologies that were done to verify the diagnosis of APS.

PAST MEDICAL HISTORY
Multiple myocardial infarctions, pulmonary involute, history of antiphospholipid syndrome, hemochromatosis diagnosed in 1996 requiring intermittent phlebotomy. Her last phlebotomy was 6 months ago. She also has a history of ventricular tachycardia, sick sinus syndrome, status post permanent pacemaker, history of Sjögren, history of osteoporosis, congestive heart failure, GERD, diabetes, and osteoarthritis.

PAST SURGICAL HISTORY
Status post total abdominal hysterectomy in 1950, status post permanent pacemaker in 2002.

(continued)

REVIEW OF SYSTEMS

She denies night sweats. She does note weight loss with diuretics, positive chest pain, positive shortness of breath, positive edema. She denies any visual changes, problems with chewing, scalp tenderness, palpitations, hearing loss, or soar throat. She does note intermittent dysphasia to solids, requiring liquids to swallow.

MEDICATIONS

1. Bactrim DS 1 b.i.d.
2. Advair 250/50 mg b.i.d.
3. Spiriva inhaler daily.
4. Lovenox 100 mg subcutaneous b.i.d.
5. Prednisone 10 mg a day.
6. Amlodipine 10 mg a day.
7. Alprazolam 0.25 mg daily.
8. Lasik 40 mg daily.
9. Endure 30 mg daily.
10. Metoprolol 100 mg b.i.d.
11. Pantoprazole 40 mg daily.
12. Potassium chloride 10 mEq daily.
13. Crestor 10 mg q.h.s.
14. Torsemide 50 mg daily.

ALLERGIES

PENICILLIN AND LEVAQUIN, WHICH CAUSE A RASH.

SOCIAL HISTORY

She is married. She lives with her husband. She has 4 daughters. Prior tobacco use of 40 years. She quit 8 years ago. No alcohol or IV drug use.

FAMILY HISTORY

Mother with hemochromatosis. No history of autoimmune disorders.

PHYSICAL EXAMINATION

Temperature is 98.6, blood pressure 126/61, heart rate 62, and respiratory rate 20. Generally, a well-developed, obese female in no acute distress. HEENT examination: Normocephalic, atraumatic. The pupils are equal,

(continued)

round, and reactive to light bilaterally. No injected conjunctivae or sclerae. Oropharynx is clear. The tongue appears dry with poor saliva pulling. She has dentures in place. Neck is supple with full range of motion. No evidence of lymphadenopathy or thyromegaly. No nodules. Pulmonary examination: Normal chest wall expansion. No wheezes, rales, or rhonchi. Cardiovascular: Regular rate and rhythm, S1 and S2, no murmurs, rubs, or gallops. Abdominal examination, normal bowel sounds, soft, nontender, nondistended. No masses. Skeletomuscular examination: There was no evidence of synovitis in her hands, elbows, shoulders, knees, ankles, or feet. She does have crepitus in her knees as well as her ankles. Range of motion is within normal limits in the upper and lower extremities. No evidence of effusion. No nodules. Extremities: Slight edema in the lower extremities. Skin is warm and pink. No clubbing or cenosis. Skin examination: No evidence of rashes.

LABORATORY

White count was 11.8, hemoglobin 11.7, hematocrit 38.5, and platelets 549. CMP was within normal limits. Albumin was 3.4 and total protein 65. BMP was 130. Chest x-ray showed pacemaker present. Lungs were clear. No evidence of active disease.

ASSESSMENT/PLAN

1. Sjögren syndrome. I cannot confirm the diagnosis of Sjögren at this time as her history of dry eyes and dry mouth may be secondary to medications, diabetes, or other factors. She has had no formal evaluation for Sjögren disease such as a salivary gland biopsy or squirmer test. As she is not very symptomatic at this time, I would recommend having her use artificial tears. In the meantime, I will check an antinuclear antibody, anti-SFA and anti-SFB antibodies, erythrocyte sedimentation rate, and T-reactive protein to see if she has any evidence of Sjögren or inflammation.
2. Osteoarthritis. I would recommend ordering physical therapy if her stay is prolonged.
3. Neuralgia. I doubt this is secondary to an underlying connective tissue disease. Check a creatine phosphokinase to evaluate statin-induced myopathy.
4. Antiphospholipid syndrome. Continue Lovenox.

ANSWER KEYS

REVIEW QUESTIONS ANSWER KEY

1. C	6. B	11. A	16. D	21. B	26. D
2. C	7. C	12. D	17. B	22. C	27. A
3. A	8. A	13. C	18. D	23. A	28. B
4. A	9. B	14. D	19. C	24. B	29. C
5. B	10. A	15. A	20. C	25. D	30. B

PROOFREADING EXERCISE #1 KEY

Incorrect term—eyes

Incorrect term—rhinorrhea

Incorrect term—pruritus

CHIEF COMPLAINT
The patient is a 7-year-old male who presents to the emergency department today with his mother complaining of bilateral swollen thighs with drainage beginning this morning.

HISTORY OF PRESENT ILLNESS
The patient states that he was playing outside in a field all day yesterday. He began having mild symptoms of nasal congestion, diarrhea, and watery eyes. The patient states he woke up this morning with puffiness around the eyes and scant drainage or discharge from both eyes. The patient states that the puffiness has improved and he no longer has pleuritis or drainage from the eyes but he still has mild nasal congestion, which has continuously improved throughout the morning. The patient denies fevers, sweats, or chills, nausea, vomiting, diarrhea, constipation, or any trauma to the face or eye area. He denies any change in vision, and he denies difficulty breathing or shortness of breath. Finally, he denies wheezing.

PAST MEDICAL/SURGICAL HISTORY
The patient has no significant past medical history.

ALLERGIES
No known drug allergies.

CURRENT MEDICATIONS
He is not currently taking any medication.

IMMUNIZATIONS
Up-to-date.

PHYSICAL EXAMINATION
VITAL SIGNS: Temperature is 98.6, pulse 72, respirations 20, blood pressure 110/57.

Incorrect age—7-year-old

Incorrect term—turgor

Incorrect term—injection

Requires plural—conjunctivae

Incorrect term—Nares

Incorrect term—mandibular

Incorrect term—rhonchi

Incorrect term—bronchitis

Incorrect dose—10 mg

GENERAL: The patient is a well-developed, well-nourished 77-year-old male in no acute distress.
SKIN: Warm and dry with normal fervor and normal pigmentation. No rashes or lesions are noted. He appears well hydrated.
HEENT: Head is normocephalic, atraumatic, and nontender. Eyes: There is mild puffiness in the paraorbital area and mild pruritus. There is no dejection and the conjunctiva are anicteric. There is no drainage or discharge. Pupils were equal, round, regular, and reactive to light. Extraocular movements are intact. Funduscopic examination is clear. Ears: Tympanic membranes are clear bilaterally. Nose: There is mild nasal congestion bilaterally. No drainage or discharge. Mares have a mild decrease in patency bilaterally. Throat: Oropharynx is clear.
NECK: No preauricular, cervical, or infundibular lymphadenopathy, and there is full range of motion.
CHEST: Lungs clear bilaterally. No wheezes, rales, or round eye.
HEART: Regular rate and rhythm, without murmurs, gallops, rubs, or clicks.
EXTREMITIES: The patient moves all extremities through full range of motion and is well coordinated.
NEUROLOGICAL: No focal deficits.

DIAGNOSIS

1. Allergic conjunctivitis.
2. Allergic initis.

DISCHARGE INSTRUCTIONS

Mother was given a prescription for Claritin 100 mg 1 p.o. q.d. The child was instructed to take all medication as prescribed and to follow up with his primary care physician in 3–4 days or return to the emergency department as needed.

PROOFREADING EXERCISE #2 KEY

Incorrect drug—Embrel

The patient's rheumatoid arthritis remains nicely controlled on ~~combined~~ Endal 50 mg per week and methotrexate 15 mg per week on Monday plus folic acid 4 mg per day. No current side reactions to the medications.

The patient has not had complications so far in terms of infections, lymphoma, or other tumors, though the patient does understands risks associated with these treatments. On the other hand, the risks of uncontrolled RA are so severe that the patient wants to continue this current regimen anyway.

Incorrect abbreviation—CMC

Incorrect term—in flexion

The patient does have stiffness and aching in the hands, neck, and back. The patient's first CNCs are prominent and subluxed. Grip is relatively poor, and neck mobility is somewhat limited inspection, extension, and rotation, though there is no atopy, radiculopathy, or reflex change. Color, temperature, and pulses are good.

Incorrect term—atrophy

Incorrect term—eosinophilia

The patient still has dryness, better on Evoxac. Apparent Sjögren syndrome related to the RA but not severe.

Incorrect word—living

The patient is tired, lethargic, and has poor stamina related to a degree of fibromyalgia remaining after an L-tryptophan reaction lead to hemophilia myalgia syndrome. Again, the blood elements have been normal, and there is no overt inflammatory feature. Overall, the patient functions in the home with activities of daily giving but cannot work because of the problems associated with RA, OA, and fiber myalgia.

Incorrect term—fibromyalgia

Lab to be done today and every 2 months.

PROOFREADING EXERCISE #3 KEY

Incorrect word—acute

Incorrect term—bronchial

Incorrect word—nebulizer

Incorrect term—accessory

Incorrect word—breath

Incorrect term—syncopal

Incorrect word—productive

Incorrect word—updraft

REASON FOR ADMISSION
A cute asthmatic attack.

HISTORY OF PRESENT ILLNESS
The patient is a 22-year-old male with a history of brachial asthma who presented to the emergency room complaining of wheezing, shortness of breath, and cough for a few days. The patient stated that the extreme heat caused him to have an asthmatic attack. Extreme temperatures, both cold and hot, usually exacerbate his asthma. He uses his red lighter at home, but his symptoms got progressively worse. He was wheezing and was using excess muscles of respiration. He had difficulty catching his breadth and, therefore, he presented to the emergency room.

The patient denied any cynical episodes. He also reports a cough with some conductive sputum of whitish coloration. He denied any fevers or chills. The patient was seen in the emergency room where he was evaluated. He had several up graft treatments, but he was subsequently wheezing and was using accessory muscles for respiration. Therefore, he was admitted.

PAST MEDICAL/SURGICAL HISTORY
Positive for bronchial asthma. The patient has had several admissions in the past for management of his asthmatic attacks.

ALLERGIES
No known drug allergies.

MEDICATIONS
Multivitamins only.

SOCIAL HISTORY
The patient is unemployed. He denied any elicit drug or alcohol use.

Incorrect word—illicit

FAMILY HISTORY
Noncontributory.

REVIEW OF SYSTEMS
Significant for shortness of breath, associated wheezing and the use of accessory muscles for respiration. He also reports a cough with some productive sputum but denied any fever or chills.

PHYSICAL EXAMINATION
GENERAL: This is a medium-built male who is wheezing; however, he is alert and responsive.
VITAL SIGNS: Temperature is 97, pulse is 128, respiratory rate 22, and blood pressure is 143/108.
HEENT: The head is atraumatic without any lesions. Pupils are equally round and reactive to light and accommodation, extraocular muscles are intact.
LUNGS: The lungs showed diffuse exploratory and inventory wheezing throughout his lungs with diffuse breathe sounds at the bases.
CARDIOVASCULAR: Normal sinus rhythm, without any gallops or murmurs.
ABDOMEN: Soft and bowel sounds are present.
EXTREMITIES: No edema. Pulses are equal and symmetrical.
NEUROLOGICAL: There are no focal deficits.

Incorrect term—inspiratory

Incorrect term—expiratory

Incorrect spelling—breath

IMPRESSION
1. Acute asthmatic attack, likely secondary to extreme temperatures.
2. Asthmatic bronchitis.

PLAN
The plan is to admit the patient for management. The patient will be given atenolol updraft treatments, and we will also start the patient on prednisone. We will follow his arterial blood gases, and further management will depend upon the patient's clinical course.

Incorrect drug—albuterol

PROOFREADING EXERCISE #4 KEY

REASON FOR CONSULTATION
Evaluation and management of show grin as well as arthritis.

HISTORY OF PRESENT ILLNESS
The patient is a 76-year-old Caucasian female with a history of coronary artery disease, status post PTCH x3 and stinting, history of multiple pulmonary emboli, antiphospholipid syndrome, Sjögren syndrome, and osteoarthritis. She stated that she was diagnosed with Sjögren syndrome 7 years ago based on dry mouth and dry eye symptoms. She denied any blood tests or autopsy to confirm this diagnosis. She states that she has been using eyedrops as needed for her high eyes and drinking fluids, especially water, when her mouth becomes dry. With regard to her arthritis, she states that she has been having joint pains for a number of years, mainly effecting her ankles and her knees, and occasionally her hands. She states that sometimes her joints will swell. Morning stiffness lasts less than 5 minutes. Joint pain is worse with significant activity. She denied any nodules, molar rash or other rashes, photosensitivity, aural or vaginal ulcers, and Ray nod phenomenon, but she did report fatigue, some hair loss, and upper body myalgias. With regard to her antiphospholipid syndrome (AVS), she was diagnosed in 1996 after having suffered from a myocardial infraction as well as pulmonary embolus. She has been on chronic Coumadin therapy for several years now. There is no documentation of serologies that were done to verify the diagnosis of APS.

Incorrect word—Sjögren

Incorrect abbreviation—PTCA

Incorrect spelling—stenting

Incorrect term—biopsy

Incorrect word—dry

Incorrect spelling—affecting

Incorrect term—malar

Incorrect term—oral

Incorrect words—Raynaud

Incorrect abbreviation—APS

Incorrect spelling—infarction

Incorrect term—embolus

PAST MEDICAL HISTORY
Multiple myocardial infarctions, pulmonary involute, history of antiphospholipid syndrome, hemochromatosis diagnosed in 1996 requiring intermittent phlebotomy. Her last phlebotomy was 6 months ago. She also has a history of ventricular tachycardia, sick sinus syndrome, status post permanent pacemaker, history of Sjögren, history of osteoporosis, congestive heart failure, GERD, diabetes, and osteoarthritis.

PAST SURGICAL HISTORY
Status post total abdominal hysterectomy in 1950, status post permanent pacemaker in 2002.

Incorrect spelling—sore

REVIEW OF SYSTEMS
She denies night sweats. She does note weight loss with diuretics, positive chest pain, positive shortness of breath, positive edema. She denies any visual changes, problems with chewing, scalp tenderness, palpitations, hearing loss, or soar throat. She does note intermittent dysphasia to solids, requiring liquids to swallow.

Incorrect term—Lasix

Incorrect spelling—dysphagia

MEDICATIONS
1. Advair 250/50 mg b.i.d.
2. Spiriva inhaler daily.
3. Lovenox 100 mg subcutaneous b.i.d.
4. Prednisone 10 mg a day.
5. Amlodipine 10 mg a day.
6. Alprazolam 0.25 mg daily.
7. Lasik 40 mg daily.
8. Endure 30 mg daily.
9. Metoprolol 100 mg b.i.d.
10. Pantoprazole 40 mg daily.
11. Potassium chloride 10 mEq daily.

Incorrect term—Imdur

ALLERGIES
PENICILLIN AND LEVAQUIN WHICH CAUSE A RASH.

Incorrect word—pooling

SOCIAL HISTORY
She is married. She lives with her husband. She has 4 daughters. Prior tobacco use of 40 years. She quit 8 years ago. No alcohol or IV drug use.

FAMILY HISTORY
Mother with hemochromatosis. No history of autoimmune disorders.

PHYSICAL EXAMINATION
Temperature is 98.6, blood pressure 126/61, heart rate 62, and respiratory rate 20. Generally, a well-developed, obese female in no acute distress. HEENT examination: Normocephalic, atraumatic. The pupils are equal, round, and reactive to light bilaterally. No injected conjunctivae or sclerae. Oropharynx is clear. The tongue appears dry with poor saliva pulling. She has dentures in place. Neck is supple with full range of motion. No evidence of lymphadenopathy or thyromegaly. No nodules. Pulmonary examination: Normal chest wall expansion. No wheezes, rales, or rhonchi. Cardiovascular: Regular rate and rhythm, S1 and S2, no murmurs, rubs, or gallops. Abdominal examination, normal bowel sounds, soft, nontender, nondistended. No masses. Skeletomuscular examination: There was no evidence of synovitis in her hands, elbows, shoulders, knees, ankles, or feet. She does have crepitus in her knees as well as her ankles. Range of motion is within normal limits in the upper and lower extremities. No evidence of effusion. No nodules. Extremities: Slight edema in the lower extremities. Skin is warm and pink. No clubbing or cenosis. Skin examination: No evidence of rashes.

Incorrect term—cyanosis

LABORATORY
White count was 11.8, hemoglobin 11.7, hematocrit 38.5, and platelets 549. CMP was within normal limits. Albumin was 3.4 and total protein 65. BMP was 130. Chest x-ray showed pacemaker present. Lungs were clear. No evidence of active disease.

Flag—improbable value for protein

Incorrect abbreviation—BNP (single value not a panel)

ASSESSMENT/PLAN

1. Sjögren syndrome. I cannot confirm the diagnosis of Sjögren at this time as her history of dry eyes and dry mouth may be secondary to medications, diabetes, or other factors. She has had no formal evaluation for Sjögren disease such as a salivary gland biopsy or squirmer test. As she is not very symptomatic at this time, I would recommend having her use artificial tears. In the meantime, I will check an antinuclear antibody, anti-SFA and anti-SFB antibodies, erythrocyte sedimentation rate, and T-reactive protein to see if she has any evidence of Sjögren or inflammation.
2. Osteoarthritis. I would recommend ordering physical therapy if her stay is prolonged.
3. Neuralgia. I doubt this is secondary to an underlying connective tissue disease. Check a creatine phosphokinase to evaluate statin-induced myopathy.
4. Antiphospholipid syndrome. Continue Lovenox.

Incorrect term—Schirmer

Incorrect abbreviation—anti-SSA

Incorrect abbreviation—anti-SSB

Incorrect letter—C-reactive

Incorrect term—Myalgia

CHAPTER 9

Infectious Disease

OBJECTIVES CHECKLIST

A prepared exam candidate will know:

- ❑ Combining forms, prefixes, and suffixes related to the study of microbiology.
- ❑ Imaging and diagnostic studies used in the identification and treatment of infectious diseases.
- ❑ Laboratory studies related to the diagnosis and treatment of infectious diseases.
- ❑ Nomenclature and classification of infectious agents.
- ❑ Modes of transmission related to the spread of infectious disease.
- ❑ Common medications indicated and prescribed for infectious diseases.
- ❑ Transcription standards pertaining to infectious agents (genus and species) and infectious diseases.

RESOURCES FOR STUDY

1. *The Language of Medicine*
   Chapter 14: Lymphatic and Immune Systems (immunity, antigens, and antibodies), pp. 529–558.
2. *Disease: Identification, Prevention, and Control*
   Unit 2: Infectious Diseases.
3. *Human Diseases*
   Chapter 3: Infectious Diseases, pp. 27–42.
4. *Laboratory Tests & Diagnostic Procedures in Medicine*
   Chapter 21: Microbiology, pp. 401–410.
5. *Understanding Pharmacology for Health Professionals*
   Chapter 27: Anti-Infective Drugs, pp. 311–322.
   Chapter 28: AIDS Drugs and Antiviral Drugs, pp. 323–333.
   Chapter 29: Anti-Fungal Drugs, pp. 334–336.
6. *The AAMT Book of Style for Medical Transcription*
   Blood counts, differential, p. 39.
   Genus names, pp. 188–190.
   Gram stain, p. 195.
   Hepatitis nomenclature, pp. 201–202.
   Lymphocytes, pp. 245–246.
   Virus names, pp. 419–420.

SAMPLE REPORTS

The following five reports are examples of reports you might encounter while transcribing reports involving infectious diseases.

HISTORY & PHYSICAL

HISTORY OF PRESENT ILLNESS
This is a 30-year-old female with history of HIV infection diagnosed 5 years ago with an unknown CD4 count and viral load and a history of opportunistic infections. The patient presented with fever of 102.2 degrees of 5 days' duration. She also had abdominal pain and vomiting. She has developed a large mass lesion in the right submandibular area that, according to her own report, comes and goes.

The patient was placed on IV ceftriaxone and then clindamycin by Dr. Smith. The patient denies cough, sputum production, or shortness of breath. There are no other concomitant symptoms.

ALLERGIES
No known allergies.

MEDICATIONS
Her current medications include Cefepime, fluconazole, Lasix, clindamycin, Demerol, and Ambien.

PHYSICAL EXAMINATION
GENERAL: Examination reveals a chronically ill-appearing female, lying in bed in no apparent distress.
HEENT: Pupils are reactive to light and accommodation. Mouth is moist. Throat has evidence of erythema.
NECK: Supple. There are at least 2 rounded lesions in the right submandibular area that are mildly tender to palpation. They may correspond to lymphadenopathy.
LUNGS: Clear to auscultation and percussion.
CARDIOVASCULAR: Normal S1 and S2. Regular rate and rhythm.
ABDOMEN: Soft and nontender. Good bowel sounds.
EXTREMITIES: No clubbing, cyanosis, or edema.
NEUROLOGIC: Grossly nonfocal.

DIAGNOSTIC STUDIES
She had a V/Q scan that showed no evidence of pulmonary embolism. She had a chest x-ray that showed no evidence of acute pulmonary disease.

LABORATORY DATA
Her initial white count was 8900 and currently is 4900, with 63% neutrophils, 5% bands, 20% lymphocytes, and 11% monocytes. Creatinine was 1.8 and now is 1.4.

MICROBIOLOGY DATA
Remarkable for a urine culture collected on 08/11/04 that showed 100,000 colonies of E. coli. She had 90 wbc's on urinalysis. Blood culture showed no growth after 24 hours.

(continued)

IMPRESSION

1. Neck mass, likely secondary to lymphadenopathy. Differential diagnosis includes:
   a. Bacterial infectious process.
   b. Mycobacterial disease such as mycobacterial tuberculosis versus atypical mycobacteria.
   c. Neoplastic process such as lymphoma.
   d. Other unusual infections cannot be excluded. I did not think that this patient had parotitis; however, a CT scan of the neck clearly indicates same. An ENT consultation was advised.
2. Urinary tract infection.
3. HIV/AIDS.
4. Renal insufficiency, improving.
5. Anemia.

PLAN

1. Obtain a CT scan.
2. Schedule lymph node biopsy, based on review of CT scan.
3. Give a PPD.
4. Agree with current antibiotics.

CONSULTATION

HISTORY OF PRESENT ILLNESS
This is a 74-year-old black female who was recently admitted for pneumonia and hypertension. Apparently, the patient came to the emergency department with a 1-day history of shortness of breath. She had a minimal cough. She did admit to chest pain, stomach pain, and back pain. She describes the chest pain as being along the rib area, perhaps related to coughing. No diaphoresis, nausea, vomiting, or diarrhea. No other concomitant symptoms.

On initial evaluation, the patient was found to have bilateral infiltrates in both lung bases for which she was placed on empiric antibiotics, including IV vancomycin and levofloxacin. Currently, the patient is alert and interactive. She does not look toxic. She has been afebrile since admission.

ALLERGIES
No known allergies.

CURRENT MEDICATIONS
Ferrous sulfate, docusate sodium, Lasix, Nitro-Dur, Lovenox, Ecotrin, Protonix, Zithromax, Catapres, albuterol, vancomycin, and levofloxacin.

PHYSICAL EXAMINATION
GENERAL: Elderly female in no apparent distress.
HEENT: Pupils are reactive to light and accommodation. Mouth is moist.
NECK: Supple. No JVD or bruits.
CARDIOVASCULAR: Normal S1 and S2. Regular rate and rhythm.
LUNGS: Bibasilar crackles.
ABDOMEN: Soft and nontender. Positive bowel sounds.
EXTREMITIES: No cyanosis, clubbing, or edema.
NEUROLOGICAL: Grossly nonfocal.

LABORATORY DATA
Chest x-ray shows bibasilar crackles. White count is 22,800. Her BNP was 928 on 08/10/04. In addition, two out of two blood cultures grew out gram-positive cocci in pairs on the second day after blood culture collection.

IMPRESSION
1. Bibasilar pneumonia adequately treated with Levaquin.
2. Gram-positive organisms in blood cultures growing 2 days after collection, which may suggest contamination rather than infection. The patient had been treated with IV vancomycin that should cover for possible bacteremia. I will request another 2 sets of blood cultures. We will formulate further recommendations once bacteriology is finalized.
3. Congestive heart failure.
4. Respiratory insufficiency.
5. Status post myocardial infarction.

PLAN
1. We will be following along with you.
2. Continue current therapy.

CONSULTATION

HISTORY OF PRESENT ILLNESS
This is a 63-year-old male with multiple medical problems including hypertension, diabetes mellitus, and end-stage renal disease, on hemodialysis. The patient apparently was referred from home with an acute change in his mental status.

On initial evaluation in the ER, he was very agitated. It was initially reported that the patient was throwing things at home. His initial vital signs were remarkable for a temperature of 95.6, respiratory rate of 18, pulse of 94, and a blood pressure of 170/87. The patient was admitted to intensive care with a working diagnosis of sepsis syndrome, rule out acute myocardial infarction, and end-stage renal disease on dialysis.

Currently, the patient is lethargic but can be aroused. He mumbles some words. He is unable to provide any further history. The patient has a dialysis catheter in the right side of his neck. He states that there is no tenderness. There is a complaint of shaking chills.

ALLERGIES
No known allergies.

PAST MEDICAL HISTORY
This is reflected in the first paragraph.

PHYSICAL EXAMINATION
GENERAL: Elderly male, chronically and acutely ill-appearing and lying in bed in no apparent distress.
HEENT: Pupils are reactive to light and accommodation. Mouth is slightly dry.
NECK: Supple; no JVD or bruits.
CARDIOVASCULAR: Normal S1 and S2; regular rate and rhythm.
CHEST: Normal expansion. There is a dialysis catheter on the right side. There is no evidence of erythema or tenderness.
ABDOMEN: Soft and nontender; positive bowel sounds.
EXTREMITIES: No clubbing, cyanosis, or edema.
NEUROLOGIC: The patient is alert and able to be aroused but lethargic, and he moves all 4 extremities.

RADIOLOGICAL DATA
Initial chest x-ray is consistent with CHF changes. A CT scan of the brain was reportedly negative.

LABORATORY DATA
Remarkable for blood cultures collected on August 14 that are negative so far. Creatinine 7.6. Initial white count 11,900 with 76% neutrophils, 2% bands, and 5% lymphocytes. PT 13, INR 1.07, and D-dimer 1.1.

(continued)

IMPRESSION

1. Patient with altered mental status and multiple medical problems. Admitted to the intensive care unit. Working diagnosis is sepsis. The patient does not have fever or an elevated white count on initial evaluation. He does not have hypotension or any other features of sepsis. However, being immunosuppressed from dialysis, some of these features may be masked and develop in subsequent days. Therefore, I would support empiric antibiotics until further diagnostic testing is completed. Cefepime seems to be adequate coverage. Since there is no evidence of gram-positive cocci in the blood cultures, I do not see a need for methicillin-resistant Staphylococcus aureus coverage with Vancomycin or other antibiotics.
2. Encephalopathy, likely multifactorial.
3. End-stage renal disease on dialysis.
4. Rule out acute myocardial infarction. Management as per Dr. Smith.
5. Uncontrolled hypertension.
6. Anemia.

RECOMMENDATION

The patient is critically ill. I agree with ICU monitoring. For the time being I would recommend continuation of his current antibiotics.

CONSULTATION

REASON FOR CONSULTATION
Fungemia history.

HISTORY OF PRESENT ILLNESS
The patient is a 59-year-old African-American male recently diagnosed with a squamous cell carcinoma of the piriform sinus, status post tracheostomy, who has now developed complications including colocutaneous and enterocutaneous fistulae. He has been in the hospital since his original initiation of treatment. He was transferred back here with increasing abdominal pain and evidence of feculent drainage from his abdominal wound, and he was started on ertapenem. Antibiotics were discontinued yesterday, but last night he spiked a temperature and was placed back on Primaxin. Blood cultures were drawn and are already positive for yeast. He has been receiving TPN for about a week and bowel rest for treatment of his enterocutaneous fistula, which was demonstrated on fistulogram. He has now been transferred to the step-down unit, and Infectious Disease is consulted regarding management of fungemia. He is currently awake and does answer some questions, but he is lethargic and somewhat uncooperative. He denies significant pain and states his pain is well controlled. No shortness of breath or chest pain.

PAST MEDICAL HISTORY
1. Metastatic squamous cell carcinoma of the piriform sinus, diagnosed 1 month ago. He was admitted with stridor and had an emergent tracheostomy. Workup revealed metastatic carcinoma, and he had a gastrostomy tube placed. His postoperative course was complicated by development of a colocutaneous fistula, which was repaired, but he has now developed an enterocutaneous fistula, as per history of present illness. He has been receiving radiation therapy and chemotherapy over at Kindred.
2. Hypertension.
3. Benign prostatic hypertrophy.
4. Tracheostomy.
5. Gastrostomy.
6. Enterocutaneous fistula repair.

MEDICATIONS
1. Epoetin.
2. Protonix.
3. Primaxin 1 g IV q. 8h.
4. Caspofungin 50 mg IV daily.
5. Morphine.
6. Zofran.

ALLERGIES
PENICILLIN causes a rash.

REVIEW OF SYSTEMS
Limited due to communication issues and mental status.

FAMILY HISTORY
Noncontributory.

(continued)

SOCIAL HISTORY
He is an ex-smoker.

PHYSICAL EXAMINATION
T-max 103.5, blood pressure 84/60, respiratory rate 18, and heart rate 84. In general, he is a lethargic, uncomfortable-appearing African-American male. He is thin and appears chronically ill. HEENT exam is unremarkable, other than tracheostomy site, which is clean. Neck is supple. Heart exam with normal S1 and S2. No murmurs, clicks, or rubs. Regular rate and rhythm. Lungs are clear. Abdomen is soft with mild tenderness. He has an open wound, which is covered by an ostomy bag. Extremities without edema or rash. He has intact distal pulses.

LABORATORY DATA
White count 3.23 with 79% polys. Hematocrit 33.4, platelets 114. Creatinine 0.6. Electrolytes unremarkable. AST 13, ALT 27. Blood cultures from 10/29/2004 show no growth. Blood cultures from 11/08/2004 have 1 out of 2 sets with budding yeast at 24 hours. Urine culture with greater than 10,000 colonies of yeast as well.

RADIOLOGY
Chest x-ray with no focal consolidation.

IMPRESSION
A 59-year-old African-American male with metastatic squamous cell carcinoma of the piriform sinus. Now re-admitted with enterocutaneous fistula. New blood cultures are showing fungemia quickly.

RECOMMENDATIONS
I think we have an explanation for the fever spike yesterday. Caspofungin is an appropriate choice for empiric antifungal therapy in this case. He could certainly have a non-albicans Candida. I do not have adequate records to tell if he has received Diflucan, but if he did, that would increase his chance of having an azole-resistant organism. Regardless, the main benefit of using an azole is to use oral therapy, and he is not a candidate right now for oral fluconazole, so caspofungin is most appropriate. He should have his port removed. He will need an ophthalmologic exam to rule out an ophthalmitis at some point. There is no evidence on cardiac exam of endocarditis. If he rapidly clears this fungemia, and the port is removed, then 2 weeks of antifungal therapy should be appropriate. He should have his LFTs checked within the first few days of starting caspofungin.

CONSULTATION

HISTORY OF PRESENT ILLNESS
This is a 48-year-old male without any past medical history who presented with a 2-day history of fevers and headaches. The patient is a poor historian. Apparently, he has been experiencing a cough that is nonproductive. He has nausea and vomiting as well. He is fairly weak but has no other symptoms. In the ER, he was noted to have a temperature of 101.2, pulse of 94, blood pressure 94/53, and a respiratory rate 18.

ALLERGIES
No known allergies.

PAST MEDICAL HISTORY
Negative.

PAST SURGICAL HISTORY
Tonsillectomy.

REVIEW OF SYSTEMS
Weakness, myalgias, cough, wheezing, nausea, vomiting, occasional confusion and headaches.

PHYSICAL EXAMINATION
GENERAL: The patient is a middle-aged man, lying in bed in no apparent distress.
HEENT: Pupils are equal, round, reactive to light and accommodation. Mouth is moist.
NECK: Supple. There is no JVD.
LUNGS: No wheezing. Clear to auscultation and percussion.
HEART: Normal S1 and S2. Regular rate and rhythm.
ABDOMEN: Soft, nontender. Positive bowel sounds.
EXTREMITIES: No clubbing, cyanosis, or edema.
NEUROLOGIC: Grossly non-focal.

RADIOLOGICAL DATA
Chest x-ray changes are consistent with COPD. There are no infiltrates.

DIAGNOSTIC DATA
A CT scan of the brain was negative.

LABORATORY DATA
White count 8800, lymphocytes 21, monocytes 9, and eosinophils 2. Normal PT/PTT and INR. LDH 243 and creatinine 1. Liver function tests were within normal limits. CSF showed negative agglutination for bacteria or pathogens. Gram stain showed no white blood cells. No organisms were seen. CSF revealed 12 wbc's, 2 rbc's, 0% segmented neutrophils, 100% lymphocytes, glucose 50, and protein 87. The urine culture was negative.

(continued)

IMPRESSION

1. Aseptic meningitis. The differential diagnoses would include viral pathogens such as enterovirus, including St. Louis encephalitis, and West Nile virus needs to be excluded in the end since Florida has become an endemic area.
2. Rule out HIV.
3. A parameningeal infection cannot be excluded.
4. The patient has already received 2 g of Rocephin that would provide coverage for the next 24 hours. My suspicion for bacterial meningitis is very low. The patient is to be ruled out for HIV.

RECOMMENDATION

I recommend sending serologies for all the above-mentioned pathogens. Specimens should be sent to the health department for further testing.

REVIEW QUESTIONS

The goal of these questions is to test your knowledge in the area of infectious disease.

Directions: Select the correct answer for each of the multiple-choice questions provided below. *Answers are provided at the end of this chapter.*

1. A patient with VRE (vancomycin-resistant enterococcus) would likely be treated with:
   A. Lidex
   B. Zovirax
   C. Zyvox
   D. Frova
2. Often infectious processes are diagnosed using:
   A. Serologic techniques
   B. Sonograms
   C. X-rays
   D. CT scans
3. A child comes into the emergency room febrile and lethargic. The doctor suspects meningitis. Which of these abnormal physical findings is classic?
   A. Stridor
   B. Coryza
   C. Stiff neck
   D. Hyperreflexia
4. CD4 counts are used to:
   A. Assess the degree of visual loss caused by Chlamydia trachomatis
   B. Monitor the efficacy of antibiotics in meningitis
   C. Test antibiotic sensitivity of Chlamydia trachomatis
   D. Monitor AIDS patients and efficacy of treatment
5. Which of the following is a sequela to bacterial endocarditis?
   A. Altered mentation
   B. Valvular vegetations
   C. Myocardial degeneration
   D. Idiopathic thrombocytic purpura
6. A patient with a severe infection of this type may require radical debridement of skin, subcutaneous tissue, and muscle:
   A. Erysipelas secondary to streptococcus
   B. Cellulitis secondary to Staphylococcus epidermidis
   C. Necrotizing fasciitis secondary to Clostridium perfringens
   D. Acanthosis nigricans secondary to diabetes
7. Which of these indicates infection?
   A. Anemia
   B. Left shift
   C. Thrombocytopenia
   D. Hyperkalemia
8. Which choice below would be a method of hepatitis C transmission?
   A. Blood transfusions
   B. Improperly cooked pork
   C. Stepping on a rusty nail
   D. Aerosol droplets from an infected individual
9. The common term for varicella is:
   A. Roseola
   B. Rubella
   C. Chicken pox
   D. Pertussis
10. Hepatitis A is frequently spread via:
    A. Sexual contact
    B. Sneezing
    C. The fecal-oral route
    D. IV drug abuse

11. Hepatitis B can be spread via:
    A. Sexual contact
    B. Improperly prepared red meat
    C. The fecal-oral route
    D. Casual contact with an infected person

12. The Western blot test is used to
    A. Assess efficacy of antibiotic treatment
    B. Confirm HIV infection
    C. Test clotting and bleeding times
    D. Trace a viral infection to its origin

13. Primary syphilis is characterized by the presence of a:
    A. Sore throat
    B. Headache
    C. Chancre
    D. Purulent discharge

14. The human papillomavirus (HPV) causes:
    A. Herpes
    B. Gonorrhea
    C. Genital warts
    D. Chlamydia

15. Mycobacteria are:
    A. Acid-fast bacteria
    B. Gram-positive cocci
    C. Gram-negative cocci
    D. Gram-positive rods

16. Bacteria which require oxygen in order to thrive are called:
    A. Aerobic
    B. Anaerobic
    C. Mycobacteria
    D. Obligate anaerobes

17. A physician orders a C&S. What information is he looking for?
    A. A list of antigens the patient is allergic to
    B. The causative infective agent and a list of antibiotics to use for treatment
    C. The causative agent in aseptic meningitis
    D. A list of antibiotics the patient is allergic to

18. How much time is typically required to culture and identify mycobacteria?
    A. 6–8 hours
    B. 6–8 days
    C. 6–8 weeks
    D. 6–8 months

19. Which of the following is not used to treat malaria?
    A. Primaquine
    B. Mefloquine
    C. Chloroquine
    D. Cephalosporin

20. Opportunistic infections:
    A. Affect immunocompromised patients
    B. Can only be treated during the initial phase of infection
    C. Affect the general population
    D. Are caused by rare infectious agents

21. When labeling tetracycline for treatment of Lyme disease, the pharmacist will add a warning to the bottle for the patient to:
    A. Avoid salty foods
    B. Avoid cola drinks
    C. Avoid dairy products
    D. Avoid eggs

22. Sulfonamides, which are frequently prescribed to treat UTIs, are also prescribed to treat:
    A. Skin, bone, and joint infections
    B. Prostatitis
    C. Herpes virus, types 1 and 2
    D. Pneumocystis carinii pneumonia

23. An AIDS patient is diagnosed with MAC, which is the abbreviation for:
    A. Multiple antiviral contraindications
    B. Multiple autoimmune complexes
    C. Mycobacterium avium complex
    D. Multidrug adverse contraindications

24. Which of the following classifications includes Trichomonas vaginalis?
    A. Fungi
    B. Bacteria
    C. Protozoa
    D. Viruses

25. An example of a helminth would be:
- **A.** Flukes
- **B.** Spirilla
- **C.** Cocci
- **D.** Bacilli

26. Diflucan is an example of:
- **A.** An antibacterial medication
- **B.** An antifungal medication
- **C.** An antiviral medication
- **D.** A chemotherapy drug

27. A high anti-streptolysin O titer would indicate:
- **A.** Therapeutic levels of antibiotics
- **B.** Acute staphylococcal infection
- **C.** Acute streptococcal infection
- **D.** Immunity to streptococcal pharyngitis

28. CMV (cytomegalovirus) causes:
- **A.** A respiratory infection only seen in AIDS patients
- **B.** A life-threatening infection only seen in newborns
- **C.** An uncommon viral infection causing pneumonia
- **D.** A common, mild or subclinical infection in the general population

29. Mycoplasma pneumoniae causes a pneumonia commonly referred to as:
- **A.** Walking pneumonia
- **B.** TB
- **C.** Consumption
- **D.** Double pneumonia

30. TB is usually treated with a combination of drugs including:
- **A.** Amoxicillin and clavulanic acid
- **B.** Isoniazid and rifampin
- **C.** Trimethoprim and sulfamethoxazole
- **D.** Erythromycin and sulfasoxazole

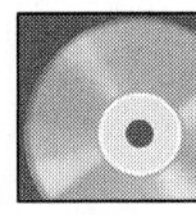

Please see the accompanying CD for additional review materials for this section.

PROOFREADING EXERCISES

These four proofreading exercises are provided to improve your skills in the areas of editing and effective identification and correction of errors in the medical record.

Directions: Identify and correct the transcription errors found in the exercises below. *Answers are provided at the end of this chapter.*

PROOFREADING EXERCISE #1

REASON FOR CONSULTATION
MRFA breast abscess.

HISTORY
The patient is a 32-year-old African-American female admitted through the emergency room yesterday with a left breast abscess. She says she first noticed a small bite or pimple-like lesion on the left breast last Thursday. Over the weekend, she developed increasing breast pain, left maxillary pain, and swelling in the left arm. By Sunday it was unbearable, so she presented to the emergency room, where she had a bedside incision and drainage performed and then was discharged on doxycycline. She took the doxycycline as instructed. She did not have rank fevers, chills, or other systemic symptoms, although she reports a little bit of mal haze on Sunday. She had been instructed that if she did not improve to come back in 2 days, which she did. She was admitted through the emergency room last night and placed on vancomycin and Levaquin. A wound swab culture of the draining breast lesion last night noted no Paulies, rare Graham-positive cocci, and rare Graham-negative pods. Culture today is growing MRSA. She has had HIV tests in the past, which were negative.

SOCIAL HISTORY
She is sexually active. She has no children. She has no breast implants.

PAST MEDICAL HISTORY
Notable for allergic rhinitis. She had a remote ectopic pregnancy and a remote pilon nodal cyst abscess.

FAMILY HISTORY
Notable for diabetes and hypertension.

(continued)

SOCIAL HISTORY
She is a part-time hairdresser. She does not wear gloves unless she is using heavy chemicals. She is single and has a boyfriend. She lives with her mother or her boyfriend. No children. Nonsmoker, no drug abuse.

ALLERGIES
No known drug allergies.

MEDICATIONS
Doxycycline and Vicodin from the ER.

REVIEW OF SYSTEMS
Negative except for history of present illness. No GI or GU symptoms.

PHYSICAL EXAMINATION
General: She is a well-appearing black female in no acute distress. Vital signs: Afebrile. Heart rate 60, respiratory rate 18, blood pressure 129/66. HEENT: Unremarkable. The neck is supple. Lungs are clear. She has no axillary lymphadenopathy. Her left breast exam is notable for a 3 cm, indurated area in the 10 o'clock position with surrounding erythema. The central induration is tender. I cannot actually feel fluctuance. There is a central lacerated area with purulent drainage. Not able to express much. The entire breast is mildly edematous compared to the right. Cardiac: Regular rate and rhythm. Abdomen: Nontender. Extremities: No rash or edema.

LABORATORY DATA
Gram stain had no polys, rare gram-positive cocci, and rare gram-negative odds from a left breast swab. Culture growing many presumptive penicillin-resistant Staphylococcus auris. Beta hCG negative. Chemistries unremarkable. Normal CBC. HIV screen is pending. LFCs are normal.

IMPRESSION
A 32-year-old black female presents with a left breast abscess due to penicillin-resistant Staphylococcus aureus.

RECOMMENDATIONS
I agree with the current antimicrobial coverage. If the cultures grow only staphylococcus, I will discontinue the Levaquin and chose an oral agent based on the MICs. She needs contract isolation.

PROOFREADING EXERCISE #2

REASON FOR CONSULTATION
Sepsis.

HISTORY
The patient is a 75-year-old white female who is a resident of Village Nursing Home since November with a history of Parkinson disease and recurrent urinary tract infections. She was found with altered level of consciousness this morning by her routine caregiver. Her last antibiotics were during a hospital stay in the fall for a UCI. Her caregiver has not noticed any diarrhea, cough, shortness of breath, skin rash, or other findings in the last few days. When EMS arrived, her blood pressure was 68 over palp. She received a fluid bullous. She was 91% saturated on nonrebreather. On arrival to the emergency room her temperature was 101.5, blood pressure 72/46. She had urgent volume resuscitation, a right subclavian line placed, a CT of the head, with the results pending. She was brought to the ICU and incubated. She is now on Levophed in the ICU.

PAST MEDICAL HISTORY
1. Parkinson disease.
2. Possible cerebrovascular ascent. Details are unclear. Her family is not aware of it.
3. Recurrent urinary track infections.

ALLERGIES
No known drug allergies.

MEDICATIONS
Medications at home: Protonics, Fosamax, aspirin, Zyrtec, Celebrex, Parlodel, Lexapro, and Artane.

SOCIAL HISTORY
She is a nursing home resident.

FAMILY HISTORY
Noncontributory.

(continued)

REVIEW OF SYSTEMS

Unobtainable.

PHYSICAL EXAMINATION

Blood pressure 114/50 on 10 mcg of Levophed, heart rate 96. She is on the ventilator on 70% with a pH of 7299, pCO_2 of 39, pO_2 of 128. HEENT exam is unrevealing. Sclerae anicteric. Lungs are clear. Cardiac exam has regular rate and rhythm, tachycardic. Abdomen is soft, quiet. Extremities without clubbing, cyanosis, rash, or edema. She has minimal, very dark urine in her holy catheter. A new central venous catheter in right subclavian position.

LABORATORY DATA

White count 25,000, hematocrit 42, platelets 147. Electrolytes notable for potassium of 3.9, creatinine 2.9, alkaline phosphatase 361, AST 203, ALT 38, bilirubin 1.0, total protein 5.8, albumin 31. Urinalysis 470 white cells, 1000 red cells. Troponin of 0.4, total CK 211, NB 2.5. Lipase is normal. Urine sodium is 45.

IMPRESSION

Elderly white female arrives with altered mental status and appears to be in peptic shock. She is being ruled out for myocardial infarction, but her electrocardiogram showed no evidence of myocardial infarction. I see no evidence of pneumonia on her chest x-ray, and her symptom complex is not appropriate. I will agree that this is probably ureal sepsis. She has marked pyuria and appears to be in acute frenal failure. She will be a Xigris candidate if there is no traumatic turnaround in the next few hours. She is getting aggressive fluid resuscitation, and the central venous pressure (CVP) monitor is in place. She is on a fluid sliding scale. She has already received Levaquin in the emergency room, and I have added Zosyn. I cannot rule out a belly source, and thus we will provide appropriate coverage for cholecystitis or bacteremia secondary to diverticulitis.

PROOFREADING EXERCISE #3

HISTORY OF PRESENT ILLNESS
This is a 62-year-old male with history of hypertension and congestive heart disease who presented with a chief complaint of shortness of breath. According to his own report, he was feeling sick for the last week or so with cold-like symptoms. He describes these as a nonproductive cough and shortness of breath on exertion occurring over the last 24 hours to the point that he was brought to the emergency room for further evaluation and management.

On initial evaluation, he was found to have a blood pressure of 155/111, pulse 124, respirations of 30, O_2 sack of 82%, and a temperature of 99. He was confused at the time. His ABC revealed a large A-a gradient. He was placed on Bye PAP and initiated on diuretics and a nitro glycerin drip. He received Zithromax and ceftriaxone after culture collection and was transferred to the intensive care unit.

Currently the patient remains alert and interactive. He is breathing on 50% oxygen by mass. His sensorium is much sharper. He is able to give me more details of his history.

The patient states that he has been noting yellow eyes for the last year or so. He does not know why. He denies nausea, vomiting, abdominal pain, diarrhea, or any other concordant symptoms. He denies shaking chills.

ALLERGIES
No known allergies.

PAST MEDICAL HISTORY
Remarkable for hypertension and CHS. He was hospitalized a year ago with a CHS exacerbation.

SOCIAL HISTORY
The patient admits to drinking alcohol.

PHYSICAL EXAMINATION
GENERAL: The patient is an elderly male in moderate respiratory distress.
HEENT: Pupils equal, round, and sluggishly reactive to light and accommodation. Mouth is moist.

(continued)

NECK: Supple without JVD, bruits, or limp nodes.
HEART: Normal S1 and S2. Regular rate and rhythm.
LUNGS: Pour inspiratory effort. Minimal crackles in the basis.
ABDOMEN: Soft and nontender. No organomegaly.
EXTREMITIES: No clubbing, cyanosis, or edema.
NEUROLOGIC: Grossly non-focal.

RADIOLOGICAL DATA
Chest x-ray showed right-middle to right-lower lung and filtrates and reportedly congestive changes.

LABORATORY DATA
AST 98, ALT 52, albumin 3.5, calcium 7.8, alk phos 66, sodium 135, potassium 3.9, chloride 100, CO_2 of 25, BUN 31, and creatinine 1.8. Bilirubin 4.0. Glucose is 98. ABG from yesterday showed a pH of 7.34, pCO_2 of 36, and pO_2 of 95. CPK 624, troponin 1.15. BNP 1690. E timer was 4.9. PT 20.9. INR 251. Amylase 125 and lipase 6. White count 7100 with 85% neutrophils, 10% lymphocytes, and 6% mono types. Blood cultures collected yesterday show no growth so far. Urine culture is negative so far. Sputum culture pending.

IMPRESSION
1. Multilevel pneumonia. Needs Rod's system antibiotics. The patient seems to be adequately covered with ceftriaxone and Zithromax.
2. Hypobilirubinemia. Repeat bilirubin with fractions. Direct is more prominent than imaging studies indicate. We recommend a liver and gallbladder sonogram.
3. Colopathy with abnormal PT.
4. Congestive heart failure.
5. Respiratory insufficiency.
6. Renal insufficiency, multifactorial.

RECOMMENDATIONS
Continue Zithromax and ceftriaxone. Obtain a biliary gallbladder sonogram as mentioned above.

PROOFREADING EXERCISE #4

REASON FOR CONSULTATION
HIV and sepsis.

HISTORY
The patient is a 39-year-old African-American male with AIDS who presented to the emergency room today after being found with altered mental status by a friend. We have few details of his recent history but do know that he is on heart therapy and PPP prophylaxis. When he presented to the emergency room today, he was febrile. He was hypoglycemic en route and received 1 ampule of P50. His respiratory rate was in the 50s; he was hypotensive. His friends and family reported several days of increasing cough and fever with dark brown sputum production. He was noted to be very dry and was aggressively volume resuscitated and received one dose of vancomycin, Rocephin, and ampicillin, and he was admitted to the ICU. Through the day his respiratory status continued to deteriorate, requiring mechanical ventilation. He has had over 7 L of fluid and is making very little urine and requiring pressor support. He is ruling in for myocardial infarction with markedly elevated serum troponin and has acute renal failure with a creatinine of 4.2 on arrival followed by 4.6. An infectious disease consultation is requested regarding further management.

PAST MEDICAL HISTORY
1. Acquired immune sufficiency syndrome. No details on recent CD4 viral load.
2. Recent hospitalization for respiratory infection in Tyler.
3. Anemia.
4. Diabetes.
5. Chronic diarrhea.

HOME MEDICATIONS
1. Abacavir 300 mg 2 p.o. daily.
2. Tenofovir 300 mg p.o. daily.
3. Nelfinavir 1000 mg p.o. b.i.d.
4. Lamivudine 150 mg p.o. b.i.d.
5. Lamus insulin.
6. Lisinopril 20 mg p.o. daily.

(continued)

7. Valcyte.
8. Imodium.
9. Diflucan 20 mg p.o. daily.
10. Bactrim DS 1 p.o. daily.

ALLERGIES

He has no known drug allergies.

SOCIAL HISTORY

Unobtainable since the patient is intubated.

REVIEW OF SYSTEMS

Unobtainable since the patient is intubated.

PHYSICAL EXAMINATION

The patient is intubated, sedated, and on 100% FIO_2, and therefore unresponsive on exam. His AVG earlier in the day was pH 7.42, pCO_2 16, pO_2 of 82 on room air. Status post intubation on 100%, pH of 7.3, pCO_2 of 25, pO_2 of 142 with an A-a gradient of 540. He is thin and appears chronically ill. HEENT exam is unremarkable. He has an ET tube in place. The neck is supple. He has coarse bilateral breath sounds with prominent crackles in the right base and consolation in the right middle upper lung fields. He is tachycardic with regular rate and rhythm. No pericardial rub. The abdomen is soft, nontender, nondistended, and quiet. Extremities without clubbing, cyanosis, edema, or rash. He has a serpiginous ulceration on his left buttock and perirectal region, without vesicals or purulent drainage. Neurologic exam is limited secondary to sedation and intubation.

RADIOLOGY

The chest x-ray notes a progressive right upper lobe infiltrate with bilateral patchy lower lobe infiltrates as well, which have progressed over the afternoon. Lower extremity Doppler examinations are negative for DDT. The head CT was unremarkable.

LABORATORY DATA

White count 1.34 with 38% segs, hemoglobin 11, platelets 59,000. Potassium 2.2, bicarbonate 15, and creatinine 4.2, with a repeat of 4.6. Blood glucose after D50 was 188. INR was 2 before and then 2 after 2 units

(continued)

of flash frozen plasma. Urine pneumococcal antigen was negative. RPR was nonreactive. Troponin was 145 with repeat value of 127. Serum lactate was 4.53. BNP was 1629. MB fraction was 8.3. Urine chloride was 18 and urine sodium was 29. The urinalysis had 22 white cells and 11 red cells. AST was 108, ALT 41, alkaline phosphatase 102, bilirubin 1.1.

ELECTROCARDIOGRAM
EKG shows sinus tachycardia with poor R-wave progression.

IMPRESSION
Critically ill, 39-year-old African-American male with acquired immunodeficiency syndrome, on highly active antiretroviral therapy (HAART) with unclear spiral control, who presents with a severe pneumonia. He has rapidly deteriorated over the course of the day. The differential diagnosis in terms of etiology of his pneumonia includes typical and atypical causes of commonly-acquired pneumonia, and because of his recent hospitalization, nodal coma pathogens as well. His Gram stain is showing many gram-negative rods, which puts pseudocoma and enteral bacteria at the top of list. This also could be hematogenous influenzae. He is at risk for Legionella as well. I doubt this is Pneumocystis pneumoniae or disseminated fungal infection, but those remain on the differential.

RECOMMENDATIONS
He meets criteria for Xigris infusion. If his repeat platelet count is adequate (i.e. greater than 40,000), I would proceed with Xigris. In terms of antimicrobial coverage, I agree with cefepime and quinolone that has been initiated for both broader gram-negative coverage and coverage of atypical agents. I agree with AFV precautions, even though I think mycobacteria is low on the differential. Also agree with continuing the Bactrim until we are sure of our diagnosis. His chest x-ray does not have a typical pattern for pneumocystic pneumonia. I would not use enteric antifungals. I would restart his heart therapy as well. I would consider new gin as well, given his leukopenia.

ANSWER KEYS

REVIEW QUESTIONS ANSWER KEY

1. C
2. A
3. C
4. D
5. B
6. C
7. B
8. A
9. C
10. C
11. A
12. B
13. C
14. C
15. A
16. A
17. B
18. C
19. D
20. A
21. C
22. D
23. C
24. C
25. A
26. B
27. C
28. D
29. A
30. B

PROOFREADING EXERCISE #1 KEY

Incorrect abbreviation—MRSA

Incorrect term—axillary

Incorrect word—frank

Incorrect term—malaise

Incorrect term—polys

Incorrect spelling—gram

Incorrect spelling—gram

Incorrect word—rods

Incorrect term—pilonidal

REASON FOR CONSULTATION

MRFA breast abscess.

HISTORY

The patient is a 32-year-old African-American female admitted through the emergency room yesterday with a left breast abscess. She says she first noticed a small bite or pimple-like lesion on the left breast last Thursday. Over the weekend, she developed increasing breast pain, left maxillary pain, and swelling in the left arm. By Sunday it was unbearable, so she presented to the emergency room, where she had a bedside incision and drainage performed and then was discharged on doxycycline. She took the doxycycline as instructed. She did not have rank fevers, chills, or other systemic symptoms, although she reports a little bit of mal haze on Sunday. She had been instructed that if she did not improve to come back in 2 days, which she did. She was admitted through the emergency room last night and placed on vancomycin and Levaquin. A wound swab culture of the draining breast lesion last night noted no Paulies, rare Graham-positive cocci, and rare Graham-negative pods. Culture today is growing MRSA. She has had HIV tests in the past, which were negative.

SOCIAL HISTORY

She is sexually active. She has no children. She has no breast implants.

PAST MEDICAL HISTORY

Notable for allergic rhinitis. She had a remote ectopic pregnancy and a remote pilon nodal cyst abscess.

FAMILY HISTORY

Notable for diabetes and hypertension.

SOCIAL HISTORY
She is a part-time hairdresser. She does not wear gloves unless she is using heavy chemicals. She is single and has a boyfriend. She lives with her mother or her boyfriend. No children. Nonsmoker, no drug abuse.

ALLERGIES
No known drug allergies.

MEDICATIONS
Doxycycline and Vicodin from the ER.

REVIEW OF SYSTEMS
Negative except for history of present illness. No GI or GU symptoms.

PHYSICAL EXAMINATION
General: She is a well-appearing black female in no acute distress. Vital signs: Afebrile. Heart rate 60, respiratory rate 18, blood pressure 129/66. HEENT: Unremarkable. The neck is supple. Lungs are clear. She has no axillary lymphadenopathy. Her left breast exam is notable for a 3 cm, indurated area in the 10 o'clock position with surrounding erythema. The central induration is tender. I cannot actually feel fluctuance. There is a central lacerated area with purulent drainage. Not able to express much. The entire breast is mildly edematous compared to the right. Cardiac: Regular rate and rhythm. Abdomen: Nontender. Extremities: No rash or edema.

Incorrect term—macerated

LABORATORY DATA
Gram stain had no polys, rare gram-positive cocci, and rare gram-negative odds from a left breast swab. Culture growing many presumptive penicillin-resistant Staphylococcus auris. Beta hCG negative. Chemistries unremarkable. Normal CBC. HIV screen is pending. LFCs are normal.

IMPRESSION
A 32-year-old black female presents with a left breast abscess due to penicillin-resistant Staphylococcus aureus.

RECOMMENDATIONS
I agree with the current antimicrobial coverage. If the cultures grow only staphylococcus, I will discontinue the Levaquin and chose an oral agent based on the MICs. She needs contract isolation.

Incorrect word—rods

Incorrect term—aureus

Incorrect drug—methicillin

Incorrect abbreviation—LFTs

Incorrect spelling—choose

Incorrect word—contact

PROOFREADING EXERCISE #2 KEY

Incorrect abbreviation—UTI

Improper abbreviation—spell out palpable

Incorrect term—intubated

Incorrect word—tract

Incorrect spelling—Protonix

Incorrect term—bolus

Incorrect word—accident

REASON FOR CONSULTATION
Sepsis.

HISTORY
The patient is a 75-year-old white female who is a resident of Village Nursing Home since November with a history of Parkinson disease and recurrent urinary tract infections. She was found with altered level of consciousness this morning by her routine caregiver. Her last antibiotics were during a hospital stay in the fall for a UCI. Her caregiver has not noticed any diarrhea, cough, shortness of breath, skin rash, or other findings in the last few days. When EMS arrived, her blood pressure was 68 over palp. She received a fluid bullous. She was 91% saturated on nonrebreather. On arrival to the emergency room her temperature was 101.5, blood pressure 72/46. She had urgent volume resuscitation, a right subclavian line placed, a CT of the head, with the results pending. She was brought to the ICU and incubated. She is now on Levophed in the ICU.

PAST MEDICAL HISTORY
1. Parkinson disease.
2. Possible cerebrovascular ascent. Details are unclear. Her family is not aware of it.
3. Recurrent urinary track infections.

ALLERGIES
No known drug allergies.

MEDICATIONS
Medications at home: Protonics, Fosamax, aspirin, Zyrtec, Celebrex, Parlodel, Lexapro, and Artane.

SOCIAL HISTORY
She is a nursing home resident.

FAMILY HISTORY
Noncontributory.

REVIEW OF SYSTEMS
Unobtainable.

PHYSICAL EXAMINATION
Blood pressure 114/50 on 10 mcg of Levophed, heart rate 96. She is on the ventilator on 70% with a pH of 7299, pCO_2 of 39, pO_2 of 128. HEENT exam is unrevealing. Sclerae anicteric. Lungs are clear. Cardiac exam has regular rate and rhythm, tachycardic. Abdomen is soft, quiet. Extremities without clubbing, cyanosis, rash, or edema. She has minimal, very dark urine in her holy catheter. A new central venous catheter in right subclavian position.

LABORATORY DATA
White count 25,000, hematocrit 42, platelets 147. Electrolytes notable for potassium of 3.9, creatinine 2.9, alkaline phosphatase 361, AST 203, ALT 38, bilirubin 1.0, total protein 5.8, albumin 31. Urinalysis 470 white cells, 1000 red cells. Troponin of 0.4, total CK 211, NB 2.5. Lipase is normal. Urine sodium is 45.

IMPRESSION
Elderly white female arrives with altered mental status and appears to be in peptic shock. She is being ruled out for myocardial infarction, but her electrocardiogram showed no evidence of myocardial infarction. I see no evidence of pneumonia on her chest x-ray, and her symptom complex is not appropriate. I will agree that this is probably ureal sepsis. She has marked pyuria and appears to be in acute frenal failure. She will be a Xigris candidate if there is no traumatic turnaround in the next few hours. She is getting aggressive fluid resuscitation, and the central venous pressure (CVP) monitor is in place. She is on a fluid sliding scale. She has already received Levaquin in the emergency room, and I have added Zosyn. I cannot rule out a belly source, and thus we will provide appropriate coverage for cholecystitis or bacteremia secondary to diverticulitis.

Missing decimal—7.299

Incorrect word—Foley

Flag—albumin value cannot exceed total protein

Incorrect abbreviation—MB (CK-MB)

Incorrect term—septic

Incorrect term—renal

Incorrect term—urosepsis

Incorrect word—dramatic

PROOFREADING EXERCISE #3 KEY

Incorrect term—"sat", spell out saturation

Incorrect abbreviation —ABG

Incorrect word— concomitant

Incorrect term—BiPAP

Use combining form— nitroglycerin

Incorrect word—mask

Incorrect abbreviation —CHF

HISTORY OF PRESENT ILLNESS
This is a 62-year-old male with history of hypertension and congestive heart disease who presented with a chief complaint of shortness of breath. According to his own report, he was feeling sick for the last week or so with cold-like symptoms. He describes these as a nonproductive cough and shortness of breath on exertion occurring over the last 24 hours to the point that he was brought to the emergency room for further evaluation and management.

On initial evaluation, he was found to have a blood pressure of 155/111, pulse 124, respirations of 30, O_2 sack of 82% and a temperature of 99. He was confused at the time. His ABC revealed a large A-a gradient. He was placed on Bye PAP and initiated on diuretics and a nitro glycerin drip. He received Zithromax and ceftriaxone after culture collection, and was transferred to the intensive care unit.

Currently the patient remains alert and interactive. He is breathing on 50% oxygen by mass. His sensorium is much sharper. He is able to give me more details of his history.

The patient states that he has been noting yellow eyes for the last year or so. He does not know why. He denies nausea, vomiting, abdominal pain, diarrhea, or any other concordant symptoms. He denies shaking chills.

ALLERGIES
No known allergies.

PAST MEDICAL HISTORY
Remarkable for hypertension and CHS. He was hospitalized a year ago with a CHS exacerbation.

SOCIAL HISTORY
The patient admits to drinking alcohol.

PHYSICAL EXAMINATION
GENERAL: The patient is an elderly male in moderate respiratory distress.
HEENT: Pupils equal, round, and sluggishly reactive to light and accommodation. Mouth is moist.
NECK: Supple without JVD, bruits, or limp nodes.
HEART: Normal S1 and S2. Regular rate and rhythm.
LUNGS: Pour inspiratory effort. Minimal crackles in the basis.
ABDOMEN: Soft and nontender. No organomegaly.
EXTREMITIES: No clubbing, cyanosis, or edema.
NEUROLOGIC: Grossly non-focal.

RADIOLOGICAL DATA
Chest x-ray showed right-middle to right-lower lung and filtrates and reportedly congestive changes.

LABORATORY DATA
AST 98, ALT 52, albumin 3.5, calcium 7.8, alk phos 66, sodium 135, potassium 3.9, chloride 100, CO_2 of 25, BUN 31, and creatinine 1.8. Bilirubin 4.0. Glucose is 98. ABG from yesterday showed a pH of 7.34, pCO_2 of 36, and pO_2 of 95. CPK 624, troponin 1.15. BNP 1690. E timer was 4.9. PT 20.9. INR 251. Amylase 125 and lipase 6. White count 7100 with 85% neutrophils, 10% lymphocytes, and 6% mono types. Blood cultures collected yesterday show no growth so far. Urine culture is negative so far. Sputum culture pending.

IMPRESSION
1. Multilevel pneumonia. Needs Rod's system antibiotics. The patient seems to be adequately covered with ceftriaxone and Zithromax.

Incorrect spelling—poor

Incorrect term—lymph

Incorrect word—bases

Incorrect term—infiltrates

Spell out—alkaline phosphatase

Flag—inappropriate value for INR

Incorrect term—D-dimer

Incorrect term—monocytes

Incorrect phrase—broad spectrum

Incorrect term—multilobar

Incorrect prefix—hyperbilirubinemia

Incorrect term—coagulopathy

2. Hypobilirubinemia. Repeat bilirubin with fractions. Direct is more prominent than imaging studies indicate. We recommend a liver and gallbladder sonogram.
3. Colopathy with abnormal PT.
4. Congestive heart failure.
5. Respiratory insufficiency.
6. Renal insufficiency, multifactorial.

RECOMMENDATIONS

Continue Zithromax and ceftriaxone. Obtain a biliary gallbladder sonogram as mentioned above.

PROOFREADING EXERCISE #4 KEY

Incorrect abbreviation—PCP

Incorrect term—HAART

Incorrect abbreviation—D50

Incorrect term—immunodeficiency

Missing word—CD4 and viral

REASON FOR CONSULTATION
HIV and sepsis.

HISTORY
The patient is a 39-year-old African-American male with AIDS who presented to the emergency room today after being found with altered mental status by a friend. We have few details of his recent history but do know that he is on heart therapy and PPP prophylaxis. When he presented to the emergency room today, he was febrile. He was hypoglycemic en route and received 1 ampule of P50. His respiratory rate was in the 50s; he was hypotensive. His friends and family reported several days of increasing cough and fever with dark brown sputum production. He was noted to be very dry and was aggressively volume resuscitated and received one dose of vancomycin, Rocephin, and ampicillin, and he was admitted to the ICU. Through the day his respiratory status continued to deteriorate, requiring mechanical ventilation. He has had over 7 L of fluid and is making very little urine and requiring pressor support. He is ruling in for myocardial infarction with markedly elevated serum troponin and has acute renal failure with a creatinine of 4.2 on arrival followed by 4.6. An infectious disease consultation is requested regarding further management.

PAST MEDICAL HISTORY
1. Acquired immune sufficiency syndrome. No details on recent CD4 viral load.
2. Recent hospitalization for respiratory infection in Tyler.
3. Anemia.
4. Diabetes.
5. Chronic diarrhea.

Incorrect term—Lantus

Incorrect dose—200 mg

Incorrect abbreviation—ABG

Incorrect term—consolidation

Incorrect spelling—vesicles

HOME MEDICATIONS

1. Abacavir 300 mg 2 p.o. daily.
2. Tenofovir 300 mg p.o. daily.
3. Nelfinavir 1000 mg p.o. b.i.d.
4. Lamivudine 150 mg p.o. b.i.d.
5. Lamus insulin.
6. Lisinopril 20 mg p.o. daily.
7. Valcyte.
8. Imodium.
9. Diflucan 20 mg p.o. daily.
10. Bactrim DS 1 p.o. daily.

ALLERGIES
He has no known drug allergies.

SOCIAL HISTORY
Unobtainable since the patient is intubated.

REVIEW OF SYSTEMS
Unobtainable since the patient is intubated.

PHYSICAL EXAMINATION
The patient is intubated, sedated, and on 100% FIO_2, and therefore unresponsive on exam. His AVG earlier in the day was pH 7.42, pCO_2 16, pO_2 of 82 on room air. Status post intubation on 100%, pH of 7.3, pCO_2 of 25, pO_2 of 142 with an A-a gradient of 540. He is thin and appears chronically ill. HEENT exam is unremarkable. He has an ET tube in place. The neck is supple. He has coarse bilateral breath sounds with prominent crackles in the right base and consolation in the right middle upper lung fields. He is tachycardic with regular rate and rhythm. No pericardial rub. The abdomen is soft, nontender, nondistended, and quiet. Extremities without clubbing, cyanosis, edema, or rash. He has a serpiginous ulceration on his left buttock and perirectal region, without vesicals or purulent drainage. Neurologic exam is limited secondary to sedation and intubation.

Incorrect abbreviation—DVT

RADIOLOGY
The chest x-ray notes a progressive right upper lobe infiltrate with bilateral patchy lower lobe infiltrates as well, which have progressed over the afternoon. Lower extremity Doppler examinations are negative for DDT. The head CT was unremarkable.

Incorrect value—2.4

Incorrect word—fresh

LABORATORY DATA
White count 1.34 with 38% segs, hemoglobin 11, platelets 59,000. Potassium 2.2, bicarbonate 15, and creatinine 4.2, with a repeat of 4.6. Blood glucose after D50 was 188. INR was 2 before and decreased to 2.1 after 2 units of flash frozen plasma. Urine pneumococcal antigen was negative. RPR was nonreactive. Troponin was 145 with repeat value of 127. Serum lactate was 4.53. BNP was 1629. MB fraction was 8.3. Urine chloride was 18 and urine sodium was 29. The urinalysis had 22 white cells and 11 red cells. AST was 108, ALT 41, alkaline phosphatase 102, bilirubin 1.1.

ELECTROCARDIOGRAM
EKG shows sinus tachycardia with poor R-wave progression.

Incorrect term—viral

Incorrect term—community

Incorrect term—nosocomial

Incorrect term—Enterobacteriaceae

Incorrect term—Pseudomonas

Incorrect term—Haemophilus

Incorrect spelling—pneumonia (not the species)

IMPRESSION
Critically ill, 39-year-old African-American male with acquired immunodeficiency syndrome, on highly active antiretroviral therapy (HAART) with unclear spiral control, who presents with a severe pneumonia. He has rapidly deteriorated over the course of the day. The differential diagnoses in terms of etiology of his pneumonia include typical and atypical causes of commonly-acquired pneumonia, and because of his recent hospitalization, nodal coma pathogens as well. His Gram stain is showing many gram-negative rods, which puts pseudocoma and enteral bacteria at the top of list. This also could be hematogenous influenzae. He is at risk for Legionella as well. I doubt this is Pneumocystis pneumoniae or disseminated fungal infection, but those remain on the differential.

RECOMMENDATIONS

He meets criteria for Xigris infusion. If his repeat platelet count is adequate (i.e. greater than 40,000), I would proceed with Xigris. In terms of antimicrobial coverage, I agree with cefepime and quinolone that has been initiated for both broader gram-negative coverage and coverage of atypical agents. I agree with AFV precautions, even though I think mycobacteria is low on the differential. Also agree with continuing the Bactrim until we are sure of our diagnosis. His chest x-ray does not have a typical pattern for pneumocystic pneumonia. I would not use enteric antifungals. I would restart his heart therapy as well. I would consider new gin as well, given his leukopenia.

Incorrect abbreviation —AFB

Incorrect term—empiric

Incorrect term—HAART

Incorrect term—Neupogen

CHAPTER 10

Otorhinolaryngology

OBJECTIVES CHECKLIST

A prepared exam candidate will know the:

- ❑ Combining forms, prefixes, and suffixes related to the body system.
- ❑ Anatomical structures of the outer, middle, and inner ear.
- ❑ Physiologic process of identifying sound, including the pathway of sound vibration from the pinna to the cerebral cortex.
- ❑ Anatomical structures of the nose and throat and the role of each in respiration and speech.
- ❑ Abnormal and pathologic conditions related to the ear, nose, and throat.
- ❑ Clinical procedures utilized to identify and treat diseases and abnormalities of the ear, nose, and throat.
- ❑ Common medications used to treat diseases and abnormalities of the ear, nose, and throat.

RESOURCES FOR STUDY

1. *The Language of Medicine*
   Chapter 5: Digestive System, Pharynx, pp. 143–144.
   Chapter 12: Respiratory System, Section II. Anatomy and Physiology of Respiration, pp. 442–443, 446–452.
   Chapter 17: Sense Organs: The Eye and the Ear, pp. 689–698, 705–707.
2. *H&P: A Nonphysician's Guide to the Medical History and Physical Examination*
   Chapter 7: Review of Systems: Head, Eyes, Ears, Nose, Throat, Mouth, Teeth, pp. 59–70.
   Chapter 20: Examination of the Ears, pp. 189–198.
   Chapter 21: Examination of the Nose, Throat, Mouth and Teeth, pp. 199–208.
3. *Human Diseases*
   Chapter 9: Diseases of the Ear, Nose and Throat, pp. 127–140.
4. *Laboratory Tests & Diagnostic Procedures in Medicine*
   Chapter 3: Measurement of Vision and Hearing, pp. 29–38.
   Chapter 7: Endoscopy: Visual Examination of the Eyes, Ears, Nose, and Respiratory Tract, pp. 95–106.
5. *Understanding Pharmacology for Health Professionals*
   Chapter 19: Ear, Nose and Throat Drugs, pp. 205–216.

SAMPLE REPORTS

The following four reports are examples of reports you might encounter while transcribing oto-rhinolaryngology.

HISTORY AND PHYSICAL

HISTORY
The patient presents with a chronic history of nasion pressure, frequent upper respiratory infections, occasional bronchitis, cough, sneezing, and possible incipient asthma. For many years, she has also had a postnasal drip. Her nasal obstruction is noted to be bilateral and equal and is associated with sneezing and a clear rhinorrhea. She has no abnormal sensation of smell but breathes through her mouth and nose. There has been no nasal trauma and she is aware of pressure in the nasion area. She also snores. There is itching of the throat, occasional postnasal drip, and clearing of her throat. It was felt that she had a possible reflux problem. She was given information on reflux and placed on Nexium, which does help her. She also has a history of significant heartburn and gastritis with a history of ulcer disease, for which she takes Librax.

The patient wears glasses for reading and distance but notes itching and tearing of her eyes when her nasal symptoms are active. There is no significant hearing loss. She does occasionally have balance and tinnitus problems. When she has respiratory symptoms, she notes pressure in her ear, but otherwise her hearing is unremarkable. As noted, for the past year, she has had occasional wheezing. One year ago, she had pneumonia. She has had episodes of bronchitis but has never been diagnosed as an asthmatic. She smokes and drinks alcohol on a social basis only. Headaches, as described above, are treated with over-the-counter medication, such as ibuprofen and Aleve. There are no cardiovascular disorders. The patient has no history of thyroid disease, diabetes, or anemia. There is no osteoporosis.

Head and neck surgery is limited to a tonsillectomy in New Jersey in 1978. There are no specific drug allergies. Her mother and sister both have sinus problems. The patient was given Astelin by Dr. Jones, which seems to have helped her. She has not used any of the newer antihistamines on a regular basis. Three or 4 years ago, she was tested in Florida for inhalant allergies and told that no significant findings were uncovered. The patient has no pets and notes no reactions from animals. She is aware that her symptoms increase with weather changes, and dust causes significant nasal symptoms, including sneezing and rhinorrhea.

A CT scan of the sinuses was ordered and was completely normal, only showing a left septal deviation. A culture of the nose at the time was negative as well.

PHYSICAL EXAMINATION
Examination reveals a comfortable lady in no distress with multiple upper respiratory complaints. The oropharyngeal examination is unremarkable. The teeth are in a good state of repair. The oral mucosa is well hydrated. There are large residual tonsil tags, despite the history of a tonsillectomy. The intranasal inspection shows hypertrophy of the turbinates with a purplish appearance and bilateral septal spurs widening the septum and resulting in a decreased nasal airway. There is no evidence of rhinorrhea or polyps. There is no sinus percussive tenderness. It is noted that the patient has prominent allergic shiners and Dennie lines. She is breathing through her nose and

(continued)

mouth. The otoscopic visualization shows intact tympanic membranes and auditory canals. There is no cerumen accumulation. There is no evidence of middle ear disease. Palpation of the neck elicits no tenderness or adenopathy. The carotid pulses are full and equal. The thyroid is not palpable. There is normal laryngeal crepitus, and the salivary glands are unremarkable. The patient's facial movements are normal. There are no temporomandibular joint findings.

The patient's history and examination are strongly suggestive of an underlying allergic diathesis, especially with a normal CT scan of the sinuses and culture of the nasal mucus. She notes some relief with the Astelin spray and will continue this. I have added Zyrtec-D and Zyrtec tablets to the regimen. I have scheduled her for intradermal allergy testing. She is very interested in possibly having septum and turbinate surgery to improve her nasal airway. This will be addressed after the completion of the allergy testing and the trial of medications.

OPERATIVE REPORT

PREOPERATIVE DIAGNOSES

1. Obstructive sleep apnea.
2. Tonsillar hypertrophy.
3. Oropharyngeal obstruction.
4. Tongue base hypertrophy.

POSTOPERATIVE DIAGNOSES

1. Obstructive sleep apnea.
2. Tonsillar hypertrophy.
3. Oropharyngeal obstruction.
4. Tongue base hypertrophy.

PROCEDURES PERFORMED

1. Uvulopalatopharyngoplasty.
2. Partial resection of the tongue base by radiofrequency.
3. Tonsillectomy.

SURGEON

John Smith, MD.

ANESTHESIA

General anesthesia.

HISTORY

This is a 33-year-old who has a history of obstructive sleep apnea, intolerant to CPAP, with tonsillar hypertrophy, redundant uvula and soft palate, and prominent tongue base.

PROCEDURE

The patient was taken to the operating room and placed on the table in the supine position. Satisfactory general anesthesia was administered via endotracheal tube. The patient was placed in the Rose tonsil position. The Crowe-Davis mouth gag was introduced into the patient's mouth and suspended from the Mayo stand. The soft palate was elevated with a red rubber catheter.

The tonsils were dissected from the tonsillar fossae bilaterally, along with resection of a small cuff of anterior tonsillar pillar mucosa using the suction cautery. The posterior tonsillar pillars were then rotated laterally and anteriorly and sutured to the anterior tonsillar pillar mucosa with interrupted 3-0 Vicryl sutures. This was performed bilaterally.

Incision was then made across the soft palate, resecting the musculus uvuli and a small cuff of anterior mucosa of the margin of the soft palate. The posterior mucosa was preserved, and bilateral diagonal relaxing incisions were made at the junction of the soft palate and the superior tonsillar pole. Flaps were rotated laterally and superiorly and secured with 3-0 Vicryl, and the posterior mucosa of the soft palate was rotated anteriorly and secured to the anterior mucosa using 3-0 Vicryl interrupted sutures. Adequate soft palate length was preserved for velopharyngeal competence, and then the mouth gag was removed.

(continued)

A side-biting mouth gag was introduced into the patient's mouth. The mouth was irrigated with Betadine and then the tongue was brought forward. The tongue base was visualized using the Somnos 2-channel tongue base probe. Four passes at the tongue base at 1500 joules per pass were then performed, 2 on the right and 2 on the left, anterior and posterior to the circumvallate papillae. Prior to each lesion, approximately 4 mL of normal saline was injected into the site. A total of 6000 joules was delivered to the tongue base.

The patient was awakened, extubated, and taken to the recovery room in satisfactory condition.

OPERATIVE REPORT

PREOPERATIVE DIAGNOSES
1. Nasal airway obstruction.
2. Nasal septal deformity.
3. Inferior turbinate hypertrophy.

POSTOPERATIVE DIAGNOSES
1. Nasal airway obstruction.
2. Nasal septal deformity.
3. Inferior turbinate hypertrophy.

OPERATION
1. Septoplasty.
2. Bilateral submucous resection of the inferior turbinates.

SURGEON
John Smith, MD.

ANESTHESIA
General via endotracheal tube.

PROCEDURE
The patient was taken to the operating room and placed on the table in the supine position. Satisfactory general anesthesia was administered via endotracheal tube. The nose was cocainized and injected with 1% Xylocaine with epinephrine for local anesthesia.

Following adequate prepping and draping, a right hemitransfixion incision was made. A left mucoperichondrial tunnel was elevated over the cartilage to the bony cartilaginous junction. The cartilage was separated from the bone. Bilateral posterior tunnels were elevated. Severely deviated bony septum was resected. The cartilage was freed up off the maxillary crest, and a large maxillary crest spur was resected. The maxillary crest was then fractured back to the midline. The cartilage was shortened inferiorly to fit back on the maxillary crest, and the hemitransfixion incision was closed with 4-0 chromic.

The inferior turbinate was injected with 1% Xylocaine with epinephrine. Then, using the turbinate microdebrider blade through an anterior stab incision, bilateral submucosal resection of the inferior turbinates was performed bilaterally, and remaining turbinate tissue was out-fractured.

The nose was then packed with hydrocolloid gel packs. The patient was awakened and taken to the recovery room in satisfactory condition.

CONSULTATION

CHIEF COMPLAINT
Vertigo and questionable sleep apnea.

HISTORY OF PRESENT ILLNESS
This is a 43-year-old Caucasian female who came down with rotational vertigo in January. This occurred over the course of the day and was severe for about 3 days. She presented to Dr. Smith and had blood work performed which was reportedly normal. She had questionable blood pressure elevation at that time and was followed up by Dr. Jones, at which time she states her blood pressure was 160/115 and she was placed on Tiazac. She continued to have a feeling of rotational vertigo, worse with eyes closed, and accompanied by nausea but no vomiting. The acute symptoms lasted for approximately 8 days, and she did as much activity as she could. She had significant improvement at that point, just noting that her symptoms return when she is tired or while watching TV. She has avoided skiing or other athletic activity for fear it would aggravate her symptoms again. She had a prior episode of vertigo 3 years ago which lasted for 4 days, rotational, continuous, with nausea and vomiting. Two years ago, she had a similar episode, although it was of less magnitude and resulted in minimal debility. She has never had any significant fluctuation in hearing or tinnitus. She denies any vision problems. Did have mild blurring initially. No recent upper respiratory symptoms. She is also concerned about possible apnea, as on several occasions she has been told by friends and family that she has a peculiar breathing pattern in which she will suddenly stop, and they are afraid she is not going to start breathing again. She has some daytime fatigue but does not nap and is functioning well. She has recently started a new business in addition to her real estate business which is taking a lot of time. Moderate stress but nothing that she feels is unusual. She has had a 20-pound weight gain in the last year. Always wakes in the morning with a dry mouth. No history of head injury or chronic medical illness.

PAST MEDICAL HISTORY
Nausea with codeine and other pain medications. Hospitalized for a broken wrist in 1996 and nasal fracture in 1979.

CURRENT MEDICATIONS
Paxil 20 mg daily, and Tiazac 180 mg p.o. daily for hypertension, still in her first week of treatment.

SOCIAL HISTORY
She has smoked a 1/2 pack of cigarettes a day for the past 27 years. She drinks 2–4 glasses of wine a day.

FAMILY HISTORY
Parents in good health. Father with heart disease and multiple family members are hypertensive.

REVIEW OF SYSTEMS
Positive for cervical degenerative joint disease and recent hypertension and depression. No cardiac disease, GI or GU problems, easy bleeding or bruising, diabetes, endocrine or metabolic disease, or neurologic illness.

(continued)

PHYSICAL EXAMINATION

Alert Caucasian female. Blood pressure 156/88, pulse 77. No cervical adenopathy or masses. Well-defined cervical triangle. Thyroid is normal, trachea midline. External ears, canals, and tympanic membranes unremarkable. Deviated nasal septum to the left, mild. No polyps, drainage, or inflammation. Lips and teeth unremarkable. Palate, tongue, floor of mouth normal. Grade 2 soft palate ptosis. Atrophic tonsils. Nasopharynx and hypopharynx clear. Pupils round and reactive to light, extraocular muscles are intact. No nystagmus. In 3-inch heels, patient performs Romberg, tandem gait, and stands on 1 foot, all without any difficulty. Cranial nerves II through XII grossly intact.

Audiogram shows normal hearing bilaterally with 5 dB SRT on the right with 96% discrimination, 5 dB SRT on the left with 100% discrimination. Impedance testing and reflex are normal.

IMPRESSION

1. Vestibular neuronitis, symptomatically resolved.
2. Erratic nocturnal respiratory pattern. Rule out obstructive sleep apnea.

PLAN

1. Polysomnography.
2. Maximize visual and environmental clues to optimize balance.
3. Continue antihypertensive. Follow up with Dr. Jones. Recheck after polysomnography.

REVIEW QUESTIONS

The goal of these questions is to test your knowledge in the area of otorhinolaryngology.

Directions: Select the correct answer for each of the multiple-choice questions provided below. *Answers are provided at the end of this chapter.*

1. Which would indicate normal hearing on a Rinne test?
   A. Air conduction greater than bone conduction
   B. Bone conduction greater than air conduction
   C. Bone and air conduction equal
   D. Negative bone conduction
2. The HIB (Haemophilus influenzae type B) vaccine has significantly reduced the incidence of:
   A. Epiglottitis
   B. Meningitis
   C. Laryngitis
   D. A and B
3. A puncture of the tympanic membrane to aspirate fluid from the middle ear is called:
   A. Hemotympanum
   B. Tympanocentesis
   C. Tympanoplasty
   D. Pneumotympanum
4. Which of the following is correct?
   A. AD=right ear; AS=left ear; AU=both/each ear
   B. AD=left ear; AS=right ear; AU=both ears
   C. AD=right ear, AS=left ear; AU=neither ear
   D. None of the above
5. Epistaxis may be treated using:
   A. Anterior nasal packing
   B. Silver nitrate cautery
   C. Topical vasoconstrictor
   D. All of the above
6. The incus, stapes, and ossicles are located in the:
   A. Inner ear
   B. Nasal cavity
   C. Middle ear
   D. Oropharynx
7. The organ of Corti is located:
   A. In the outer ear
   B. In the paranasal sinuses
   C. In the inner ear
   D. In the cerebral cortex
8. The projecting portion of the outer ear is called the:
   A. Eustachian tube
   B. Pinna
   C. Ossicles
   D. Stapes
9. A Weber test is performed and the results are dictated, "Weber lateralizes to the left." What can be said about this patient?
   A. The patient has some hearing loss
   B. The patient has fluid in the left middle ear
   C. The patient has nystagmus
   D. This is a normal finding
10. What is the name of the membrane between the external auditory canal and the middle ear?
    A. Oval window
    B. Mastoid process
    C. Tympanic
    D. Choroid

11. A cyst-like mass containing cholesterol that is most commonly found in the middle ear and mastoid region is called:
    A. Schwannoma
    B. Neuroma
    C. Keratoma
    D. Cholesteatoma

12. The medical term for tone deafness is:
    A. Dysgeusia
    B. Anosmia
    C. Sensory amusia
    D. Dysphonia

13. Endolymphatic hydrops is:
    A. Another name for Ménière disease
    B. Distention of the membranous labyrinth
    C. Lymphadenopathy around the pharynx and ears
    D. A & B

14. The medical term for hearing loss occurring with age is:
    A. Anacusis
    B. Presbycusis
    C. Nosoacusis
    D. Paracusis

15. Myringotomy is a surgical incision into the:
    A. Tympanic membrane
    B. Cochlea
    C. Pinna
    D. Larynx

16. A procedure to help correct snoring is called:
    A. Tympanoplasty
    B. Uvulopalatopharyngoplasty
    C. Laryngectomy
    D. Mandibuloplasty

17. The Mallampati classification measures:
    A. Tongue size relative to pharyngeal size
    B. Size of the sinuses
    C. Tonsillar size
    D. Length of the eustachian tube

18. A patient is brought from the sitting position to the supine position with head hanging over the edge of the exam table and turned to the left or right. This test is called:
    A. Dix-Hallpike Maneuver
    B. Weber test
    C. Rinne test
    D. ENG

19. Inflammation of the nasal mucosa secondary to excessive or improper topical medication is called:
    A. Crista nasalis
    B. Samter syndrome
    C. Rhinitis medicamentosa
    D. Rhinenchysis

20. Ringing in the ears is also known as:
    A. Dysacusis
    B. Tenonitis
    C. Tinnitus
    D. Barotitis

21. What is the commonly used name for the pharyngeal tonsil?
    A. Tonsil
    B. Parotid gland
    C. Salivary gland
    D. Adenoid

22. Difficulty swallowing is:
    A. Dysphagia
    B. Dysphasia
    C. Deglutition
    D. Odynophagia

23. Where is the arytenoid cartilage located?
    A. Larynx
    B. Pharynx
    C. Nasopharynx
    D. Between the sinuses

24. The word piriform means:
    A. Pea-shaped
    B. Pear-shaped
    C. Spiral shaped
    D. Chain-like

25. What is concha bullosa?
    A. An abnormality of the middle turbinate
    B. A type of pharyngitis
    C. A form of laryngitis
    D. An infection of the pinna

26. Barany caloric test is performed:
    A. By irrigating the EAC with warm and cold water
    B. To test for vestibular function
    C. By limiting caloric intake to determine effect on the inner ear
    D. A & B

27. The medical term for a nosebleed is:
    A. Apostaxis
    B. Hematemesis
    C. Epistaxis
    D. Hematostaxis

28. The patient is referred for polysomnography with symptoms of lethargy and memory problems. It is likely she is going to be evaluated for:
    A. Arrhythmia
    B. Obstructive sleep apnea
    C. Sleeping sickness
    D. Epilepsy

29. A nasal smear taken from a patient suffering from seasonal allergy may show:
    A. Monocytes
    B. Yeast
    C. Eosinophils
    D. A & B

30. ENG is the abbreviation for:
    A. Electroneurogram
    B. Electronic night guard
    C. Electronystagmogram
    D. Endoscopic nasal galvanometer

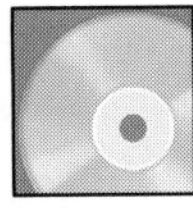

Please see the accompanying CD for additional review materials for this section.

PROOFREADING EXERCISES

These three proofreading exercises are provided to improve your skills in the areas of editing and effective identification and correction of errors in the medical record.

Directions: Identify and correct the transcription errors found in the exercises below. *Answers are provided at the end of this chapter.*

PROOFREADING EXERCISE #1

PREOPERATIVE DIAGNOSIS
Bilateral splenoid and frontal sinusitis.

POSTOPERATIVE DIAGNOSIS
Bilateral splenoid and frontal sinusitis.

OPERATION
Bilateral endoscopic sinus surgery with image guidance, including:
1. Bilateral frontal sinusotomy by endoscopy.
2. Bilateral sphenoidotomy with removal of tissue from sphenoid sinus by endoscopy.
3. Bilateral maxillary gastrostomy.
4. Ethmoidectomy.

SURGEON
John Smith, MD.

ANESTHESIA
General endotracheal.

HISTORY
This is a 27-year-old gentleman who has a history of previous sphenoid sinusitis and now has recurrence of sphenoid sinusitis with opacification of the sphenoids bilaterally and frontal sinusitis as well. Due to sphenoid and frontal involvement, and revision nature of surgery, the surgery was done with image guidance.

PROCEDURE
The patient was taken to the operating room and placed on the table in the supine position. Satisfactory general anesthesia was administered via

(continued)

endotracheal tube. The nose was congested with topical cocaine and injected with 1% Xylocaine with ephedrine for local anesthesia. The Landmark image-guided CT scan was downloaded into the image-guided system, and corresponding registration points marked on the computer-generated model.

The head frame was placed on the patient. Corresponding registration points were marked on the patient, and endoscopic visualization of the left side of the nose was obtained. The left middle turbulent was fractured medially, and the maxillary ostium was opened, and with back-fracture and resection of the uncinate process, the nasal frontal area was identified. Azure nasi cells were taken down. The nasal frontal duct was cannulated with the aid of image guidance. The ethmoid air sails were taken down back to the sphenoid. The sphenoid opening had polypoid mucosa around the opening. This was resected using the micro-debrider, and the sphenoid ostium was identified. This had been previously opened and the opening was enlarged inferiorly by drilling down the inferior crest of the sphenoid ostium to enlarge the opening. There was some thick debris in the sinus which was suctioned, and some tissue was sent for pathology as well as special strains for fungus. The sinus was suctioned, and it primarily consisted of hyperemic mucosa.

The procedure was repeated on the right side.

Hemostasis was then obtained with adrenalin pellets and bipolar cautery. A hydrocolloid gel packing was placed in the ethmoid cavities bilaterally, and the patient was awakened, extubated, and taken to the recovery room in satisfactory condition.

PROOFREADING EXERCISE #2

CHIEF COMPLAINT
Tinnitus.

HISTORY OF PRESENT ILLNESS
2-year-old Caucasian male who had a severe fall while skiing approximately 3 weeks ago. He did a back flip and landed on his back and neck and fractured some ribs. He was able to get up and ski off the mountain but was extremely soar and in relative shock about 5 hours later. He required no hospitalization or other treatment but noticed some global tinnitus approximately 2 weeks ago, which has continued today. It is annoying but has not interfered with auditory perception or routine activity. Had tinnitus in the passed following a head injury in 1995 accompanied by CSS leak requiring a craniotomy for repair. Wife was concerned this may be happening again. Patient has noted no drainage from the nose and does not complain of headaches. No salty taste. He only took a couple of Tylenol after his fall and reports no other analgesic use. Has noted no change in hearing or dizziness. No loss of consciousness associated with injury.

PAST MEDICAL HISTORY
No allergy to medications and no current medications. Treated for severe left hemifacial spasm 1989 with occipital craniotomy. Skull fracture, post traumatic, 1995, with CSF leak repair 5 months later.

SOCIAL HISTORY
No tobacco or alcohol use. Patient is married and retired.

REVIEW OF SYSTEMS
Positive for prostatic problems and hypercholesterolemia. Significant noise exposure at the steal mill when a young man with documented high-frequency loss. Denies cardiac or pulmonary disease, GI problems, easy bleeding or bruising, visual change, change in hearing, fluctuation in hearing, dizziness, or other neurologic symptoms.

(continued)

PHYSICAL EXAMINATION
Reveals alert Caucasian male in no distress. Well-heeled anterior and occipital craniotomy. No cervical adenopathy or masses. External ears, canals, and tympanic membranes unremarkable. Turning fork 512: Difference left, Webber right, air conduction greater than bone conduction bilaterally. Nose: Deviated nasal septum markedly to the right. No drainage or polyps. Lips and teeth unremarkable. Plate, tongue, floor of mouth normal with 1+ tonsils. Nasopharynx and hypopharynx clear. Rhomboid stable. Tandem gait and single-foot standing normal.

Audiogram reveals bilateral high-frequency and moderately severe sensorineural hearing loss: 15 dB SRT AD with 100% scrim; 10 dB SRT AS with 96% scrim.

IMPRESSION
High-frequency sensory neural hearing loss with posttraumatic global tinnitus secondary to concussion. No CSF leak.

PLAN
Multivitamin with sink. Reassurance. Recheck p.r.n.

PROOFREADING EXERCISE #3

PREOPERATIVE DIAGNOSES
1. Chronic hoarseness.
2. History of spasmodic dysphonia.
3. Probable reflux laryngitis.
4. Allergic rhinitis.

POSTOPERATIVE DIAGNOSES
Same.

PROCEDURE PERFORMED
Flexible fiberoptic nasopharyngolaryngoscopy.

ANESTHESIA
Xylocaine 4%.

ESTIMATED BLOOD LOSS
None.

INDICATIONS FOR PROCEDURE
The patient returns for follow up. She has had hoarseness on and off for quiet some time but her hoarseness has gotten worse in the past few weeks. A fiberoptic examination is undertaken because of the chronicity of her symptoms and acute exacerbation in a lady who has no established history of dysphoria.

PROCEDURE IN DETAIL
After adequate application of topical anesthetic to the nose and throat with 40% Xylocaine solution and after decongesting the nose, the Olympus scope is introduced into the left nasal cavity. No blood is seen in the nasal cavity. Septal spurring is appreciated. The septum is otherwise relatively straight. Septal and turbinate mucosa are healthy. The sinus orifices are clear. The scope is taken back to the nasal pharynx where the posterior, superior, and lateral nasal pharyngeal walls are clear. No mass, lesion, or ulcer noted. The posterior aspect of the soft palate and uvula, and the posterior and lateral oropharyngeal walls demonstrate no ulcer, erosion, or mass. The base of tongue, trabecula, lateral pharyngeal band,

(continued)

epiglottis, aryepiglottic folds, pure form, and postcricoid areas are systematically seen and these are all within normal limits. No mass, lesion, ulcer, pooling of secretions, blood, or other abnormalities are noted. The arytenoids are moderately boggy and there is mucosal edema. There is some scarring and bridging across the posterior commissure and interarytenoid space. There was no leukoplakia seen.

Chord mobility is completely intact. The false chords and true chords are healthy in appearance and chord mobility is intact. The subglottis is clear.

The scope was then backed out and advanced into the contra lateral nasal cavity. Septal and turbinate mucosa are healthy. No other mass or lesion is noted. The scope is removed. The patient tolerated the procedure well without complications.

RECOMMENDATIONS
At this point, I have asked her to start Nexium daily and she also has some over the counter allergy remedies at home, but she does not recall the names. I have asked her to take both, and we will see her back in about 4 or 5 weeks to see how she does on this regime.

ANSWER KEYS

REVIEW QUESTIONS ANSWER KEY

1. A
2. D
3. B
4. A
5. D
6. C
7. C
8. B
9. A
10. C
11. D
12. C
13. D
14. B
15. A
16. B
17. A
18. A
19. C
20. C
21. D
22. A
23. A
24. B
25. A
26. D
27. C
28. B
29. C
30. C

PROOFREADING EXERCISE #1 KEY

Incorrect term—sphenoid

PREOPERATIVE DIAGNOSIS
Bilateral splenoid and frontal sinusitis.

POSTOPERATIVE DIAGNOSIS
Bilateral splenoid and frontal sinusitis.

OPERATION
Bilateral endoscopic sinus surgery with image guidance, including:

1. Bilateral frontal sinusotomy by endoscopy.
2. Bilateral sphenoidotomy with removal of tissue from sphenoid sinus by endoscopy.
3. Bilateral maxillary gastrostomy.
4. Ethmoidectomy.

Incorrect term—antrostomy

SURGEON
John Smith, MD.

ANESTHESIA
General endotracheal.

HISTORY
This is a 27-year-old gentleman who has a history of previous sphenoid sinusitis and now has recurrence of sphenoid sinusitis with opacification of the sphenoids bilaterally and frontal sinusitis as well. Due to sphenoid and frontal involvement, and revision nature of surgery, the surgery was done with image guidance.

PROCEDURE
The patient was taken to the operating room and placed on the table in the supine position. Satisfactory general anesthesia was administered via endotracheal tube. The nose was congested with topical cocaine and injected with 1% Xylocaine with ephedrine for local anesthesia. The Landmark image-guided CT scan was downloaded into the image-guided system, and corresponding

Needs prefix—decongested

Incorrect drug—epinephrine

registration points marked on the computer-generated model.

The head frame was placed on the patient. Corresponding registration points were marked on the patient, and endoscopic visualization of the left side of the nose was obtained. The left middle turbulent was fractured medially, and the maxillary ostium was opened, and with back-fracture and resection of the uncinate process, the nasal frontal area was identified. Azure nasi cells were taken down. The nasal frontal duct was cannulated with the aid of image guidance. The ethmoid air sails were taken down back to the sphenoid. The sphenoid opening had polypoid mucosa around the opening. This was resected using the micro-debrider, and the sphenoid ostium was identified. This had been previously opened and the opening was enlarged inferiorly by drilling down the inferior crest of the sphenoid ostium to enlarge the opening. There was some thick debris in the sinus which was suctioned, and some tissue was sent for pathology as well as special strains for fungus. The sinus was suctioned, and it primarily consisted of hyperemic mucosa.

The procedure was repeated on the right side.

Hemostasis was then obtained with adrenalin pellets and bipolar cautery. A hydrocolloid gel packing was placed in the ethmoid cavities bilaterally, and the patient was awakened, extubated, and taken to the recovery room in satisfactory condition.

Incorrect term—turbinate

Incorrect term—Agger

Incorrect word—cells

Incorrect word—stains

Incorrect term—pledgets

PROOFREADING EXERCISE #2 KEY

Flag age—inconsistent with remainder of report; also, do not begin sentences with numerals—add "A" or "This is a"

Incorrect spelling—sore

Incorrect spelling—past

Incorrect abbreviation—CSF

Use combined form—posttraumatic

CHIEF COMPLAINT
Tinnitus.

HISTORY OF PRESENT ILLNESS
2-year-old Caucasian male who had a severe fall while skiing approximately 3 weeks ago. He did a back flip and landed on his back and neck and fractured some ribs. He was able to get up and ski off the mountain but was extremely soar ~~and~~ in relative shock about 5 hours later. He required no hospitalization or other treatment but noticed some global tinnitus approximately 2 weeks ago, which has continued today. It is annoying but has not interfered with auditory perception or routine activity. Had tinnitus in the passed ~~following~~ a head injury in 1995 ~~accompanied by~~ CSS leak requiring a craniotomy for repair. Wife was concerned this may be happening again. Patient has noted no drainage from the nose and does not complain of headaches. No salty taste. He only took a couple of Tylenol after his fall and reports no other analgesic use. Has noted no change in hearing or dizziness. No loss of consciousness associated with injury.

PAST MEDICAL HISTORY
No allergy to medications and no current medications. Treated for severe left hemifacial spasm 1989 with occipital craniotomy. ~~Skull~~ fracture, post traumatic~~, 1995~~, with CSF leak repair 5 months later.

SOCIAL HISTORY
No tobacco or alcohol use. Patient is married and retired.

REVIEW OF SYSTEMS
Positive for prostatic problems and hypercholesterolemia. Significant noise exposure at

the steal mill when a young man with documented high-frequency loss. Denies cardiac or pulmonary disease, GI problems, easy bleeding or bruising, visual change, change in hearing, fluctuation in hearing, dizziness, or other neurologic symptoms.

PHYSICAL EXAMINATION

Reveals alert Caucasian male in no distress. Well-heeled anterior and occipital craniotomy. No cervical adenopathy or masses. External ears, canals, and tympanic membranes unremarkable. Turning fork 512: Difference left, Webber right, air conduction greater than bone conduction bilaterally. Nose: Deviated nasal septum markedly to the right. No drainage or polyps. Lips and teeth unremarkable. Plate, tongue, floor of mouth normal with 1+ tonsils. Nasopharynx and hypopharynx clear. Rhomboid stable. Tandem gait and single-foot standing normal.

Audiogram reveals bilateral high-frequency and moderately severe sensorineural hearing loss: 15 dB SRT AD with 100 % scrim; 10 dB SRT AS with 96% scrim.

IMPRESSION

High-frequency sensory neural hearing loss with posttraumatic global tinnitus secondary to concussion. No CSF leak.

PLAN

Multivitamin with sink. Reassurance. Recheck p.r.n.

Incorrect spelling—steel

Incorrect spelling—healed

Incorrect word—tuning

Incorrect spelling—Weber

Incorrect word—palate

Incorrect term—Romberg

Dangerous abbreviations—spell out right ear and left ear

Spell out entire word—discrimination

Use combined form—sensorineural

Incorrect term—zinc

PROOFREADING EXERCISE #3 KEY

PREOPERATIVE DIAGNOSES
1. Chronic hoarseness.
2. History of spasmodic dysphonia.
3. Probable reflux laryngitis.
4. Allergic rhinitis.

POSTOPERATIVE DIAGNOSES
Same.

Repeat full text of diagnoses

PROCEDURE PERFORMED
Flexible fiberoptic nasopharyngolaryngoscopy.

ANESTHESIA
Xylocaine 4%.

ESTIMATED BLOOD LOSS
None.

INDICATIONS FOR PROCEDURE
The patient returns for follow up. She has had hoarseness on and off for quiet some time but her hoarseness has gotten worse in the past few weeks. A fiberoptic examination is undertaken because of the chronicity of her symptoms and acute exacerbation in a lady who has no established history of dysphoria.

One word—followup

Incorrect word—quite

Incorrect term—dysphonia

PROCEDURE IN DETAIL
After adequate application of topical anesthetic to the nose and throat with 40% Xylocaine solution and after decongesting the nose, the Olympus scope is introduced into the left nasal cavity. No blood is seen in the nasal cavity. Septal spurring is appreciated. The septum is otherwise relatively straight. Septal and turbinate mucosa are healthy. The sinus orifices are clear. The scope is taken back to the nasal pharynx where the posterior, superior, and lateral nasal pharyngeal walls are clear. No mass, lesion, or ulcer noted. The posterior aspect of

Incorrect percentage—4%

Use combined form—nasopharynx

Use combined form—nasopharyngeal

Incorrect term—piriform

Incorrect term—vallecula

the soft palate and uvula, and the posterior and lateral oropharyngeal walls demonstrate no ulcer, erosion, or mass. The base of tongue, trabecula, lateral pharyngeal band, epiglottis, aryepiglottic folds, pure form, and postcricoid areas are systematically seen and these are all within normal limits. No mass, lesion, ulcer, pooling of secretions, blood, or other abnormalities are noted. The arytenoids are moderately boggy and there is mucosal edema. There is some scarring and bridging across the posterior commissure and interarytenoid space. There was no leukoplakia seen.

Incorrect spelling—cord

Chord mobility is completely intact. The false chords and true chords are healthy in appearance and chord mobility is intact. The subglottis is clear.

Use combined form—contralateral

The scope was then backed out and advanced into the contra lateral nasal cavity. Septal and turbinate mucosa are healthy. No other mass or lesion is noted. The scope is removed. The patient tolerated the procedure well without complications.

RECOMMENDATIONS

Hyphenate over-the-counter

Incorrect word—regimen

At this point, I have asked her to start Nexium daily and she also has some over the counter allergy remedies at home, but she does not recall the names. I have asked her to take both, and we will see her back in about 4 or 5 weeks to see how she does on this regime.

CHAPTER

11

Dermatology

OBJECTIVES CHECKLIST

A prepared exam candidate will know:

- ❑ All combining forms, prefixes, and suffixes related to dermatology.
- ❑ Layers of the skin and the role/function of each.
- ❑ Anatomy and function of the accessory organs of the skin (hair, nails, and glands).
- ❑ Definitions and attributes of all lesion types.
- ❑ Signs, symptoms, and diseases related to the skin and accessory organs.
- ❑ Laboratory studies related to the diagnosis and treatment of dermatologic dysfunction and disease.
- ❑ Common medications prescribed for dermatologic symptoms and diseases.
- ❑ Transcription standards pertaining to allergies, immunologic disorders, and lymphocytes.

RESOURCES FOR STUDY

1. *The Language of Medicine*
   Chapter 16: Skin, pp. 629–668.
2. *H&P: A Nonphysician's Guide to the Medical History and Physical Examination*
   Chapter 14: Review of Systems: Skin, pp. 125–130.
   Chapter 17: Examination of the Skin, pp. 157–168.
3. *Human Diseases*
   Chapter 7: Diseases of the Skin: pp. 87–104.
4. *Laboratory Tests & Diagnostic Procedures in Medicine*
   Chapter 16: Normal Anatomy and Histology, pp. 225–250.
   Chapter 17: Procedures and Practice in Anatomic Pathology, pp. 251–278.
5. *Understanding Pharmacology for Health Professionals*
   Chapter 11: Dermatologic Drugs, pp. 82–101.
6. *The AAMT Book of Style for Medical Transcription*
   Clark level, pp. 51–52.

SAMPLE REPORTS

The following four reports are examples of reports you might encounter while transcribing dermatology.

OFFICE NOTE

HISTORY
A 68-year-old man has a 10-month history of an intermittent, itchy rash on his right thigh. This settles with a topical steroid, and between episodes the skin is normal. He occasionally has a similar eruption on his left chest but has had no rashes anywhere else.

SOCIAL HISTORY
He works part time as a bookmaker's assistant. He smokes a pipe, but his personal and family history is otherwise noncontributory.

PHYSICAL EXAMINATION
Shows eczematous rash with redness, weeping, scaling, and vesiculation on the anterior thighs. Some lichenification is present. There were no abnormal findings elsewhere on general examination.

Patch test was performed and was positive for acrylates.

ASSESSMENT
Allergic contact dermatitis. He does not have a history of joint replacement to account for his exposure to acrylates, and after extensive interviewing, we suspect the causative agent is from his work environment. He often carries bank notes in his pants pockets and sometimes in his shirt pocket.

PLAN
1. Avoid carrying papers in pockets.
2. Return p.r.n.

OFFICE NOTE

HISTORY
The patient presents for assessment of pigmented lesions developing on the trunk and extremities. The patient has no previous history of skin cancer. She states she has had previous nevi excised. She has had significant sun exposure in the past and likes to tan using indoor tanning beds.

PAST MEDICAL HISTORY
Hypothyroidism, on replacement; otherwise, no health problems.

CURRENT MEDICATIONS
Synthroid.

PHYSICAL EXAMINATION
Revealed several seborrheic keratoses and lentigines on the trunk and upper extremities. A small actinic keratosis was seen on the right forehead. Erythematous lichenoid keratoses were present on the left lower leg.

ASSESSMENT
1. Actinic keratosis of right forehead.
2. Lichenoid keratoses of left lower leg.

PLAN
1. Liquid nitrogen cryotherapy.
2. Return p.r.n.

HISTORY AND PHYSICAL

HISTORY OF PRESENT ILLNESS
The patient is seen today for an initial evaluation. She is a very pleasant 50-year-old female with a history of anxiety, hypercholesterolemia, and recent skin loss on her arms and legs as well as a recurring lesion on the lower back area. She also has multiple general complaints.

CURRENT MEDICATIONS
She is on Paxil, Ambien, Lopid, Premarin, and another medicine that I cannot read.

ALLERGIES
She is allergic to ASPIRIN.

PAST MEDICAL HISTORY
There is no diabetes, hepatitis, heart disease, or recent blood transfusion. She is a nonsmoker.

DIAGNOSES
1. Skin loss areas on the arms and legs consistent with idiopathic guttate hypomelanosis.
2. A recurring eruption on the lower back, upper buttock area. She has post-inflammatory changes as well, but no active rash is seen. We have to consider herpes simplex.

PLAN
She will return to the office right away the next time the rash occurs.

OFFICE NOTE

HISTORY

The patient presents for assessment of acne symptoms. She develops papules and pustules as well as inflammatory nodules. She has taken systemic antibiotic therapy, including erythromycin, which she took for 2 months. She has also used Retin-A but found this to be too irritating. Her menstrual cycles are regular and she is on birth control pills. She also gives a history of easy flushing and blushing of the face.

PHYSICAL EXAMINATION

Revealed papules and pustules distributed on the forehead, cheeks, and chin. Only a slight comedone component was present.

ASSESSMENT

Combination of both rosacea and acne vulgaris.

PLAN

1. Doxycycline 100 mg daily.
2. Hydrocortisone 1%, clindamycin 1%, and metronidazole 1% in Complex 15 lotion applied twice a day.

REVIEW QUESTIONS

The goal of these questions is to test your knowledge in the area of dermatology.

Directions: Select the correct answer for each of the multiple-choice questions provided below. *Answers are provided at the end of this chapter.*

1. What procedure is utilized for the destruction of tissue by high-frequency electric sparks?
   A. Dermabrasion
   B. Fulguration
   C. Mohs micrographic surgery
   D. Radiotherapy
2. Abnormal dilation of small blood vessels under the skin is called:
   A. Telangiectasias
   B. Verrucae
   C. Seborrheic dermatitis
   D. Ecchymosis
3. A superficial squamous cell carcinoma in situ which occurs as one or more sharply defined, red-brown, thickened, scaly, crusty plaques is:
   A. Bowen disease
   B. Pyogenic granuloma
   C. Keratosis pilaris
   D. Keratoacanthoma
4. The highly contagious skin disease caused by a female mite burrowing under the skin resulting in intense pruritus and secondary infection is called:
   A. Pediculosis
   B. Tinea unguium
   C. Scabies
   D. Erythrasma
5. A Wood lamp is an ultraviolet light used to diagnose:
   A. Onychomycosis
   B. Urticaria
   C. Fungal infections
   D. Ecchymosis
6. What cancer classification is utilized to designate malignant melanoma of the skin?
   A. CIN grade
   B. Gleason score
   C. Dukes classification
   D. Clark level
7. The removal of scab tissue resulting from burns or other skin injuries is known as:
   A. Diascopy
   B. Escharotomy
   C. Dermatoplasty
   D. Cauterization
8. A thickened area of the epidermis caused by excessive exposure to light is:
   A. Actinic keratosis
   B. Callus
   C. Keloid
   D. Leukoplakia
9. One type of skin cancer is:
   A. Urticaria
   B. Scabies
   C. Basal cell
   D. Leiomyoma
10. The medical term for hives is:
    A. Psoriasis
    B. Eczema
    C. Urticaria
    D. Scabies
11. Contact dermatitis may be caused by:
    A. Laundry soap
    B. Exposure to the sun
    C. Overdose of vitamin C
    D. A bee sting

12. The medical term for severe itching is:
    A. Pruritus
    B. Eczema
    C. Erythema
    D. Papilledema

13. A closed comedo is also known as a:
    A. Whitehead
    B. Pustule
    C. Blackhead
    D. Papule

14. A circumscribed, raised skin lesion filled with pus is a:
    A. Papule
    B. Macule
    C. Pustule
    D. Wheal

15. The medical term for warts is:
    A. Verrucae
    B. Stratum corneum
    C. Scleroderma
    D. DLE

16. Which of these combining forms mean yellow, red, and black (respectively)?
    A. Jaund/o, erythr/o, melan/o
    B. Albin/o, anthrac/o, chlor/o
    C. Poli/o, xantho/o, cyan/o
    D. Eosin/o, cirrh/o, leuk/o

17. Which classification is used to indicate the thickness of a melanoma tumor?
    A. Mohs
    B. Breslow
    C. FAB
    D. Gleason

18. Which of the following terms is not related to dermatology?
    A. Cicatrix
    B. Dermographia
    C. Pityriasis
    D. Calices

19. Which of these are signs of subcutaneous infection?
    A. Rubor, dolor, and calor
    B. Jaundice, hyperbilirubinemia, and colic
    C. Miosis, ptosis, and anhidrosis
    D. Hypesthesia, proprioception, and xerostomia

20. A disease manifested by patchy areas of epidermal hypopigmentation:
    A. Vertigo
    B. Vitiligo
    C. Ecchymosis
    D. Eczema

21. The patient is a 54-year-old diabetic woman who is being discharged home from the hospital where she had been admitted for diabetic ketoacidosis. She has also complained of having some problems with intertrigo. Other than insulin, what other medication is likely to be prescribed for her on discharge?
    A. Lamictal
    B. Lupron
    C. Lomotil
    D. Lamisil

22. A person who bites his nails might develop a condition known as:
    A. Paronychia
    B. Psittacosis
    C. Parenchyma
    D. Parotitis

23. Freckles result from a concentration of:
    A. Leukocytes
    B. Keratin
    C. Melanin
    D. Blasts

24. The outer layer of the skin is termed the:
    A. Dermis
    B. Cutaneous tissue
    C. Epidermis
    D. Stratum germinativum

25. Treatment of warts may include:
   A. Cryotherapy
   B. Electrodesiccation
   C. Keratolysis
   D. Electrocautery

26. An adult form of acne commonly treated with metronidazole (MetroGel) is called
   A. Acne rosacea
   B. Acne vulgaris
   C. Bullae
   D. Cystic acne vulgaris

27. Impetigo is a contagious, superficial skin infection usually caused by:
   A. Candida albicans
   B. HSV
   C. Verruca vulgaris
   D. Staphylococcus aureus

28. Which of the following is the most lethal form of skin cancer?
   A. Basal cell
   B. Squamous cell
   C. Melanoma
   D. Scleroderma

29. A malignant vascular neoplastic growth associated with AIDS is:
   A. Kaposi sarcoma
   B. Basal cell carcinoma
   C. Melanoma
   D. Angioma:

30. Which of these is a topical anesthetic?
   A. EMLA
   B. Lindane
   C. Silvadene
   D. MetroGel

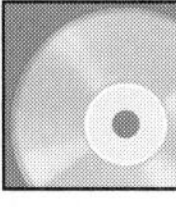

Please see the accompanying CD for additional review materials for this section.

PROOFREADING EXERCISES

These three proofreading exercises are provided to improve your skills in the areas of editing and effective identification and correction of errors in the medical record.

Directions: Identify and correct the transcription errors found in the exercises below. *Answers are provided at the end of this chapter.*

PROOFREADING EXERCISE #1

PREOPERATIVE DIAGNOSIS
Melanemia, left cheek.

POSTOPERATIVE DIAGNOSIS
Melanemia, left cheek.

SURGEON
John Smith, MD.

PROCEDURE
Excision of melanoma, left cheek, 1 cm, and complex repair 5 cm.

ANESTHESIA
IP Sedation.

INDICATION
This 58-year-old woman had a biopsy-proven melanoma, Clarks level 1, in sight of the left cheek and was advised to have this excised. She was agreeable to this and was aware that she might have more melanoma found in the remainder of the specimen, but would proceed with that if she needed to.

DETAILS OF PROCEDURE
After intravenous sedation, the patient was prepped with Betadine and draped in the usual sterile manner. The lesion was then filtrated with a mixture of 1% Xylocaine plane and 0.5% Marcaine with epinephrine. After allowing 10 minutes for the anesthetic effect of the metanephrine, the lesion was excised in an illogical fashion. With the scalpel and the Bovie coagulator, the skin edges were undermined widely. The area was closed with 5-0 Monocryl interrupted subcuticular sutures and 6-0 protein interrupted skin sutures. The wound was banded with mast and all and supported with Steri-Strips. The patient tolerated this well and left the operating room in good condition.

PROOFREADING EXERCISE #2

HISTORY
This 35-year-old woman has a 5-year history of an intensely itchy rash on her limbs. Strong tropical steroids have not helped and she finds it virtually impossible to stop scratching.

PAST MEDICAL HISTORY
There is no medical history of note and she is generally healthy. She takes no medications and there are no known allergies or allergic contract factors.

SOCIAL HISTORY
She immigrated from Asia 5 years ago. She runs her own business but does not feel that she is under any stress.

PHYSICAL EXAMINATION
On her upper back there were signs of rippled pigmentation.

Biopsy showed amorphous globular highland material in the pupillary dermis, widening the rete ridges. Bongo red staining was positive.

ASSESSMENT
Liken amyloidosis caused by myeloid deposits resulting from chronic fiction.

PLAN
1. Activate 0.05% twice a day until symptoms resolve.
2. Desquam-E topical karyolytic agent.
3. Symptomatic relief with topical Elidel.

PROOFREADING EXERCISE #3

PREOPERATIVE DIAGNOSIS
Wound right nose.

POSTOPERATIVE DIAGNOSIS
Wound right nose.

SURGEON
John Smith, MD.

PROCEDURE
Full-thickness skin graph from right clavicle to right nose 12 cm^2.

ANESTHESIA
General.

INDICATION
This 58-year-old man had a large basil cell carcinoma on the right side of his nose. Earlier in the week, he had moss surgery and was left with a 4 x 3 cm defect on the right side of his nose. The basal musculature and auricularis muscle were left intact, and it was felt this was too large for flap reconstruction, but with sufficient bed for skin graph. The patient was willing to accept this and knew the donor sight would be from similar skin.

DETAILS OF PROCEDURE
After induction of general anesthesia, the right face and right chest were prepped with Betadine and draped in a sterile manner. A 3-cm white full-thickness elliptical skin graft was harvested from the right clavicular area matching like skin with similar tension lines. This was excised with the scalpel after the area had been infiltrated with 5 percent Marcaine with epinephrine. The skin graft was set aside. The skin edges were undermined with a Bovie coagulator. Hemostasis was obtained with a Bovie coagulator and the donor site closed with 4-0 Monocryl interrupted subcuticular suture and then painted with Mastisol and supported with Steri-Strips, Telfa, and Tegaderm. The chin graft was defatted. The base of the wound was cleansed and hemostasis was obtained with a Bovie coagulator. Skin graft was placed over the defect and tailored to fit

(continued)

without any tension. Then, it was sewn in place with 5-0 Prolene interrupted sutures. Ten of the sutures were left long and then the graft was irrigated with saline underneath and then dressed with a bolus dressing of zero form, which was held in place with 10 tie-over stitches. This wound was dressed with Bacitracin ointment.

The patient tolerated the procedure well with minimal blood loss and was transferred to the recovery room in stable condition.

ANSWER KEYS

REVIEW QUESTIONS ANSWER KEY

1. B
2. A
3. A
4. A
5. C
6. D
7. B
8. A
9. C
10. C
11. A
12. A
13. A
14. C
15. A
16. A
17. B
18. D
19. A
20. B
21. D
22. A
23. C
24. C
25. A
26. A
27. D
28. C
29. A
30. A

PROOFREADING EXERCISE #1 KEY

Incorrect term—melanoma

Melanemia, left cheek.

POSTOPERATIVE DIAGNOSIS
Melanemia, left cheek.

SURGEON
John Smith, MD.

PROCEDURE
Excision of melanoma, left cheek, 1 cm, and complex repair 5 cm.

Incorrect term—IV

ANESTHESIA
IP sedation.

INDICATION
This 58-year-old woman had a biopsy-proven melanoma, Clarks level 1, in sight of the left cheek and was advised to have this excised. She was agreeable to this and was aware that she might have more melanoma found in the remainder of the specimen, but would proceed with that if she needed to.

Incorrect word—situ

Incorrect format—Clark level I

DETAILS OF PROCEDURE
After intravenous sedation, the patient was prepped with Betadine and draped in the usual sterile manner. The lesion was then filtrated with a mixture of 1% Xylocaine plane and 0.5% Marcaine with epinephrine. After allowing 10 minutes for the anesthetic effect of the metanephrine, the lesion was excised in an illogical fashion. With the scalpel and the Bovie coagulator, the skin edges were undermined widely. The area was closed with 5-0 Monocryl interrupted subcuticular sutures and 6-0 protein interrupted skin sutures. The wound was banded with mast and all and supported with Steri-Strips. The patient tolerated this well and left the operating room in good condition.

Incorrect term—infiltrated

Incorrect spelling—plain

Incorrect term—epinephrine

Incorrect term—elliptical

Incorrect term—Prolene

Incorrect term—Mastisol

PROOFREADING EXERCISE #2 KEY

HISTORY
This 35-year-old woman has a 5-year history of an intensely itchy rash on her limbs. Strong tropical steroids have not helped and she finds it virtually impossible to stop scratching.

PAST MEDICAL HISTORY
There is no medical history of note and she is generally healthy. She takes no medications and there are no known allergies or allergic contract factors.

SOCIAL HISTORY
She immigrated from Asia 5 years ago. She runs her own business but does not feel that she is under any stress.

PHYSICAL EXAMINATION
On her upper back there were signs of rippled pigmentation.

Biopsy showed amorphous globular highland material in the pupillary dermis, widening the rete ridges. Bongo red staining was positive.

ASSESSMENT
Liken amyloidosis caused by myeloid deposits resulting from chronic fiction.

PLAN
1. Activate 0.05% twice a day until symptoms resolve.
2. Desquam-E topical karyolytic agent.
3. Symptomatic relief with topical Elidel.

Incorrect word—topical

Incorrect word—contact

Incorrect term—papillary

Incorrect term—hyaline

Incorrect term—Congo

Incorrect term—amyloid

Incorrect term—lichen

Incorrect word—friction

Incorrect drug—Aclovate

Incorrect term—keratolytic

PROOFREADING EXERCISE #3 KEY

Incorrect term—graft

PREOPERATIVE DIAGNOSIS
Wound right nose.

POSTOPERATIVE DIAGNOSIS
Wound right nose.

SURGEON
John Smith, MD.

PROCEDURE
Full-thickness skin graph from right clavicle to right nose 12 cm^2.

ANESTHESIA
General.

INDICATION
This 58-year-old man had a large basil ~~cell~~ carcinoma on the right side of his nose. Earlier in the week, he ~~had~~ moss surgery and was left with a 4 x 3 cm defect on the right side of his nose. The basal musculature and auricularis ~~muscle~~ were left intact, and it was felt this was too large for flap reconstruction, but with sufficient bed for skin graph. The patient was willing to accept this and knew the donor sight ~~would~~ be from similar skin.

Incorrect word—basal

Incorrect term—Mohs

Incorrect term—nasal

Incorrect term—orbicularis

Incorrect term—graft

Incorrect word—site

DETAILS OF PROCEDURE
After induction of general anesthesia, the right face and right chest were prepped with Betadine and draped in a sterile manner. A 3-cm white ~~full~~-thickness elliptical skin graft was harvested from the right clavicular area matching like skin with similar tension lines. This was excised with the scalpel after the area had been infiltrated with 5 percent Marcaine with epinephrine. The skin graft was set aside. The skin edges were undermined with a Bovie coagulator. Hemostasis

Incorrect concentration and format—0.5%

Incorrect word—wide

Incorrect word—skin

Incorrect term—Xeroform

was obtained with a Bovie coagulator and the donor site closed with 4-0 Monocryl interrupted subcuticular suture and then painted with Mastisol and supported with Steri-Strips, Telfa, and Tegaderm. The chin graft was defatted. The base of the wound was cleansed and hemostasis was obtained with a Bovie coagulator. Skin graft was placed over the defect and tailored to fit without any tension. Then, it was sewn in place with 5-0 Prolene interrupted sutures. Ten of the sutures were left long and then the graft was irrigated with saline underneath and then dressed with a bolus dressing of zero form, which was held in place with 10 tie-over stitches. This wound was dressed with Bacitracin ointment.

The patient tolerated the procedure well with minimal blood loss and was transferred to the recovery room in stable condition.

CHAPTER 12

General Surgery/Plastic Surgery

OBJECTIVES CHECKLIST

A prepared exam candidate will know:

- ❑ Common terminology related to surgical intervention and fundamentals of the surgical process.
- ❑ Fundamental terminology related to muscular and skeletal anatomy.
- ❑ Fundamental terminology related to all dermatologic, subcutaneous, and fascial layers for the purposes of surgical entry, repair, and closure.
- ❑ Procedures associated with surgical incisions, hemostasis, and wound closure, including bandages and dressings.
- ❑ Risk management issues pertaining to the documentation of surgical treatment, including blood loss and material counts.
- ❑ Common terminology related to surgical instrumentation, including but not limited to: catheters, forceps, blades, elevators, drains, curettes, tubes, tenaculums, scopes, sutures, stents, screws, wires, pins, scissors, rongeurs, rasps, rods, retractors, needles, lasers, clamps, knives, and guides.
- ❑ Medications administered before, during, and after surgical intervention for sedation, pain control, nausea, etc.

RESOURCES FOR STUDY

1. *The Language of Medicine*
   Chapter 5: Digestive System, pp. 145–169.
   Chapter 6: Addition Suffixes and Digestive System Terminology, pp. 185–196.
   Chapter 7: Urinary Anatomy, pp. 215–227.
   Chapter 8: Female Reproductive Anatomy, pp. 254–261, 273–274.
   Chapter 9: Male Reproductive Anatomy, pp. 306–311.
   Chapter 15: Musculoskeletal System Anatomy, pp. 563–573, 593–594.
   Chapter 16: Skin, pp. 630–632.
2. *Laboratory Tests & Diagnostic Procedures in Medicine*
   Chapter 16: Normal Anatomy and Histology, pp. 225–250.
3. *Understanding Pharmacology for Health Professionals*
   Chapter 31: Anesthetics, pp. 365–372.
   Chapter 32: Intravenous Fluids and Blood Products, pp. 373–280.
4. *The AAMT Book of Style for Medical Transcription*
   Sutures, pp. 380–381.
5. *Prentice Hall Health's Complete Review of Surgery Technology*
6. *Introduction to Surgery*
7. *Berry & Kohn's Operating Room Technique*

SAMPLE REPORTS

The following three reports are examples of reports you might encounter while transcribing general and plastic surgery.

OPERATIVE REPORT

DATE OF PROCEDURE
04/08/05

PREOPERATIVE DIAGNOSIS
Recurrent pregnancy loss.

POSTOPERATIVE DIAGNOSES
Recurrent pregnancy loss, small septate uterus, and partial right hydrosalpinx.

SURGEON
John Cutem, MD.

PROCEDURE
1. Hysteroscopy.
2. Incision of uterine septum (septoplasty).
3. Hysterosalpingogram.
4. Endometrial biopsy with cultures.

COMPLICATIONS
None.

ESTIMATED BLOOD LOSS
Minimal.

ANESTHESIA
IV sedation.

FINDINGS AT SURGERY
On hysteroscopy, the patient had a small septate uterus, which was incised. This was rather a small to moderate-sized septum. The uterine cavity itself otherwise was within normal limits without any evidence of any indentations from fibroids, and she did not have any polyps. She does have intramural fibroids, but they do not appear to be impinging on the uterine cavity. Endometrial biopsy was taken for cultures. Hysterosalpingogram was performed that showed the uterus to have an arcuate shape. The left tube was patent with some delay of dye coming out the distal end of the tube. The right tube was dilated. There was some dye extruding from the tube; therefore it was not completely occluded. However, it is a partial hydrosalpinx.

DETAILS OF PROCEDURE
The patient was prepped and draped in sterile fashion and placed in dorsal lithotomy position. Next, a speculum was placed in the vagina, and the anterior lip of the cervix was grasped with a single-toothed tenaculum. Cervix was gently dilated and hysteroscope was introduced into the endometrial cavity. Using saline as distention media, the endometrial cavity was inspected. A small

(continued)

septum was visualized, and scissors were used to excise it. The remainder of the cavity was within normal limits. After this, the hysteroscope was removed, and a curette was placed. A small specimen of the endometrium was removed and sent for anaerobic and aerobic cultures. Next, a balloon catheter was placed in the endometrial cavity, and hysterosalpingogram was performed.

The uterus appeared to be of approximately normal contour and shape, with small arcuate configuration at the fundal aspect of the uterus. The left tube was first filled with a moderate amount of dye and spill was visualized. Rugae were not clearly visualized. There appeared to be some delay of spill of the tube after 5 minutes. The right tube was with some delayed fill. After a fair amount of dye was placed in the tube, there was some extrusion of dye. She had a slight hydrosalpinx of the right side based on 5-minute film. The dye was delayed in the right fallopian tube. At 5 minutes, there was no dye left in the uterus.

The patient tolerated the procedure well. All instruments and sponge counts were correct. The patient was sent to recovery room in stable condition.

OPERATIVE REPORT

PREOPERATIVE DIAGNOSIS
Left inguinal hernia.

POSTOPERATIVE DIAGNOSIS
Left direct inguinal hernia.

SURGEON
John Cutem, MD.

PROCEDURE
Cooper ligament repair of left direct inguinal hernia with Marlex mesh.

ANESTHESIA
General.

DETAILS OF PROCEDURE
The patient was placed in the supine position and his left groin was prepped and draped. An oblique incision was made in the left groin and carried down through the external oblique fascia. The spermatic cord was mobilized and the floor of the canal was cleaned out. The ilioinguinal and iliohypogastric nerves were mobilized and resected out of the field. The cremasteric fibers were divided and ligated with silk ties, and the cord was skeletonized. A cord lipoma was also removed. There was no indirect hernia, but there was a moderately large direct hernia coming out medial to the epigastric vessels. I then incised the transversalis fascia from the pubic tubercle out to the internal ring without dividing the inferior epigastric vessels. The Cooper ligament was cleaned off from the pubic tubercle out to and including the medial wall of the femoral vein. The conjoined tendon was cleaned off above and mobilized with a relaxing incision in the usual place. A Cooper ligament repair was then done with interrupted 0 silk sutures, bringing the conjoined tendon down to the Cooper ligament out to the femoral space. Two transition stitches were placed from the Cooper ligament up to the anterior femoral sheath to close off the femoral space. The conjoined tendon did come down to the Cooper ligament with a minimal amount of tension. The remainder of the stitch brought the conjoined tendon down to the shelving edge of the Cooper ligament out to the internal ring. After tying and cutting all the stitches, I could place only a Kelly clamp on the internal ring. A piece of Marlex mesh was soaked in antibiotic solution, cut to size, and sutured into the relaxing incision defect with a running Prolene stitch. The external oblique fascia was then closed over the cord with a running chromic stitch. The subcutaneous was irrigated and closed with interrupted chromic stitches. The wound was closed with staples and was injected with 10 mL of 0.5% Marcaine with epinephrine during closure.

A dressing was placed, and the patient was taken to recovery in stable condition.

OPERATIVE REPORT

PREOPERATIVE DIAGNOSES
Bilateral hypermastia, neck ache, backache, intertrigo, and breast asymmetry.

POSTOPERATIVE DIAGNOSES
Bilateral hypermastia, neck ache, backache, intertrigo, and breast asymmetry.

SURGEON
John Cutem, MD.

PROCEDURE
Bilateral reduction mammoplasties.

ANESTHESIA
General.

DRAINS
15-mm Blake.

ESTIMATED BLOOD LOSS
200 mL.

INDICATIONS
This is a 49-year-old female with worsening problems of backache and neck ache because of the size of her breasts. She tried nonoperative measures without success. Plan today was for bilateral breast reduction. I discussed with her the options that were available, the risks, the benefits, and alternatives, including no treatment, and possible consequences.

DETAILS OF PROCEDURE
After adequate anesthesia, the patient was prepped and draped in the usual sterile fashion. She had been marked in the sitting position. She had a modified inferomedial pedicle created with epithelialization. She then had resection of tissue, mostly laterally and minimal superiorly. Once this had been accomplished, the nipple-areola was on the pedicle and it was about 42–44 mm in diameter. Bleeders were controlled with an electrocoagulation unit. A couple of bleeders had to be ligated with 3-0 Vicryl suture.

After this had been completed, she was closed with inverted 2-0 PDS, inverted 3-0 Vicryl, and subcuticular pullout 4-0 Vicryl. She had a few interrupted 4-0 Prolene stitches. Nipple was inset with inverted using 3-0 Vicryl and subcuticular pullout 4-0 Monocryl. Each side had been irrigated with saline. She had 15-French round Blake drain placed. It was sutured in with 4-0 Prolene. Same was done on the contralateral side. On her left side, she had 965 g removed; on her right side, she had 761 g removed. She was placed in the upright position. She was about equal in size. She then had her chest dressed with Adaptic, 4 x 4, slough, soft Kling, and an Ace bandage. The patient tolerated the procedure well. She was taken to postanesthesia care area in satisfactory condition.

REVIEW QUESTIONS

The goal of these questions is to test your knowledge in the areas of general and plastic surgery.

Directions: Select the correct answer for each of the multiple-choice questions provided below. *Answers are provided at the end of this chapter.*

1. Which of the following is a bariatric procedure?
   A. Amputation of the great toe
   B. Hyperbaric oxygen therapy for wound healing
   C. Gastric bypass surgery
   D. Gamma-knife surgery

2. Kelly, Kocher, mosquito, and Crile are examples of:
   A. Trocars
   B. Forceps
   C. Elevators
   D. Catheters

3. Universal precautions are intended to protect people from:
   A. Needle sticks
   B. Radiation
   C. Aerosolized pathogens
   D. Bloodborne pathogens

4. Jackson-Pratt and Penrose are examples of surgical:
   A. Drains
   B. Sutures
   C. Scissors
   D. Needles

5. Which of the following are catheters?
   A. Catgut, Prolene, silk
   B. Kelly, Charnley, Kocher
   C. Swan-Ganz, coude tip, double-lumen
   D. Metzenbaum, Army-Navy, DeBakey

6. Bard-Parker is a common:
   A. Bougie
   B. Surgical blade
   C. Scissor
   D. Clamp

7. Which of these is correct?
   A. Allis clamp
   B. Alice clamp
   C. Forcep
   D. None of these

8. The surgeon dictated, "There is an indurated area noted over the calf." What does indurated mean?
   A. Hardened
   B. Fluctuant
   C. Containing pus
   D. Scabbed over

9. An Esmarch bandage is used to:
   A. Cover an abdominal wound
   B. Exsanguinate a limb before surgery
   C. Cover a wound before casting
   D. Cover the skull following intracranial surgery

10. A surgical instrument shaped like a spoon and used to remove material from a cavity is called a:
    A. Bur
    B. Hemostat
    C. Cannula
    D. Curette

11. Which of the following is an example of a local anesthetic?
    A. Halothane
    B. Xylocaine
    C. Curare
    D. Benzodiazepine

12. The removal of dead or necrotic tissue from a wound is termed:
    A. Electrodesiccation
    B. Keratolysis
    C. Debridement
    D. Electrocautery

13. A stone-like formation in the appendix is called a:
    A. Urolith
    B. Gallstone
    C. Lithotripsy
    D. Fecalith

14. A surgical incision made at the McBurney point is usually for performance of a/an:
    A. Hemicolectomy
    B. Cholecystectomy
    C. Appendectomy
    D. Hysterectomy

15. Which type of hernia may cause intestinal contents to prolapse into the scrotum?
    A. Umbilical hernia
    B. Diaphragmatic hernia
    C. Inguinal hernia
    D. Hiatal hernia

16. Which of these is correctly matched to its plural form?
    A. Apex – apices
    B. Diverticulum – diverticuli
    C. Petechium – petechia
    D. Ramus – rama

17. Which of these is correctly stated?
    A. The abdomen was insufflated to 15 degrees of pressure
    B. The patient's hematocrit was 42 grams
    C. Cardioversion was achieved at 300 joules
    D. The doctor said to give 8 mg of regular insulin subcu

18. Feeding a patient through a PEG tube is also known as:
    A. Antrectomy
    B. Gavage feeding
    C. Gastric lavage
    D. Nasogastric intubation

19. Removal of the right or left side of the colon is called a/an:
    A. Ileostomy
    B. Billroth II procedure
    C. Colectomy
    D. Hemicolectomy

20. A cardiac procedure in which a catheter is threaded into the coronary artery and an occlusion is eliminated by inflation of a balloon, thus improving blood flow, is called a/an:
    A. PTCA
    B. CABG
    C. VAD
    D. AAA

21. The surgical procedure used to remove acne scars, for example, is called:
    A. Mohs micrograph surgery
    B. Cryosurgery
    C. Dermabrasion
    D. Argon laser surgery

22. A rongeur is used to:
    A. Nip away at bone
    B. Close an incision
    C. Cut ligaments
    D. Dissect muscle

23. A TRAM flap procedure is sometimes done following:
    A. Abdominoplasty
    B. Mastectomy
    C. Augmentation mammoplasty
    D. Bariatric surgery

24. Halothane, Diprivan, and etomidate are examples of:
    A. General anesthesia
    B. Local anesthetics
    C. Antibiotics
    D. None of these

25. An elongated cylindrical instrument used for calibrating the lumen of a body cavity is called a/an:
    A. Cannula
    B. Tenaculum
    C. Sound
    D. Catheter

26. An instrument used for prying up or raising tissues is called a/an:
    A. Caliper
    B. Elevator
    C. Dissector
    D. Sound

27. MAC is an abbreviation used to describe:
   A. General anesthesia
   B. Local anesthesia
   C. A type of cannula
   D. A type of clamp

28. An instrument used to expose the opening of a canal in order to inspect the interior is called a:
   A. Trocar
   B. Retractor
   C. Tenaculum
   D. Speculum

29. Which of the following are not surgical sutures?
   A. Mattress, figure-of-8
   B. Subcuticular, apposition
   C. Nonabsorbable, pledgetted
   D. Hemostatic, bougie

30. Which of these medications might be given before or during surgery to prevent nausea?
   A. Anzemet
   B. Duragesic
   C. Brevital
   D. Demerol

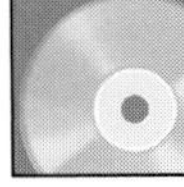

Please see the accompanying CD for additional review materials for this section.

PROOFREADING EXERCISES

These three proofreading exercises are provided to improve your skills in the areas of editing and effective identification and correction of errors in the medical record.

Directions: Identify and correct the transcription errors found in the exercises below. *Answers are provided at the end of this chapter.*

PROOFREADING EXERCISE #1

PREOPERATIVE DIAGNOSIS
Localized fat deposits and an acceptable appearance.

POSTOPERATIVE DIAGNOSIS
Localized fat deposits and an acceptable appearance.

SURGEON
John Cutum, MD.

PROCEDURE
Ultrasonic-assisted and suction-assisted lithectomy of breast and flanks.

ANESTHESIA
General.

INDICATIONS
This 45-year-old woman had a massive weight loss and has subsequently had areas of localized fat deposit even after skin reduction with the circumferential abdominoplasty and a breast reduction. These were localized to the lateral breast and laryngismus area and the flank. She is aware that this might loosen the skin more and she is willing to accept that.

DETAILS OF PROCEDURE
In the holding area, in the standing position, the areas of localized fat were marked on the lateral breast, latissimus, and flank. She was then brought to the operating room and general anesthesia was induced. She was placed in the prone position and the back was prepped with Betadine and draped in asterol manner. In the latissimus area on the left, 640 mL of

(continued)

tumescent solution consisting of 1 liter of Ringers lactate, 30 mL of lidocaine, and 1 mL of 1:1000 epinephrine was infiltrated; 640 mL on the left side and 650 mL on the right side. Then in the flank areas, 200 mL was injected on the left and 200 mL on the right. Following injection of the tumescent solution and time for the hemostatic effect, and beginning with the left latissimus area, the ultra sonic machine was used for 2 minutes and 46 seconds and 100 mL of fluid was removed. Attention was then turned to the right latissimus area and the ultrasonic was used for 3 minutes and 19 seconds and 125 mL was removed. Following this, these areas were touched up with traditional liposuction and 500 mL was removed from the left and 200 mL from the right for a total of 600 mL on the left and 3.25 mL on the right. Attention was then turned to the flank. On the left, 53 seconds of ultrasonic time was used with 75 mL removed and then 175 mL of fat for a total of 250 mL. On the right side, where there was more fat, 1 minute and 28 seconds was used and 75 mL was removed and 300 mL with regular liposuction for a total of 375 mL. At this point, pinch test confirmed fairly symmetrical skin flaps on each side and the 4 incisions were closed with 5-0 Monocryl buried suture and dressed with ABGs and Mediport tape.

The patient was transferred to a stretcher and surgical garment was applied to the breast and to the abdomen. The patient tolerated this well. There was adequate in and out for the entire case, and the patient was transferred to the recovery room in stable condition.

PROOFREADING EXERCISE #2

PREOPERATIVE DIAGNOSIS
Acute appendicitis.

POSTOPERATIVE DIAGNOSIS
Acute appendicitis.

SURGEON
John Cutem, MD.

PROCEDURE
Appendectomy.

ANESTHESIA
General.

DESCRIPTION OF PROCEDURE
With the patient in the supine position and after general anesthesia had been achieved, a Rockey-Davis incision was made at the McBirney point and deepened through subcutaneous tissue. Using electrical cautery, the bleeders were cauterized. The external oblique aponeurosis was incised along the length of its fibers using the mets and balm scissors. The internal oblique and transverse abdominal muscles were split bluntly using Kelly clamps. The peritoneum was grasped with 2 Kelly clamps, raised and nicked with a scalpel. Immediately after which pus came through the incision in the peritoneum. The pus was cultured. The incision of the peritoneum was completed with mets and balm scissors.

After that had been achieved, we identified the appendix, which was grasped with 2 Babcock stamps and raised into the wound. Another Babcock was used to grasp the sebum which was mobilized toward the wound. The mesoappendix was surreally clamped, divided, and ligated with 2-0 chromic. The append seal base was clamped with straight hemostats and was ligated twice with zero chromic. The appendix was amputated, and the appendiceal stump was cauterized with electrocautery.

The abdominal cavity was copiously irrigated with kanamycin solution.

(continued)

The wound was closed in layers. The peroneum was closed in a continuous fashion using 2-0 Maxon. The transverse abdominal muscles and internal oblique were closed in an interrupted fashion using 2-0 Maxon. The external oblique aponeurosis was closed in a continuous fashion using 2-0 Maxon and the skin was closed with staples.

PROOFREADING EXERCISE #3

PREOPERATIVE DIAGNOSES

1. Pancreatic carcinoma.
2. Inadequate venus access.

POSTOPERATIVE DIAGNOSES

1. Pancreatic carcinoma.
2. Inadequate venus access.

SURGEON

John Cutem, MD.

PROCEDURE

Placement of left portal cath.

ANESTHESIA

General.

DETAILS OF PROCEDURE

The patient was placed in the supine position and the left chest wall and neck were prepped and draped. A 4-cm oblique incision was made in the left deltopectoral groove and a subcutaneous pocket based on the temporalis muscle was made. The Port-A-Catheter was soaked in antibiotic solution and the tubing was cut to length. The patient was placed in the Trendelenburg position. Using the Seldinger technique, a soft Jay-wire was placed into the right heart via a left subclavian vein puncture. The dilator and peal-away sheath were placed over the wire and the catheter tubing was threaded through the peel-away sheath as this was pulled out. There was excellent blood return through the port and it was flushed it with 1000 units of Humulin. The chamber was then secured to the pectoralis muscle with 3 sutures of 2-0 proline on all sides and a 4th suture around the neck of the chamber. We then closed the wound over the port with a running chromic stitch to the subcutaneous and a running subcuticular Velcro stitch to the skin. Fluoroscopy was obtained, which showed good positioning of the tip of the line at the junction of the superior vena cava and brachial cephalic vein.

A dressing was placed and the patient was taken to recovery in stable condition.

ANSWER KEYS

REVIEW QUESTIONS ANSWER KEY

1. C
2. B
3. D
4. A
5. C
6. B
7. A
8. A
9. B
10. D
11. B
12. C
13. D
14. B
15. C
16. A
17. C
18. B
19. D
20. A
21. C
22. A
23. B
24. A
25. C
26. B
27. A
28. D
29. D
30. A

PROOFREADING EXERCISE #1 KEY

Incorrect word—unacceptable

PREOPERATIVE DIAGNOSIS
Localized fat deposits and an acceptable appearance.

POSTOPERATIVE DIAGNOSIS
Localized fat deposits and an acceptable appearance.

SURGEON
John Cutum, MD.

PROCEDURE
Ultrasonic-assisted and suction-assisted lithectomy of breast and flanks.

Incorrect term—lipectomy

ANESTHESIA
General.

INDICATIONS
This 45-year-old woman had a massive weight loss and has subsequently had areas of localized fat deposit even after skin reduction with the circumferential abdominoplasty and a breast reduction. These were localized to the lateral breast and laryngismus area and the flank. She is aware that this might loosen the skin more and she is willing to accept that.

Incorrect term—latissimus

DETAILS OF PROCEDURE
In the holding area, in the standing position, the areas of localized fat were marked on the lateral breast, latissimus, and flank. She was then brought to the operating room and general anesthesia was induced. She was placed in the prone position and the back was prepped with Betadine and draped in asterol manner. In the latissimus area on the left, 640 mL of tumescent solution consisting of 1 liter of Ringers lactate, 30 mL of lidocaine, and 1 mL of 1:1000 epinephrine was infiltrated; 640 mL on the

Incorrect term—a sterile

Incorrect spelling—Ringer

left side and 650 mL on the right side. Then in the flank areas, 200 mL was injected on the left and 200 mL on the right. Following injection of the tumescent solution and time for the hemostatic effect, and beginning with the left latissimus area, the ultra sonic machine was used for 2 minutes and 46 seconds and 100 mL of fluid was removed. Attention was then turned to the right latissimus area and the ultrasonic was used for 3 minutes and 19 seconds and 125 mL was removed. Following this, these areas were touched up with traditional liposuction and 500 mL was removed from the left and 200 mL from the right for a total of 600 mL on the left and 3.25 mL on the right. Attention was then turned to the flank. On the left, 53 seconds of ultrasonic time was used with 75 mL removed and then 175 mL of fat for a total of 250 mL. On the right side, where there was more fat, 1 minute and 28 seconds was used and 75 mL was removed and 300 mL with regular liposuction for a total of 375 mL. At this point, pinch test confirmed fairly symmetrical skin flaps on each side and the 4 incisions were closed with 5-0 Monocryl buried suture and dressed with ABGs and Mediport tape.

The patient was transferred to a stretcher and surgical garment was applied to the breast and to the abdomen. The patient tolerated this well. There was adequate in and out for the entire case, and the patient was transferred to the recovery room in stable condition.

Use combined form—ultrasonic

No decimal needed—325 mL

Incorrect abbreviation—ABDs

Incorrect term—Medipore

PROOFREADING EXERCISE #2 KEY

PREOPERATIVE DIAGNOSIS
Acute appendicitis.

POSTOPERATIVE DIAGNOSIS
Acute appendicitis.

SURGEON
John Cutem, MD.

PROCEDURE
Appendectomy.

ANESTHESIA
General.

DESCRIPTION OF PROCEDURE
With the patient in the supine position and after general anesthesia had been achieved, a Rockey-Davis incision was made at the McBirney point and deepened through subcutaneous tissue. Using electrical cautery, the bleeders were cauterized. The external oblique aponeurosis was incised along the length of its fibers using the mets and balm scissors. The internal oblique and transverse abdominal muscles were split bluntly using Kelly clamps. The peritoneum was grasped with 2 Kelly clamps, raised and nicked with a scalpel. Immediately after which pus came through the incision in the peritoneum. The pus was cultured. The incision of the peritoneum was completed with mets and balm scissors.

After that had been achieved, we identified the appendix, which was grasped with 2 Babcock stamps and raised into the wound. Another Babcock was used to grasp the sebum which was mobilized toward the wound. The mesoappendix

Incorrect spelling—McBurney

Use combined form—electrocautery

Incorrect—Metzenbaum

Incorrect word—clamps

Incorrect term—cecum

was surreally clamped, divided, and ligated with 2-0 chromic. The append seal base was clamped with straight hemostats and was ligated twice with zero chromic. The appendix was amputated, and the appendiceal stump was cauterized with electrocautery.

The abdominal cavity was copiously irrigated with kanamycin solution. The wound was closed in layers. The peroneum was closed in a continuous fashion using 2-0 Maxon. The transverse abdominal muscles and internal oblique were closed in an interrupted fashion using 2-0 Maxon. The external oblique aponeurosis was closed in a continuous fashion using 2-0 Maxon and the skin was closed with staples.

Incorrect word—serially

Incorrect—appendiceal

Use numbers with suture material—0

Incorrect term—peritoneum

PROOFREADING EXERCISE #3 KEY

PREOPERATIVE DIAGNOSES
1. Pancreatic carcinoma.
2. Inadequate venus access.

POSTOPERATIVE DIAGNOSES
1. Pancreatic carcinoma.
2. Inadequate venus access.

SURGEON
John Cutem, MD.

PROCEDURE
Placement of left portal cath.

ANESTHESIA
General.

DETAILS OF PROCEDURE
The patient was placed in the supine position and the left chest wall and neck were prepped and draped. A 4-cm oblique incision was made in the left deltopectoral groove and a subcutaneous pocket based on the temporalis muscle was made. The Port-A-Catheter was soaked in antibiotic solution and the tubing was cut to length. The patient was placed in the Trendelenburg position. Using the Seldinger technique, a soft Jay-wire was placed into the right heart via a left subclavian vein puncture. The dilator and peal-away sheath were placed over the wire and the catheter tubing was threaded through the peel-away sheath as this was pulled out. There was excellent blood return through the port and it was flushed it with 1000 units of Humulin. The chamber was then secured to the pectoralis muscle with 3 sutures of 2-0

Incorrect spelling—venous

Incorrect—Port-a-Cath

Incorrect—Port-a-Cath

Incorrect term—pectoralis

Incorrect—J-wire

Incorrect spelling—peel

Incorrect drug—heparin

proline on all sides and a 4th suture around the neck of the chamber. We then closed the wound over the port with a running chromic stitch to the subcutaneous and a running subcuticular Velcro stitch to the skin. Fluoroscopy was obtained, which showed good positioning of the tip of the line at the junction of the superior vena cava and brachial cephalic vein.

A dressing was placed and the patient was taken to recovery in stable condition.

Incorrect spelling—Prolene

Incorrect term—Vicryl

Use combined form—brachiocephalic

CHAPTER

13

Family Medicine/Geriatrics/ Nutrition & Dietetics

OBJECTIVES CHECKLIST

A prepared exam candidate will know the:

- ❑ Unique role of family practice and geriatric care as a specialty service in health care.
- ❑ Diseases and/or conditions treated by a family practitioner, as well as health promotion and disease prevention, including routine immunizations, smoking cessation, weight control, prenatal care; minor acute injury and infection including lacerations, sprains, and strains; infections of the respiratory, gastrointestinal, and urogenital tract; and chronic diseases including COPD and asthma, hypertension, GERD, headache, and back pain.
- ❑ Diseases and/or conditions commonly seen in the elderly such as Alzheimer disease and other forms of dementia, depression, proper nutrition, Parkinson disease, osteoporosis and fractures, hearing and vision loss, arthritis, hypertension, heart disease, COPD, incontinence, constipation, and diabetes.
- ❑ Diseases and/or conditions related to nutrition and diet.
- ❑ Role of nursing homes and assisted living facilities (ALFs) in managing and coordinating care in the geriatric setting.
- ❑ Meaning, role, and implications of advance directives and DNR status.
- ❑ Medications typically prescribed for treating symptoms and diseases encountered in a family practice setting or common to the aging population.

RESOURCES FOR STUDY

1. *Understanding Pharmacology for Health Professionals*
   Chapter 24: Alzheimer and Parkinson Diseases, pp. 267–271.
   Chapter 12: Urinary Tract Drugs, pp. 103–114.
   Chapter 13: Gastrointestinal Drugs, pp. 115–135.
   Chapter 18: Pulmonary Drugs—specifically bronchodilator drugs, leukotriene receptor blockers and mast cell stabilizers, pp. 193–196.
   Chapter 23: Oral Contraceptives, pp. 248–253; PMS, pp. 254–255.
   Chapter 26: Analgesics, pp. 299–307

2. *Human Diseases*
   Chapter 4: Rheumatoid Arthritis, pg. 49.
   Chapter 10: Asthma, pg. 144.
   Chapter 12: Incontinence, pg. 180.
   Chapter 15: Diabetes, pp. 232–233.
   Chapter 17: Osteoporosis, pg. 265; Arthritis, pp. 265–267.
   Chapter 19: Parkinsonism, pg. 303; Headache, pp. 305–306.
   Chapter 20: Mood Disorders and Eating Disorders, pp. 322–323; Delirium and Dementia, pg. 326.

3. *H&P: A Nonphysician's Guide to the Medical History and Physical Examination*
   Introduction: General Principles of Physical Diagnosis, pp. 1–12.
   Chapters 2–6: Patient History (General Remarks, Current, Past, Social and Family), pp. 13–58.
   Chapter 15: General Remarks on the Physical Examination, pp. 131–146.
   Chapter 39: Diagnostic Formulations, pp. 291–293.

SAMPLE REPORTS

The following three reports are examples of reports you might encounter while transcribing family medicine, geriatrics, and nutrition and dietetics.

HISTORY & PHYSICAL

HISTORY OF PRESENT ILLNESS
This is an 89-year-old gentleman. The patient has had 2 hospitalizations recently. His last one was a short hospitalization for hypotension due to dehydration, secondary to C. difficile colitis with diarrhea. Prior to that, the patient had been hospitalized for an extended period of time with mental status changes and fever. He required an ICU stay and was discharged on oral vancomycin to treat the C. difficile colitis. Since then, he has been feeling well. His toe seems to be healing. He is not short of breath or dizzy. He is not having chest pain or palpitations.

PROBLEM LIST

1. Significant peripheral vascular disease, status post right below-knee amputation for gangrene, status post left great toe amputation for nonhealing ischemic ulcer.
2. Hypertension.
3. Coronary artery disease, status post bypass grafting, with ischemic cardiomyopathy; congestive heart failure, status post pacemaker and defibrillator placement.
4. Atrial fibrillation, chronically anticoagulated with warfarin.
5. Status post abdominal aortic aneurysm repair and left carotid endarterectomy.
6. History of bowel obstruction status post laparotomy.
7. History of right inguinal hernia repair.
8. Depression.
9. Gastroesophageal reflux disease.
10. Type 2 diabetes.
11. Osteoarthritis.
12. Benign prostatic hypertrophy.
13. Anemia.

CURRENT MEDICATIONS
Effexor 75 mg daily, Questran 2 g b.i.d., Humalog 2 units prior to meals, Neurontin 600 mg t.i.d., Lopressor 25 mg p.o. b.i.d., Lantus 10 units each evening, warfarin, vancomycin 125 mg p.o. q.6 h. p.r.n., Flomax 0.4 mg p.o. q.d., nortriptyline 25 mg p.o. q.d., Prilosec 20 mg p.o. q.d., Proscar 5 mg p.o. q.d.

ALLERGIES
No known drug allergies.

CODE STATUS
FULL CODE, HEALTHCARE PROXY.

DIET
No added salt, no concentrated sweets, regular consistency, thin liquids.

(continued)

RESTRAINTS
None.

PHYSICAL EXAMINATION
Patient is alert, oriented, and pleasant. He is not in acute distress. His lungs are clear to auscultation and percussion. Heart is irregularly irregular. Abdomen soft, nontender, normoactive bowel sounds. Left great toe seems to be healing reasonably well.

ASSESSMENT/PLAN
The patient has had a very difficult March. He has had 2 hospitalizations, the first one being quite significant. He has multiple medical morbidities and, at this point, striking a balance in terms of treating each of these is proving challenging.

1. Cut back on his insulin.
2. Because of his diabetes and congestive heart failure, the patient should be on an ACE inhibitor for his hypotension. We will start a low dose of Captopril to begin with.
3. Peripheral vascular disease, certainly problematic and will clearly pose more problems for him as time goes on. Will continue with local wound care. His amputation site looks pretty good currently.
4. Other issues are stable, and we will continue current medical regimen for these, including gastroesophageal reflux disease, depression, benign prostatic hypertrophy, atrial fibrillation on chronic anticoagulation.

PROGRESS NOTE

The patient was visited at the bedside. Her case was discussed in detail with Dr. Jones who has been seeing the patient over the last few days. She complains of soreness in her abdomen. She is refusing to eat or drink anything at this time. She has no nausea or vomiting today but still has difficulty swallowing, with frequent choking. She continues to fail the cookie-swallow test.

PHYSICAL EXAMINATION
GENERAL: This is an elderly female lying in bed and refusing to eat.
HEENT: Pupils were equal, round, and reactive to light and accommodation. Oral mucosa was dry.
NECK: Supple without jugular venous distension.
CARDIOVASCULAR: S1 and S2 with a regular rate and rhythm.
LUNGS: Clear to auscultation and percussion.
ABDOMEN: There is a PEG tube in place with no discharge and no erythema around the insertion site.

LABORATORY DATA
Cultures were reviewed, and there was growth of Enterobacter cloacae from a specimen collected yesterday. Multiple other cultures showed growth of Candida albicans.

IMPRESSION
Ascending cholangitis, polymicrobial, on adequate therapy with Levaquin, Unasyn, and Diflucan.

PLAN
We will continue the same management of total parenteral nutrition with Jevity via PEG tube. She will be provided with glycerin swabs for her lips as well as ice chips p.r.n.

CONSULTATION

HISTORY
This patient is a 14-year-old female with morbid obesity who comes in today with her mother seeking my assistance with a weight reduction program. The child has been my patient virtually since birth. She had a birthweight of 7 pounds and a length of 21 inches. I also treat the rest of her family, including her parents and younger brother.

PHYSICAL EXAMINATION
GENERAL: This is a morbidly obese teenager who appears depressed.
VITAL SIGNS: Her temperature is 97.8, pulse rate is 72, respirations are 18, and blood pressure is 110/80. Her current height is 5 feet 5 inches and her weight is 287 pounds. Her BMI is 37, which makes her morbidly obese.
HEENT: Normocephalic and atraumatic. Pupils are equal, round, and reactive to light and accommodation. No scleral icterus.
NECK: Supple. No jugular venous distension.
CHEST: Symmetrical. Breath sounds are equal bilaterally.
HEART: Regular sinus rhythm. No murmur, gallop, clicks, rubs, or heaves.
ABDOMEN: Pendulous. Normal bowel sounds.
EXTREMITIES: Full range of motion. Pedal pulses are palpable.
NEUROLOGICAL: The patient appears to be depressed at this time, but otherwise the neurological exam is nonfocal.

PLAN
I have provided the patient with a diet and exercise plan designed to fit the lifestyle of a teenager. I have provided her with a balanced meal plan for 3 meals and 3 snacks per day and have set her up with an exercise plan to include brisk walking for 2 miles a day, 7 days a week, and some dance routines, which she feels she would be interested in pursuing. The goal will be for her to lose 2 to 3 pounds per week until she reaches her goal weight of 130 pounds. I have also recommended that her mother look into some counseling for her daughter due to her depression.

REVIEW QUESTIONS

The goal of these questions is to test your knowledge in the areas of family medicine, geriatrics, nutrition, and dietetics.

Directions: Select the correct answer for each of the multiple-choice questions provided below. *Answers are provided at the end of this chapter.*

1. The patient has had these blood tests ordered: Ferritin level, B-12 level, folate level, and TIBC. What is the patient being worked up for?
   - A. Jaundice
   - B. Iron-deficiency anemia
   - C. Malabsorption syndrome
   - D. Chronic fatigue syndrome

2. Aciphex, Protonix, and Nexium are prescribed for:
   - A. GERD
   - B. Hyperlipidemia
   - C. Depression
   - D. Hypertension

3. Decubitus ulcers most frequently occur in individuals who are:
   - A. Paralyzed, unconscious, or elderly
   - B. Postoperative, sedated, and on pulse oximetry
   - C. Young, diabetic, and active
   - D. Psychotic, medicated, and in soft restraints

4. A constellation of symptoms preceding disease is termed:
   - A. Sequelae
   - B. Staging
   - C. Prodrome
   - D. Auscultation

5. Which of these statements is correct?
   - A. The patient will be given a quinolone antibiotic in lieu of his penicillin allergy
   - B. In lieu of her DNR status, the patient is not to be intubated
   - C. The patient's surgery was postponed in lieu of the fact that his PT was elevated
   - D. Because of her asthma, the patient will be given an ACE inhibitor in lieu of a beta-blocker

6. Which of the following would not be prescribed to prevent pregnancy?
   - A. Ortho Evra
   - B. Orth Tri-Cyclen
   - C. Evista
   - D. Yasmin

7. An electrolyte imbalance may occur with:
   - A. Constipation
   - B. Diarrhea
   - C. Glucose intolerance
   - D. Azotemia

8. A disease characterized by binging and purging is:
   - A. Anorexia
   - B. Cachexia
   - C. Bulimia nervosa
   - D. Consumption

9. A gastric bypass procedure is a type of:
   - A. Barbotage
   - B. Bariatric surgery
   - C. Hyfrecator surgery
   - D. Fallot procedure

10. Body mass index (BMI) is commonly used to:
    - A. Assess health risk and degree of obesity
    - B. Determine exercise tolerance
    - C. Determine waist/hip ratio
    - D. Decide on weight loss method

11. A BRAT diet is often prescribed for children in cases of:
    A. Tonsillitis
    B. Pneumonia
    C. Gastroenteritis
    D. Hydrocephalus

12. Which of the following would be prescribed for urinary urgency and frequency?
    A. Detrol LA
    B. Lantus
    C. Ultracet
    D. Mobic

13. Miacalcin, a medication used to treat osteoporosis, is administered:
    A. Orally in tablets
    B. Monthly by IV
    C. 70 mg weekly
    D. Via nasal spray

14. In a cachectic patient, you would see:
    A. Hilar adenopathy
    B. Mutism and avoidance behaviors
    C. Positive Babinski sign
    D. Bitemporal wasting

15. An elderly woman who fell a short while ago presents to the emergency room with severe pain and deformity of her right wrist. An x-ray reveals what type of fracture?
    A. LeFort
    B. Collie
    C. Colles
    D. Epiphysial

16. Presenile dementia is also known as:
    A. Huntington chorea
    B. Parkinson disease
    C. Alzheimer disease
    D. Psychogenic dementia

17. Which of these is a classic sign of Parkinson disease?
    A. Diaphoresis
    B. Dementia
    C. Exophthalmos
    D. Cogwheeling

18. Presbyesophagus would most likely be found in someone:
    A. Who has multiple sclerosis
    B. Who is elderly
    C. Who has a large mediastinal tumor
    D. Who has reversed position of the trachea and esophagus

19. Under which part of the physical examination would you find "edentulous"?
    A. HEENT examination
    B. Musculoskeletal examination
    C. Mental status examination
    D. Skin/integument examination

20. Which of the following is a common finding on examination of the hands of an elderly patient?
    A. Heberden nodes
    B. Senile lentigo
    C. Swan-neck deformity
    D. All of these

21. Which of these ocular findings is common in elderly patients?
    A. Argyll Robertson pupil
    B. Arcus senilis
    C. Fixed pupil
    D. AV nicking

22. A 77-year-old woman sees her primary care physician for the following complaints: Hand tremors with pill-rolling and micrographia, retropulsive gait, and some generalized body stiffness. What is a likely diagnosis?
    A. Hyperthyroidism
    B. Temporal lobe epilepsy
    C. Parkinson disease
    D. Subclinical depression

23. Metformin is the generic name of a common medication used to treat:
    A. Type 2 diabetes
    B. Hypertension
    C. Alopecia
    D. Osteoporosis

24. Ipratropium, prescribed for COPD, is administered via:
    A. A metered-dose inhaler
    B. An IV
    C. A time-release capsule
    D. A quick-dissolving tablet

25. Adipose tissue is commonly called:
    A. Phagocytes
    B. Muscle
    C. Fat
    D. Bone

26. A neonate is an infant less than:
    A. 28 days old
    B. 1 year old
    C. 6 months old
    D. 1 day old

27. Selegiline, amantadine, and levodopa are used to treat:
    A. Alzheimer disease
    B. Incontinence
    C. Memory impairment
    D. Parkinson disease

28. Analgesics such as propoxyphene are often combined with APAP, which is the abbreviation for:
    A. Aspirin
    B. Advil
    C. Acetaminophen
    D. Naproxen

29. Fosamax is prescribed in a once-weekly dose to treat:
    A. Osteoporosis
    B. Anemia
    C. BPH
    D. Hyperlipidemia

30. Immediately preceding and during pregnancy, women are advised to increase their intake of which of the following vitamins to prevent neural tube defects?
    A. Vitamin C
    B. Vitamin D
    C. Folic acid
    D. Vitamin E

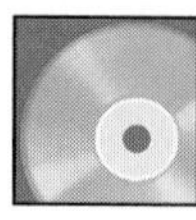

Please see the accompanying CD for additional review materials for this section.

PROOFREADING EXERCISES

These two proofreading exercises are provided to improve your skills in the areas of editing and effective identification and correction of errors in the medical record.

Directions: Identify and correct the transcription errors found in the exercises below. *Answers are provided at the end of this chapter.*

PROOFREADING EXERCISE #1

HISTORY OF PRESENT ILLNESS

This 79-year-old married white female is admitted from home for long-term placement. History includes history of chronic bronchitis, arteriosclerotic heart disease, angina, frequent falls, dementia, Type 2 diabetes, and congestive heart failure requiring diuretics and venus insufficiency in her ankles.

MEDICATIONS AT THE TIME OF TRANSFER

According to a list provided by her family, medications include Norvasc 10 mg a day, Lasix 40 mg a day, glyburide 2.5 mg a day, levothyroxine 50 mg a day, Lexapro 10 mg a day, baby aspirin 81 mg a day, Ferris sulfate 325 mg once a day, Macula Complete 3 tablets b.i.d., Zocor 20 mg a day, Toprol XL 150 mg in the evening, Aricept 10 mg a day, hydrocodone with APAP 5/500 mg 1–2 q.4 h. p.r.n. for pain, Tums 1 t.i.d., Combivent inhaler 2 puffs 4 times a day.

LABORATORY STUDIES

03/25, normal urine analysis; 03/24 blood sugar 223, BUN 78, creatinine 3.2, normal electrolytes except for a potassium of 33, albumin 3.9, total protein 8.2, calcium 9, alkaline phosphatase 55, SGOT 26, SGPT 13, bilirubin 0.4, calculated GFR 15, hemoglobin 11.6, hematocrit 33, white count 7200 and on 03/24, T_4 7.6, T_3 of 81, 3T3 2.0, TSH 1.20. A chest x-ray on 03/10 shows cardiomegaly, tortuous aorta, interstitial changes in both lung fields indicative of congestive heart failure. A chemistry profile on 03/10 showed a BUN of only 36 and creatinine 2.2. A urine culture on 12/04 grew greater than 100,000 CSU Klebsiella pneumoniae. Hemoglobin A_{1C} 12/20/04 was 5.4. An aortic ultrasound 12/22 showed a very extensive aneurysm in the upper abdominal aorta which involved

(continued)

the real arteries. A CT scan of the abdomen 02/27/04 showed an 8.5-cm infrarenal abdominal aortic aneurysm. Brain natriuretic peptide in January was elevated at 1420.

ALLERGIES
PENICILLIN.

PAST MEDICAL HISTORY
The patient is able to speak but is a very limited historian. Her history includes hypertension for 10 years, diabetes for 10 or 12 years, dementia, sleeplessness, agitation, anxiety for about 5 years. She had an appendectomy in her 40s, a hysterectomy in her 50s, a right mastectomy for cancer in 1998, a "bladder suspension" for incontinence in 2002. She has had elevated cholesterol for many years and has been bothered life-long with eczema on her arms and face. She had an abdominal aortic aneurysm repair in January, 2005. She also has an atrophic right kidney.

PERSONAL AND SOCIAL HISTORY
She has been married for 56 years. She was living at home, but her husband is apparently unable to care for her anymore because of her needs. She never smoked, never used alcohol.

PHYSICAL EXAMINATION
Height 5 feet 2 inches, weight 158 pounds (down 10 pounds from last year), temperature 98.4, pulse 82, respirations 18, blood pressure 140/82. The patient is a slightly pale, very frail, confused, befuddled white female who cannot tell me the month or the year but knows it is winter. She can repeat her own name. She is pleasant and cooperative. She is attempting to get into a wheelchair to ride to supper. She has a very unsteady, flat-footed gait. There is a coarse, red, seborrheic-type dermatitis on her face and four arms. There are no suspicious lesions. There are no significant oropharyngeal lesions. The neck is supple. Parotid pulses are symmetrical and strong. There are no bruits and no goiter. There is no lymphadenopathy. Chest is shallowly expanded, but clear. I cannot hear any rales. Left border of cardiac dullness is approximately 1 cm beyond the midclavicular line in the 5th intercostal space. Rhythm is regular. I cannot hear any murmur. Absent right breast with a mastectomy scar. The right breast is normal. The axillae is clear. Abdomen is soft. There is a right

(continued)

lower quadrant appendectomy scar and a Pfannenstiel incision underneath her abdominal panniculus, both well healed. The liver span is about 7 cm to percussion, the spleen span about 4.0 cm. Normal external female genitalia. Rectal exam shows a few small external hemorrhoids. The stool is brown and heme occult negative. Extremities showed arthritic widening of the knees and ankles. There are faint dorsalis pedis pulses bilaterally. She has bilateral varicose veins but no calf asymmetry or edema. Symmetric motor strength in major muscle groups of the upper and lower extremities. There is a rapid tremor of both hands, more pronounced on the left than the right.

IMPRESSION

1. Dementia, probably Alzheimer.
2. Noninsulin-dependent diabetes mellitus.
3. Hypertension.
4. Arteriosclerotic heart disease with angina, cardiomegaly, and recent congestive heart failure.
5. Hyperthyroidism.
6. Hyperlipidemia.
7. History of anxiety, depression, and agitation.
8. Diffuse degenerative arthritis.
9. History of recurrent urinary tract infections.
10. Chronic renal insufficiency, worsening since repair of abominable aortic aneurysm.
11. Chronic eczematoid dermatitis.
12. Limited vision due to molecular degeneration.

PLAN

I will get baseline laboratory studies next week and keep on maintenance medications as mentioned above and prescribe .1% triamcinolone cream t.i.d. for eczema. Will check stools for occult blood times three.

PROOFREADING EXERCISE #2

The patient is a 15-year-old female who presents today with her mother. She presents to my office today with the complaints of anorexia. Privately, her mother tells me the patient is abusing laxatives and has cholemia. She said the child leaves the table after eating and immediately goes to the bathroom to vomit. Mother says she also found empty boxes of additives in the girl's school bag.

On examination, her blood pressure is 112/56, pulse is 72, respiratory rate is 18, and temperature is 98.2. Her height is 5 feet 6 inches, and her weight is 84 pounds, making her obviously overweight.

I recommended to her mother that we admit the child to the hospital for IV fluids and parental nutrition. Following this, I have recommended an excellent facility for treatment of her eating disorders.

I will follow her while she is at the hospital and once she is admitted to the eating disorders facility. I explained to the mother that this condition will not get better on its own without intervention by professionals trained to deal with eating disorders. Mother agreed and will take her daughter directly to the hospital for admission.

ANSWER KEYS

REVIEW QUESTIONS ANSWER KEY

1. B
2. A
3. A
4. C
5. D
6. C
7. B
8. C
9. B
10. A
11. C
12. A
13. D
14. D
15. C
16. C
17. D
18. B
19. A
20. D
21. B
22. C
23. A
24. A
25. C
26. A
27. D
28. C
29. A
30. C

PROOFREADING EXERCISE #1 KEY

HISTORY OF PRESENT ILLNESS
This 79-year-old married white female is admitted from home for long-term placement. History includes history of chronic bronchitis, arteriosclerotic heart disease, angina, frequent falls, dementia, Type 2 diabetes, and congestive heart failure requiring diuretics and venus insufficiency in her ankles.

MEDICATIONS AT THE TIME OF TRANSFER
According to a list provided by her family, medications include Norvasc 10 mg a day, Lasix 40 mg a day, glyburide 2.5 mg a day, levothyroxine 50 mg a day, Lexapro 10 mg a day, baby aspirin 81 mg a day, Ferris sulfate 325 mg once a day, Macula Complete 3 tablets b.i.d., Zocor 20 mg a day, Toprol XL 150 mg in the evening, Aricept 10 mg a day, hydrocodone with APAP 5/500 mg 1–2 q.4 h. p.r.n. for pain, Tums 1 t.i.d., Combivent inhaler 2 puffs 4 times a day.

LABORATORY STUDIES
03/25, normal urine analysis; 03/24 blood sugar 223, BUN 78, creatinine 3.2, normal electrolytes except for a potassium of 33, albumin 3.9, total protein 8.2, calcium 9, alkaline phosphatase 55, SGOT 26, SGPT 13, bilirubin 0.4, calculated GFR 15, hemoglobin 11.6, hematocrit 33, white count 7, 200 and on 03/24, T_4 7.6, T_3 of 81, 3T3 2.0, TSH 1.20. A chest x-ray on 03/10 shows cardiomegaly, tortuous aorta, interstitial changes in both lung fields indicative of congestive heart failure. A chemistry profile on 03/10 showed a BUN of only 36 and creatinine 2.2. A urine culture on 12/04 grew greater than 100,000 CSU Klebsiella pneumoniae. Hemoglobin A_{1C} 12/20/04 was 5.4. An aortic ultrasound 12/22 showed a very extensive aneurysm in the upper abdominal aorta which

Incorrect spelling—venous

Incorrect dose—mcg

Incorrect spelling—ferrous

Use combined form—urinalysis

Flag—invalid result for potassium

Incorrect—free T_3

Incorrect abbreviation—CFU

Incorrect term—renal

~~involved the~~ real arteries. A CT scan of the abdomen 02/27/04 showed an 8.5-cm infrarenal abdominal aortic aneurysm. Brain natriuretic peptide in January was elevated at 1420.

ALLERGIES

PENICILLIN.

PAST MEDICAL HISTORY

The patient is able to speak but is a very limited historian. Her history includes hypertension for 10 years, diabetes for 10 or 12 years, dementia, sleeplessness, agitation, anxiety for about 5 years. She had an appendectomy in her 40s, a hysterectomy in her 50s, a right mastectomy for cancer in 1998, a "bladder suspension" for incontinence in 2002. She has had elevated cholesterol for many years and has been bothered life-long with eczema on her arms and face. She had an abdominal aortic aneurysm repair in January, 2005. She also has an atrophic right kidney.

PERSONAL AND SOCIAL HISTORY

She has been married for 56 years. She was living at home, but her husband is apparently unable to care for her anymore because of her needs. She never smoked, never used alcohol.

PHYSICAL EXAMINATION

Height 5 feet 2 inches, weight 158 pounds (down 10 pounds from last year), temperature 98.4, pulse 82, respirations 18, blood pressure 140/82. The patient is a slightly pale, very frail, confused, befuddled white female who cannot tell me the month or the year but knows it is winter. She can repeat her own name. She is pleasant and cooperative. She is attempting to get into a wheelchair to ride to supper. She has a very unsteady, flat-footed gait. There is a coarse, red,

Incorrect term—carotid

Flag—right breast dictated twice

Incorrect term—Hemoccult

Incorrect prefix—hypothyroidism

Incorrect word—forearms

Use plural verb—are

Incorrect format—do not type a zero following a decimal

seborrheic-type dermatitis on her face and four arms. There are no suspicious lesions. There are no significant oropharyngeal lesions. The neck is supple. Parotid pulses are symmetrical and strong. There are no bruits and no goiter. There is no lymphadenopathy. Chest is shallowly expanded, but clear. I cannot hear any rales. Left border of cardiac dullness is approximately 1 cm beyond the midclavicular line in the 5th intercostal space. Rhythm is regular. I cannot hear any murmur. Absent right breast with a mastectomy scar. The right breast is normal. The axillae is clear. Abdomen is soft. There is a right lower quadrant appendectomy scar and a Pfannenstiel incision underneath her abdominal panniculus, both well healed. The liver span is about 7 cm to percussion, the spleen span about 4.0 cm. Normal external female genitalia. Rectal exam shows a few small external hemorrhoids. The stool is brown and heme occult negative. Extremities showed arthritic widening of the knees and ankles. There are faint dorsalis pedis pulses bilaterally. She has bilateral varicose veins but no calf asymmetry or edema. Symmetric motor strength in major muscle groups of the upper and lower extremities. There is a rapid tremor of both hands, more pronounced on the left than the right.

IMPRESSION

1. Dementia, probably Alzheimer.
2. Noninsulin-dependent diabetes mellitus.
3. Hypertension.
4. Arteriosclerotic heart disease with angina, cardiomegaly, and recent congestive heart failure.
5. Hyperthyroidism.
6. Hyperlipidemia.
7. History of anxiety, depression, and agitation.
8. Diffuse degenerative arthritis.
9. History of recurrent urinary tract infections.

Incorrect word—abdominal

10. Chronic renal insufficiency, worsening since repair of abominable aortic aneurysm.
11. Chronic eczematoid dermatitis.
12. Limited vision due to molecular degeneration.

Incorrect term—macular

PLAN

I will get baseline laboratory studies next week and keep on maintenance medications as mentioned above and prescribe .1% triamcinolone cream t.i.d. for eczema. Will check stools for occult blood times three.

Incorrect format—type the leading zero (0.1%)

Incorrect format—x3

PROOFREADING EXERCISE #2 KEY

Incorrect term—bulimia

Incorrect word—laxatives

Incorrect prefix—underweight

Incorrect term—parenteral

The patient is a 15-year-old female who presents today with her mother. She presents to my office today with the complaints of anorexia. Privately, her mother tells me the patient is abusing laxatives and has cholemia. She said the child leaves the table after eating and immediately goes to the bathroom to vomit. Mother says she also found empty boxes of additives in the girl's school bag.

On examination, her blood pressure is 112/56, pulse is 72, respiratory rate is 18, and temperature is 98.2. Her height is 5 feet 6 inches, and her weight is 84 pounds, making her obviously overweight.

I recommended to her mother that we admit the child to the hospital for IV fluids and parental nutrition. Following this, I have recommended an excellent facility for treatment of her eating disorders.

I will follow her while she is at the hospital and once she is admitted to the eating disorders facility. I explained to the mother that this condition will not get better on its own without intervention by professionals trained to deal with eating disorders. Mother agreed and will take her daughter directly to the hospital for admission.

CHAPTER

14

Gastroenterology

OBJECTIVES CHECKLIST

A prepared exam candidate will know:

- ☐ All combining forms, prefixes, and suffixes related to the body system.
- ☐ Sequential structures of the digestive system, beginning with the mouth and ending with the anus.
- ☐ Primary function and role of those structures in the digestive process.
- ☐ Anatomy and function of the accessory organs, including the liver, gallbladder, and pancreas.
- ☐ Role and function of the hepatic portal system.
- ☐ Role and function of the primary digestive enzymes.
- ☐ Common gastrointestinal signs, symptoms, and disease processes.
- ☐ Imaging and diagnostic studies used in the identification and treatment of gastrointestinal disorders.
- ☐ Laboratory studies related to the diagnosis and treatment of gastrointestinal dysfunction and disease.
- ☐ Common medications indicated and prescribed for gastrointestinal symptoms and diseases.

RESOURCES FOR STUDY

1. *The Language of Medicine*
   Chapter 5: Digestive System, pp. 139–184.
   Chapter 6: Additional Suffixes and Digestive System Terminology, pp. 185–211.
2. *H&P: A Nonphysician's Guide to the Medical History and Physical Examination*
   Chapter 10: Review of Systems: Gastrointestinal, pp. 89–96.
   Chapter 25: Examination of the Abdomen, pp. 235–248.
3. *Human Diseases*
   Chapter 11: Diseases of the Digestive System, pp. 153–172.
4. *Laboratory Tests & Diagnostic Procedures in Medicine*
   Chapter 8: Examination of the Digestive Tract and Genitourinary System, pp. 107–118.
   Chapter 20: Chemical Examination of the Blood, pp. 355–400.
   Chapter 21: Microbiology (Bacteriology, Mycology, Virology and Parasitology), pp. 401–409.
   Chapter 24: Examination of Urine, Stool and Other Fluids and Materials (Laboratory Examination of Stool), pp. 442–443.
5. *Understanding Pharmacology for Health Professionals*
   Chapter 13: Gastrointestinal Drugs, pp. 115–136.

SAMPLE REPORTS

The following five reports are examples of reports you might encounter while transcribing gastroenterology.

OPERATIVE REPORT

SURGEON
John Smith, MD.

PREOPERATIVE DIAGNOSIS
Biliary atresia.

POSTOPERATIVE DIAGNOSIS
Biliary atresia.

PROCEDURES PERFORMED
1. Kasai procedure (Roux-en-Y hepatic portoenterostomy).
2. Liver biopsy.

ANESTHESIA
General endotracheal.

ESTIMATED BLOOD LOSS
Approximately 10 mL.

SPECIMENS SUBMITTED
1. Wedge liver biopsy from segment IV of the liver.
2. Gallbladder with atretic extrahepatic biliary tree.

COMPLICATIONS
None apparent.

JUSTIFICATION FOR PROCEDURE
The patient is a 7-week-old male who presented to his pediatrician with jaundice. Evaluation, including right upper quadrant ultrasound and nuclear hepatobiliary scans, revealed evidence of biliary atresia. The patient is now being taken to the operating room for exploration with confirmation of the diagnosis and a Kasai procedure.

PROCEDURE IN DETAIL
In the operating room, general endotracheal anesthesia was induced. The abdomen and chest were prepped with Betadine and draped sterilely. The initial incision was a right upper quadrant subcostal incision. The abdominal wall was traversed using the Bovie electrocautery until the peritoneal cavity was entered. The falciform ligament was divided and ligated with silk suture. The liver appeared to be congested with bile. The liver was firm but was not hard or sclerotic as would be expected with cirrhosis. The gallbladder was noted to be atretic and, upon initial observation of the hepatoduodenal ligament, the extrahepatic biliary tree was not evident.

(continued)

We now performed a liver biopsy to evaluate for the presence or absence of bile ducts. Along the free edge of segment IV of the liver, two figure-of-8 Vicryl sutures were placed in a wedge configuration for hemostasis. The segment of liver isolated by these two sutures was sharply excised with a scalpel. This segment of liver was immediately sent to pathology for evaluation. Their initial report revealed evidence of microscopic biliary radicles. Thus, the patient had evidence of microscopic bile ducts and a Kasai procedure was now the procedure of choice.

Before performing the Kasai, we performed an intraoperative cholangiogram via the atretic gallbladder to further prove that there was no patent extrahepatic biliary tree. A small hole was made in the dome of the gallbladder into which a cholangiogram catheter was placed. This catheter was secured with suture. Now, using fluoroscopic assistance, a cholangiogram was obtained. This cholangiogram failed to demonstrate evidence of an extrahepatic or intrahepatic biliary tree. Upon entering the gallbladder, a small amount of white bile was encountered, further confirming the non-patency of the biliary tree. With pressure, the contrast extravasated from the gallbladder but still failed to fill a biliary tree. Thus, with the preoperative and intraoperative data, we were confident of the diagnosis of biliary atresia and proceeded with the Kasai procedure.

The next step was dissection of the gallbladder down from its peritoneal attachments at the undersurface of the liver. The entire atretic biliary tree was dissected out on the hepatoduodenal ligament, taking care to identify and preserve the vascular structures in the hepatoduodenal ligament, including the portal vein and its bifurcation as well as the hepatic artery and its bifurcation. The dissection was carried up to the porta hepatis where a disk of liver tissue was excised in continuity with the atretic biliary tree. This disk was carved out of the inner surface of the liver, the limits of which were on the left and right hepatic artery on either side. After removing this disk of liver and sending it to pathology for evaluation, close observation revealed bile emanating from the raw surface of the liver where the disk had been excised. The drainage from the atretic right hepatic duct was brisk and, with time, the drainage from the left side also appeared to be good. Hemostasis along the raw edge of the liver was obtained with Gelfoam and thrombin.

After gaining hemostasis, we turned our attention to the construction of a Roux-en-Y limb in order to perform our portoenterostomy. A window in the small bowel mesentery was made in the mid-jejunum. The bowel was transected at this point with an Endo GIA stapler, and 45 cm distal to this staple line the bowel was marked with a silk suture, thus noting the point of construction of the Roux-en-Y. The proximal end of the stapled bowel was now brought down to the point at which we placed our tag for construction of the Roux-en-Y limb.

Silk sutures of 5-0 were used to align the two segments of bowel. The anastomosis was constructed such that it was slightly larger than the lumen of each segment of bowel. A two-layer, hand-sewn anastomosis was now performed. The outside layer was constructed of interrupted 5-0 silk sutures and the inner layer was constructed of 5-0 Vicryl sutures, with a running, locking stitch for the back row and, after turning the corner, a Connell stitch for the top row. The order of the anastomosis proceeded with placement of the silk sutures for the back row, followed by the Vicryl sutures circumferentially, followed by completion of the anastomosis by Lembert suturing the front side with the 5-0 interrupted silk suture. The anastomosis was hemostatic and widely patent. Also, there were no kinks or twists in the anastomosis.

(continued)

The small bowel was now replaced into the peritoneal cavity, and the limb was brought up to the porta for construction of our biliary anastomosis. We removed the Gelfoam from the area and found it to be hemostatic. There was good bile drainage still, as manifested by saturation of the Gelfoam and gauze with biliary fluid. The liver surface was not as fibrotic as often seen in biliary atresia, and we were able to place our sutures in the liver and Glisson's capsule circumferentially in order to perform our anastomosis.

The biliary anastomosis was constructed as a hepatic portoenterostomy, suturing the side of the Roux to the porta. The anastomosis was constructed as a single-layer, hand-sewn anastomosis using 5-0 Prolene suture in an interrupted fashion. The limits of our anastomosis medially and laterally were the left and right hepatic arteries, respectively. Posteriorly, the limit of our anastomosis was the portal vein and anteriorly, the fibrotic edge of the liver and Glisson capsule. We proceeded first by placing the back row of interrupted sutures and then, after tying these down, the front row was constructed. The anastomosis was without kinks or evidence of a leak. In order to prevent kinking of the bowel just distal to the anastomosis, the limb was tacked to the undersurface of the liver a few centimeters from our anastomosis using silk suture.

The abdominal cavity was now copiously irrigated with warmed saline solution. Wound closure was carried out in the usual fashion, and the patient was transported to the pediatric surgery special care unit in stable condition, having tolerated the procedure well.

OPERATIVE REPORT

PREOPERATIVE DIAGNOSIS
Chronic cholecystitis and cholelithiasis.

POSTOPERATIVE DIAGNOSIS
Chronic cholecystitis and cholelithiasis.

OPERATION
Laparoscopic cholecystectomy and intraoperative cholangiogram.

ANESTHESIA
General endotracheal anesthesia.

PROCEDURE IN DETAIL
With the patient in the supine position, satisfactory general anesthesia was given. The patient had a Foley catheter and sequential compression devices were in place on both legs. The patient received 2 g of Ancef intravenously. The abdomen was then prepped with Betadine and draped in the usual manner.

The Hasson technique was utilized, making a small incision below the umbilicus. Bleeders were controlled with the electrocautery. The midline was grasped with a straight Kocher and lifted upwards. The midline was identified and entered with a small hemostat. I was able to introduce my index finger and there were no adhesions around the entrance. Two sutures of 0 Vicryl were placed in each corner, and then the Hasson trocar was introduced and secured to the opening.

The next step was to place the video camera. The patient was then placed in reverse Trendelenburg position, slightly tilted to the left. The patient presented the left lobe of the liver, which appeared to be covering the gallbladder area.

The next step was to make a small incision in the epigastric area, and under direct vision, a 10-mm trocar was introduced and advanced without difficulty. The gallbladder was identified and lifted in an upward position from the fundus with the help of the dolphin dissector.

Then 2 small openings were made in the lateral abdominal wall utilizing the 5-mm trocars. Then the tissue holder was utilized to pull the gallbladder by the fundus in an upward position, and the second one was at the infundibulum of the gallbladder with a small amount of lateral traction in order to expose Calot triangle. The anatomy was identified and dissected carefully with the dolphin dissector. The cystic duct at the junction of the gallbladder was identified, and also the cystic artery was identified, and then proximal and distal control was carried out with Ligaclips and transected.

Next, utilizing the peanut pusher for gallbladder surgery, I was able to expose very well the cystic duct, and also the junction with the common bile duct was identified. The cystic duct appeared to be going around the common bile duct. The next step was to place a Ligaclip at the junction of the gallbladder with the cystic duct, and then, with the Endoshears scissors, a small opening was made in the cystic duct. The next step was to place a #14 Cholangiocath into the abdominal wall, again under direct vision, and then the Reddick catheter for intraoperative cholangiogram was utilized. I was able to introduce the catheter into the cystic duct without difficulty. The small balloon was inflated, and then the patient underwent the intraoperative cholangiogram.

(continued)

The cholangiogram showed the dye going into the duodenum very well, with no evidence of filling defects, and the upper radicles, right and left, as well. The x-rays were interpreted by the radiologist and reported as normal. The Cholangiocath was deflated and removed, and then the cystic duct was controlled with a Ligaclip and transected. The gallbladder was then removed from the liver bed with the electrocautery and removed with an Endocatch through the epigastric area.

The liver bed was then inspected and a small area of oozing was controlled at the upper aspect of the liver edge. Another area down into the lower third, lateral aspect of the liver, was controlled with a small Ligaclip. A small piece of Surgicel was also left in the area. The abdominal cavity was irrigated with a copious amount of saline and aspirated. There was no evidence of any active bleeding from the operative area during this procedure. The epigastric port and the lateral port were removed. The next step was to remove the video camera. Then the infra-umbilical incision was approached, and the fascia was closed with figure-of-8 sutures of 0 Vicryl. The subcutaneous tissue was then approximated with 3-0 chromic catgut, and then a subcuticular suture was used for the incisions at the epigastric and infraumbilical areas.

The sponge, needle and instrument counts were given as correct. Blood loss was about 50 mL. The patient was then transferred to the recovery room in stable condition.

PROGRESS NOTE

PROBLEM
Hepatitis C, genotype 1a variant.

SUBJECTIVE
The patient returns for followup evaluation of hepatitis C on Pegasys and ribavirin therapy. The patient is doing much better on therapy. His mood is better. He has fewer physical symptoms. Anorexia is still a problem. He complains of itching. He was recently seen by Dr. Smith and was started on a Medrol Dosepak and has now almost completed therapy.

OBJECTIVE
VITAL SIGNS: Within normal limits. The patient is afebrile. Weight 160 pounds.
ABDOMEN: Soft, without masses, organomegaly, or ascites.

LABORATORY DATA
The patient's hemoglobin and hematocrit on 11/22/04 were 10 and 32, respectively. The liver function tests were normal. Hepatitis C RNA titer by PCR was less than 10 IU/mL.

ASSESSMENT
Normal liver function tests and low viral titer on Pegasys and ribavirin after 12 weeks of therapy; however, I could not find a pre-treatment viral load. We will consider this an early virologic response.

PLAN
Continue treatment for another 3 months. CBC and CMP today. Follow up in 4 weeks. Will draw AFP titers to screen for hepatocellular carcinoma. I have advised the patient not to take prednisone in the future without consulting a gastroenterologist.

PROCEDURE

PROCEDURE PERFORMED
Esophagogastroduodenoscopy with gastrostomy tube placement.

INDICATIONS FOR PROCEDURE
The patient is a 79-year-old woman admitted to the hospital with generalized weakness. The patient has had very poor oral intake. Gastrostomy tube placement is requested to facilitate nutrition as well as the administration of medications.

MEDICATIONS GIVEN FOR THE PROCEDURE
Demerol 25 mg IV push plus Versed 1 mg IV push in incremental doses.

INSTRUMENT USED
Pentax EG-2901 upper endoscope.

PROCEDURE IN DETAIL
The patient was placed on her back and the above medications were given. When she appeared adequately sedated, the instrument was placed into the oral cavity and advanced beyond the upper esophageal sphincter into the stomach, into the pylorus, and into the second portion of the duodenum. The duodenal mucosa was unremarkable. The pylorus was symmetrical. The gastric body had scattered areas of erythema and old heme pigment. On retroflexion, no significant hiatal hernia was identified. The gastric mucosa was otherwise unremarkable.

GASTROSTOMY TUBE PLACEMENT
The site of the gastrostomy tube placement was determined by transillumination of the endoscope light through the anterior abdominal wall. A site was chosen in the left upper quadrant. This was confirmed by seeing an indentation of the gastric mucosa when external pressure was applied to the abdomen at that site. The area was then cleansed with Betadine and anesthetized with 1% Xylocaine. A small incision was made at the site, and then a Seldinger needle was introduced through the incision into the gastric lumen under endoscopic guidance.

A guide wire was threaded through the hub of the needle, grasped with a snare, and then pulled out through the endoscope, and the endoscope and guide wire were withdrawn from the patient. A 20-French Wilson-Cooke gastrostomy tube was then threaded over the guide wire, advanced into the oral cavity, into the stomach, and then out through the incision in the abdominal wall. When this was completed, the endoscope was reintroduced into the stomach and confirmed good placement of the inner bolster of the gastrostomy tube. The esophagus was examined as the endoscope was withdrawn, and this appeared unremarkable.

The patient tolerated the procedure well and no complications were encountered during the procedure.

IMPRESSION
1. Successful placement of a 20-French Wilson-Cooke gastrostomy tube.
2. Scattered areas of gastric mucosal erythema.

RECOMMENDATIONS
As per postprocedure orders.

PROCEDURE

PROCEDURES
Upper endoscopy and colonoscopy.

INDICATIONS FOR PROCEDURES
The patient is a 52-year-old man admitted to the hospital with anemia, diffuse abdominal pain, and diarrhea.

MEDICATIONS GIVEN FOR THE PROCEDURE
Demerol 100 mg IV push plus Versed 5 mg IV push in incremental doses.

INSTRUMENT USED
Pentax EG-2901 upper endoscope and EC-3801-L colonoscope.

PROCEDURE IN DETAIL
UPPER ENDOSCOPY: The patient was placed in the left lateral decubitus position. The above-noted medications were given. When he appeared adequately sedated, the instrument was placed into the oral cavity and advanced beyond the upper esophageal sphincter into the stomach, into the pylorus, and into the second portion of the duodenum. The duodenal mucosa was unremarkable. The pylorus was symmetrical. The gastric mucosa had a diffuse erythematous appearance with some suggestion of nodularity. This was seen primarily in the body, but the antrum and cardia were also involved. Biopsies were taken from the antrum for CLOtest and randomly from the gastric body for routine histology.

On retroflexion, a hiatal hernia was identified. The instrument was pulled back into the esophagus and the Z-line was distinct. The esophageal mucosa appeared unremarkable.

The patient tolerated the procedure well and no complications were encountered during the procedure.

IMPRESSION
1. Diffuse nodularity of upper gastric mucosa.
2. Otherwise normal upper endoscopy.

COLONOSCOPY: After the above, the patient was turned 180 degrees. The instrument was placed into the rectum and, utilizing the push-pull technique, advanced to the cecum. There was moderate tortuosity of the colonic wall.

The instrument was pulled back from the cecum with careful examination of the colonic mucosa. In the proximal portion of the colon, extending from the cecum to the proximal to midtransverse colon, the colonic mucosa was characterized by the presence of multiple, small nodular areas averaging from 3 to 5 mm in diameter. Some of these had central umbilication with focal mucosal erosion. Biopsies were taken for routine histology from some of these areas. The more distal portion of the colon had a much smaller number of these areas.

The instrument was retroflexed in the rectum and internal hemorrhoids were present.

The patient tolerated the procedure well and no complications were encountered during the procedure.

(continued)

IMPRESSION

1. Diffuse gastric mucosal erythema.
2. Hiatal hernia.
3. Proximal colonic mucosal lymphoid hyperplasia with central umbilication.
4. Internal hemorrhoids.
5. Tortuosity of colonic wall.

RECOMMENDATIONS

1. Check CLOtest and treat if this is positive.
2. Tagamet 400 mg b.i.d. for approximately 4 to 6 weeks.
3. Stool softeners as needed to avoid constipation.
4. Colonoscopy in 10 years.

REVIEW QUESTIONS

The goal of these questions is to test your knowledge in the area of gastroenterology.

Directions: Select the correct answer for each of the multiple-choice questions provided below. *Answers are provided at the end of this chapter.*

1. Small pouches in the wall of the intestine are called:
   A. Cystoceles
   B. Diverticula
   C. Rugae
   D. Ducts
2. Which of the following would not be used to decrease stomach acid?
   A. Tagamet
   B. Xanax
   C. Zantac
   D. Cimetidine
3. The pyloric sphincter is located at:
   A. The exit of the stomach
   B. The entrance to the stomach
   C. The esophagus
   D. The ileum
4. The most common cause of PUD is:
   A. *Streptococcus durans*
   B. *Helicobacter pylori*
   C. *Proteus mirabilis*
   D. *Staphylococcus aureus*
5. One class of drugs used to treat acid reflux is:
   A. HMG-CoA reductase inhibitors
   B. Proton pump inhibitors
   C. Beta blockers
   D. Antihistamines
6. Another name for celiac disease is:
   A. Inflammatory bowel disease
   B. Pancreatic ascariasis
   C. Sprue
   D. SARS
7. Which of the following signs is used to assess for appendicitis?
   A. Bamberger
   B. Kernig
   C. Brudzinski
   D. McBurney
8. A patient undergoing EGD might have which of the following tests performed?
   A. Wet prep to check for trichomonas
   B. Biopsy for HBsAg
   C. CLOtest to check for *Helicobacter pylori*
   D. CAMP test
9. An alcoholic with severe gastritis might present to the emergency room with:
   A. Hematuria
   B. Hematemesis
   C. Hemolysis
   D. Hemothorax
10. A gastrectomy removes all or part of the:
    A. Stomach
    B. Ovaries
    C. Bowel
    D. Thorax
11. Located at the end of the descending colon is the:
    A. Appendix
    B. Rectum
    C. Diaphragm
    D. Corpus callosum
12. The passage of dark, tarry stools is termed:
    A. Melanoma
    B. Leukorrhea
    C. Melena
    D. Hematemesis

13. Located at one end of the ascending colon is the:
    A. Haustra
    B. Cecum
    C. Ilium
    D. Rectum

14. Which of these adjectives refers to an abnormal sound heard on examination of the abdomen?
    A. Vesicular
    B. Adventitious
    C. Succussion
    D. Sonolucent

15. A patient with cirrhosis and portal hypertension might also have:
    A. Ulcerative colitis
    B. Esophageal varices
    C. Gallbladder disease
    D. Hemorrhoids

16. A surgeon dictating a consultation report mentions that a 53-year-old woman has a bilirubin of 13.2. What physical finding would be associated with this?
    A. Fever
    B. Asterixis
    C. Icterus
    D. Xanthelasma

17. A surgeon is dictating an open cholecystectomy and common bile duct exploration. What would be clipped and divided?
    A. The common bile duct
    B. The left hepatic duct
    C. The ampullary duct
    D. The cystic duct

18. A synonym for *laparotomy* is:
    A. Celiotomy
    B. Colliotomy
    C. Abdominoplasty
    D. Peritoneoscopy

19. A Billroth II is:
    A. An upgraded model of the Billroth I cautery unit
    B. A more severe form of Billroth I gastritis
    C. An endoscope used for gastrectomy
    D. A type of intestinal anastomosis

20. The patient is taken to the operating room with a perforated gastric ulcer. The surgeon performs a:
    A. Gastrorrhaphy
    B. Gastrostomy
    C. Gastrectomy
    D. Gastrotomy

21. You are transcribing a colonoscopy report. A large lesion is seen, and the endoscopist is having difficulty getting a biopsy as the tissue seems to be falling apart. The lesion is said to be:
    A. Piecemeal
    B. Gelatinous
    C. Friable
    D. Eroded

22. A young man comes to the ER with right-sided abdominal pain for 24 hours, fever, nausea, and vomiting. An x-ray is done but the appendix is not visualized. He is taken to the operating room at which time his inflamed appendix is found to be:
    A. Proctoscopic
    B. Retrocecal
    C. Intrathecal
    D. Retrosternal

23. Retroflexion might be done during which procedure?
    A. Colonoscopy
    B. Cardiac catheterization
    C. MRI of the spine
    D. Paracentesis

24. A patient is complaining of dysphagia and regurgitation. A possible cause seen on EGD is:
    A. Diverticula of the colon
    B. Spasm of the sphincter of Oddi
    C. Zenker diverticulum
    D. Wilms tumor
25. Bariatric surgery would be an option for:
    A. A person who scuba dives on a regular basis
    B. An elderly person who has suffered more than two strokes
    C. A toddler with club foot
    D. A person whose obesity is causing medical complications
26. A patient being treated for several weeks or months with a combination of Prilosec, Flagyl, and bismuth most likely has:
    A. *Helicobacter pylori* gastritis
    B. Meckel diverticulitis
    C. Mesenteric adenitis
    D. Ulcerative colitis
27. A barium enema test performed on a patient with Crohn disease might show:
    A. An apple core lesion
    B. Polyps
    C. String sign
    D. Peritonitis
28. GERD, left untreated, may lead to:
    A. Crohn disease
    B. Esophageal varices
    C. Pancreatitis
    D. Barrett esophagus
29. IBS is often treated with:
    A. Preparation H
    B. Activated charcoal
    C. Levsin
    D. Nexium
30. Which of the following would not necessarily be associated with pancreatitis?
    A. Diabetes mellitus
    B. Steatorrhea
    C. Hepatic cirrhosis
    D. Grey Turner sign

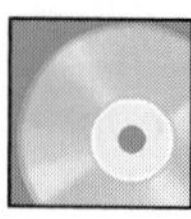

Please see the accompanying CD for additional review materials for this section.

PROOFREADING EXERCISES

These five proofreading exercises are provided to improve your skills in the areas of editing and effective identification and correction of errors in the medical record.

Directions: Identify and correct the transcription errors found in the exercises below. *Answers are provided at the end of this chapter.*

PROOFREADING EXERCISE #1

PROCEDURE
Esophagogastroduodenoscopy with biopsies.

PREPROCEDURE DIAGNOSIS
Iron deficiency anemia.

POSTPROCEDURE DIAGNOSES
1. Esophageal ulcer.
2. Garrett esophagus.
3. Hiatal hernia.

DESCRIPTION OF THE PROCEDURE
The procedure was explained to the patient and consent obtained. The patient was then sedated with Demerol 50 mg IV and versed 4 mg IV. The patient was placed in the left lateral decubitus position.

The Olympus video gastroscope was inserted under direct visualization into the esophagus. The esophageal mucosa showed an ulcer at the BE junction with Garrett esophagus extending from 23 cm down to the BE junction at 32 cm. There was a small hiatus hernia.

The scope was advanced into the stomach, which was unremarkable. The pylorus was latent and symmetric. The duodenal bulb and descending duodenum were normal. The scope was drawn back into the antrum, and retroflexed to view the angularis, fondus, and cardia. The hiatus hernia was seen again. The scope was straightened. Multiple biopsies were then taken of the esophageal ulcer and Garrett areas.

(continued)

The scope was then withdrawn. It should be noted that duodenal biopsies were also done to rule out cilia disease. The patient tolerated the procedure well.

FINDINGS

1. Esophageal ulcer.
2. Barrett esophagus.
3. Gastroesophageal reflex.
4. Hiatus hernia.

RECOMMENDATIONS

1. Check biopsies.
2. Continue antireflux diet.
3. Institute antireflux measures such as elevation of head of bed.
4. Will treat with Protonics once a day for 2 weeks.
5. Iron therapy for anemia.

PROOFREADING EXERCISE #2

PREOPERATIVE DIAGNOSES
1. Hepatitis C.
2. Alcohol-related xerosis.

POSTOPERATIVE DIAGNOSES
1. Hepatitis C.
2. Alcohol-related xerosis.

PROCEDURE
Liver transplantation (piggyback).

ANESTHESIA
General endotracheal anesthesia.

FINDINGS
A difficult but uneventful liver transplant was performed for this patient, who has hepatitis C and alcohol-related xerosis. The donor was a 22-year-old local donor who had a motorcycle accident. This appeared to be an excellent liver. It had a small amount of visible fat and the liver produced bile on the table.

DESCRIPTION OF THE PROCEDURE
The patient was supine on the operating table. After he was anesthetized, the skin was prepped and draped in the usual sterile fashion. The abdomen was entered, and approximately 10 liters of acidic was emptied. A midline incision was performed with a small right subcostal extension.

The liver was mobilized, and the hepatogastric ligament was ligated and transected. Then, the hyalin of the liver was clamped and transected. The liver was then stripped from the vena cava. The 3 suprahepatic veins were carefully preserved.

(continued)

Subsequently, the hilar dissection followed. The hepatic artery and bile duck were individually ligated and transected, as was the gastroduodenal artery. The portal vein was mobilized. Then, the new liver was brought into the field. The upper caval anastomosis was performed with 3-0 Prolene, and then the portal vein anastomosis with 5-0 Prolene. Both anastomosis appeared to be satisfactory.

After the liver was reperfused, there was a brief episode of hypertension, which was treated successfully by the anesthesiologist. The hepatic artery anastomosis was performed between the common hepatic artery of the recipient and the celiac artery of the donor using 7-0 choline. The anastomosis appeared to be satisfactory, and the liver started producing bile right away.

The co-surgeon then took over, and he will dictate his portion of the procedure, including the biliary reconstruction.

PROOFREADING EXERCISE #3

PREOPERATIVE DIAGNOSIS
Colorectal neoplasm.

POSTOPERATIVE DIAGNOSES
1. Diverticulosis of the sigmoid and distal dissenting colon.
2. Solitary internal hemorrhoid, grade 1.

PROCEDURE
Colonoscopy.

SURGEON
John Smith, MD.

EQUIPMENT
Olympus video colonoscope.

SPECIMENS
None.

PHOTOGRAPHS
None.

COMPLICATIONS
None.

PREOPERATIVE AND INTRAOPERATIVE MEDICATIONS
Demerol 65 mg and Versed 2.5 mg IV.

POSTOPERATIVE MEDICATIONS
None.

INDICATIONS FOR PROCEDURE
Family history of colorectal neoplasm.

(continued)

FINDINGS
Digital rectal examination was unremarkable. Colonoscopy to the sebum revealed mild-to-moderate diverticulosis in the sigmoid and distal descending colon without any sign of complication of diverticular disease. No other abnormalities of caliper, contour, or mucosa are seen. Withdrawal examination was confirmatory. Retroflexion within the rectum is positive for a small, salivary hemorrhoid.

PROCEDURE: The patient's fully informed consent was obtained prior to scheduling her procedure. She was incrementally sedated prior to and during the procedure as she was carefully observed and monitored. She was awake, comfortable and stable throughout. A digital spectral examination was performed. The colonoscope was introduced per rectum and advanced to the sebum with minimal difficulty, owing to tortuosity, necessitating the application of manual transabdominal pressure.

The iliotibial valve was identified. A withdrawal faze examination to the rectum followed. This was characterized by tip rotation, intermittent insertion and withdrawal, occasional washing and suctioning. Retroflexion within the rectum was accomplished. Air was evacuated from the bowel and the scope was removed. She tolerated the procedure well.

IMPRESSION
Diverticulosis. No sign of spasm in a patient with a family history of colorectal neoplasm.

RECOMMENDATIONS
Anal fecal occult blood testing and repeat colonoscopy in 3–5 years.

PROOFREADING EXERCISE #4

PROCEDURE PERFORMED
Colonoscopy.

INDICATIONS FOR PROCEDURE
Diarrhea with HIM-positive stools.

PREOPERATIVE MEDICATIONS
Demerol 75 mg, Versed 2 mg.

POSTOPERATIVE MEDICATIONS
None.

PROCEDURE IN DETAIL
After adequate sedation had been achieved, a rectal examination was performed and was found to be unremarkable. The Olympus video podiatric colonoscope was then inserted in the usual manner. Examination was completed to the cecum, and the ileocecal valve and appendiceal orifice were identified. The terminal ilium was then entered and it was normal. The cecum itself was caked with semi-solid stool. Even with washing, visualization was suboptimal, but it was felt that the cecum was somewhat nodular, and biopsies were taken through the stool. There did not appear to be a mass although, again, it was suboptimally scene. This patient had been on a 48-hour preparation with clear liquids, 2 bottles of fleet, and also magnesium caprate.

The scope was then withdrawn to the right colon, which had a mild colitis appearance, and in fact this appearance persisted throughout the colon, the hepatic flexor, transverse colon, splenic flexor, descending, sigmoid, and rectum. The appearance was edematous, with mild submucosal hemorrhage and some granularity. Biopsies were taken from the transverse colon and from the rectum. No other pathology was seen except for several diverticulum.

A retrospect view within the rectum showed small internal hemorrhoids.

At the termination of the examination, the patient was drowsy but in no apparent distress.

(continued)

FINAL IMPRESSION

Colonoscopy completed to the cecum and terminal ilium. The examination revealed diffuse colitis of a mild degree, consisting of mild submucosal hemorrhage, granularity, and edema. The cecum was somewhat suboptimally seen due to caking, although there was somewhat of a nodular appearance of some of the mucosa in the cecum. The terminal ilium was normal. Biopsies were taken from the cecum. There was mild colitis in the transverse colon and what appeared to be mild prostatitis in the rectum. There were also small internal hemorrhoids and occasional diverticula seen.

PROOFREADING EXERCISE #5

PROBLEM
Right upper quadrant pain.

SUBJECTIVE
The patient underwent esophagogastroduodenoscopy with miliary drainage to evaluate right upper quadrant pain with suspected gallbladder disease. She was given 8.5 mg CPK without evidence of biliary track emptying. There was no noticeable bile in the bile duct after 10–15 minutes postinjection. She continues to have left upper quadrant pain. There are no associated fevers or chills. A previous hyla scan was normal, as was abdominal sonogram.

OBJECTIVE
VITAL SIGNS: Within normal limits. She is afebrile.
ABDOMEN: Soft, without masses, organomegaly, or ascites. There is moderate epiblastic tenderness. Bowel sounds are normal.

ASSESSMENT
Left upper quadrant pain, etiology unclear. The findings are certainly consistent with gallbladder disease, although her workup to date has been inconclusive.

PLAN
1. Will refer the patient to Dr. Smith for surgical opinion, although there is no strong data pointing to gallbladder disease.
2. Will schedule choloscopy to rule out abnormalities in the hepatic flexure.
3. The patient will be given NuLev.

ANSWER KEYS

REVIEW QUESTIONS ANSWER KEY

1. B
2. B
3. B
4. B
5. B
6. C
7. D
8. C
9. B
10. A
11. B
12. C
13. B
14. C
15. B
16. C
17. D
18. A
19. D
20. A
21. C
22. B
23. A
24. C
25. D
26. A
27. C
28. D
29. C
30. C

PROOFREADING EXERCISE #1 KEY

Incorrect eponym—Barrett

PROCEDURE
Esophagogastroduodenoscopy with biopsies.

PREPROCEDURE DIAGNOSIS
Iron deficiency anemia.

POSTPROCEDURE DIAGNOSES
1. Esophageal ulcer.
2. Garrett esophagus.
3. Hiatal hernia.

DESCRIPTION OF THE PROCEDURE
The procedure was explained to the patient and consent obtained. The patient was then sedated with Demerol 50 mg IV and versed 4 mg IV. The patient was placed in the left lateral decubitus position.

Incorrect eponym—Barrett

Incorrect abbreviation—GE for gastroesophageal

The Olympus video gastroscope was inserted under direct visualization into the esophagus. The esophageal mucosa showed an ulcer at the DE junction with Garrett esophagus extending from 23 cm down to the DE junction at 32 cm. There was a small hiatus hernia.

Incorrect term—patent

Incorrect term—fundus

The scope was advanced into the stomach, which was unremarkable. The pylorus was latent and symmetric. The duodenal bulb and descending duodenum were normal. The scope was drawn back into the antrum, and retroflexed to view the angularis, fondus, and cardia. The hiatus hernia was seen again. The scope was straightened. Multiple biopsies were then taken of the esophageal ulcer and Garrett areas.

Incorrect eponym—Barrett

Incorrect term—celiac

The scope was then withdrawn. It should be noted that duodenal biopsies were also done to rule out cilia disease. The patient tolerated the procedure well.

FINDINGS

1. Esophageal ulcer.
2. Barrett esophagus.
3. Gastroesophageal reflex.
4. Hiatus hernia.

Incorrect term—reflux

RECOMMENDATIONS

1. Check biopsies.
2. Continue antireflux diet.
3. Institute antireflux measures such as elevation of head of bed.
4. Will treat with Protonics once a day for 2 weeks.
5. Iron therapy for anemia.

Incorrect term—Protonix

PROOFREADING EXERCISE #2 KEY

Incorrect term—cirrhosis

PREOPERATIVE DIAGNOSES

1. Hepatitis C.
2. Alcohol-related xerosis.

POSTOPERATIVE DIAGNOSES

1. Hepatitis C.
2. Alcohol-related xerosis.

PROCEDURE

Liver transplantation (piggyback).

ANESTHESIA

General endotracheal anesthesia.

FINDINGS

A difficult but uneventful liver transplant was performed for this patient, who has hepatitis C and alcohol-related xerosis. The donor was a 22-year-old local donor who had a motorcycle accident. This appeared to be an excellent liver. It had a small amount of visible fat and the liver produced bile on the table.

DESCRIPTION OF THE PROCEDURE

Incorrect term—ascites

The patient was supine on the operating table. After he was anesthetized, the skin was prepped and draped in the usual sterile fashion. The abdomen was entered, and approximately 10 liters of acidic was emptied. A midline incision was performed with a small right subcostal extension.

Incorrect term—hilum

The liver was mobilized, and the hepatogastric ligament was ligated and transected. Then, the hyalin of the liver was clamped and transected. The liver was then stripped from the vena cava. The 3 suprahepatic veins were carefully preserved.

Subsequently, the hilar dissection followed. The hepatic artery and bile duck were individually ligated and transected, as was the gastroduodenal artery. The portal vein was mobilized. Then, the new liver was brought into the field. The upper caval anastomosis was performed with 3-0 Prolene, and then the portal vein anastomosis with 5-0 Prolene. Both anastomosis appeared to be satisfactory.

After the liver was reperfused, there was a brief episode of hypertension, which was treated successfully by the anesthesiologist. The hepatic artery anastomosis was performed between the common hepatic artery of the recipient and the celiac artery of the donor using 7-0 choline. The anastomosis appeared to be satisfactory, and the liver started producing bile right away.

The co-surgeon then took over, and he will dictate his portion of the procedure, including the biliary reconstruction.

Incorrect form—plural anastomoses

Incorrect word—duct

Incorrect term—Prolene

PROOFREADING EXERCISE #3 KEY

Incorrect word—descending

PREOPERATIVE DIAGNOSIS
Colorectal neoplasm.

POSTOPERATIVE DIAGNOSES
1. Diverticulosis of the sigmoid and distal dissenting colon.
2. Solitary internal hemorrhoid, grade 1.

PROCEDURE
Colonoscopy.

SURGEON
John Smith, MD.

EQUIPMENT
Olympus video colonoscope.

SPECIMENS
None.

PHOTOGRAPHS
None.

COMPLICATIONS
None.

PREOPERATIVE AND INTRAOPERATIVE MEDICATIONS
Demerol 65 mg and Versed 2.5 mg IV.

POSTOPERATIVE MEDICATIONS
None.

INDICATIONS FOR PROCEDURE
Family history of colorectal neoplasm.

Incorrect term—cecum

Incorrect term—caliber

FINDINGS

Digital rectal examination was unremarkable. Colonoscopy to the sebum revealed mild-to-moderate diverticulosis in the sigmoid and distal descending colon without any sign of complication of diverticular disease. No other abnormalities of caliper, contour, or mucosa are seen. Withdrawal examination was confirmatory. Retroflexion within the rectum is positive for a small, salivary hemorrhoid.

Incorrect word—solitary

PROCEDURE:

Incorrect term—rectal

The patient's fully informed consent was obtained prior to scheduling her procedure. She was incrementally sedated prior to and during the procedure as she was carefully observed and monitored. She was awake, comfortable and stable throughout. A digital spectral examination was performed. The colonoscope was introduced per rectum and advanced to the sebum with minimal difficulty, owing to tortuosity, necessitating the application of manual transabdominal pressure.

Incorrect word—cecum

Incorrect term—ileocecal

The iliotibial valve was identified. A withdrawal faze examination to the rectum followed. This was characterized by tip rotation, intermittent insertion and withdrawal, occasional washing and suctioning. Retroflexion within the rectum was accomplished. Air was evacuated from the bowel and the scope was removed. She tolerated the procedure well.

Incorrect spelling—phase

IMPRESSION

Diverticulosis. No sign of spasm in a patient with a family history of colorectal neoplasm.

Incorrect term—neoplasm

RECOMMENDATIONS

Anal fecal occult blood testing and repeat colonoscopy in 3–5 years.

Incorrect word—annual

PROOFREADING EXERCISE #4 KEY

PROCEDURE PERFORMED
Colonoscopy.

INDICATIONS FOR PROCEDURE
Diarrhea with HIM-positive stools.

PREOPERATIVE MEDICATIONS
Demerol 75 mg, Versed 2 mg.

POSTOPERATIVE MEDICATIONS
None.

PROCEDURE IN DETAIL
After adequate sedation had been achieved, a rectal examination was performed and was found to be unremarkable. The Olympus video podiatric colonoscope was then inserted in the usual manner. Examination was completed to the cecum, and the ileocecal valve and appendiceal orifice were identified. The terminal ilium was then entered and it was normal. The cecum itself was caked with semi-solid stool. Even with washing, visualization was suboptimal, but it was felt that the cecum was somewhat nodular, and biopsies were taken through the stool. There did not appear to be a mass although, again, it was suboptimally scene. This patient had been on a 48-hour preparation with clear liquids, 2 bottles of fleet, and also magnesium caprate.

The scope was then withdrawn to the right colon, which had a mild colitis appearance, and in fact this appearance persisted throughout the colon, the hepatic flexor, transverse colon, splenic flexor, descending, sigmoid, and rectum. The appearance was edematous, with mild submucosal hemorrhage and some granularity. Biopsies were taken from the transverse colon and from the rectum. No other pathology was seen except for several diverticulum.

Incorrect term—heme

Incorrect term—pediatric

Incorrect spelling—ileum

Incorrect spelling—seen

Incorrect term—citrate

Capitalize product names—Fleet

Incorrect word—flexure

Plural form required—diverticula

A retrospect view within the rectum showed small internal hemorrhoids.

Incorrect term—retroflexed

At the termination of the examination, the patient was drowsy but in no apparent distress.

FINAL IMPRESSION

Colonoscopy completed to the cecum and terminal ilium. The examination revealed diffuse colitis of a mild degree, consisting of mild submucosal hemorrhage, granularity, and edema. The cecum was somewhat suboptimally seen due to caking, although there was somewhat of a nodular appearance of some of the mucosa in the cecum. The terminal ilium was normal. Biopsies were taken from the cecum. There was mild colitis in the transverse colon and what appeared to be mild prostatitis in the rectum. There were also small internal hemorrhoids and occasional diverticula seen.

Incorrect spelling—ileum

Incorrect spelling—ileum

Incorrect term—proctitis

PROOFREADING EXERCISE #5 KEY

PROBLEM
Right upper quadrant pain.

SUBJECTIVE
The patient underwent esophagogastroduodenoscopy with miliary drainage to evaluate right upper quadrant pain with suspected gallbladder disease. She was given 8.5 mg CPK without evidence of biliary track emptying. There was no noticeable bile in the bile duct after 10–15 minutes postinjection. She continues to have left upper quadrant pain. There are no associated fevers or chills. A previous hyla scan was normal, as was abdominal sonogram.

OBJECTIVE
VITAL SIGNS: Within normal limits. She is afebrile.
ABDOMEN: Soft, without masses, organomegaly, or ascites. There is moderate epiblastic tenderness. Bowel sounds are normal.

ASSESSMENT
Left upper quadrant pain, etiology unclear. The findings are certainly consistent with gallbladder disease, although her workup to date has been inconclusive.

PLAN
1. Will refer the patient to Dr. Smith for surgical opinion, although there is no strong data pointing to gallbladder disease.
2. Will schedule choloscopy to rule out abnormalities in the hepatic flexure.
3. The patient will be given NuLev.

Incorrect term—biliary

Incorrect abbreviation—CCK

Incorrect word—tract

Incorrect side—right

Incorrect term—HIDA

Incorrect term—epigastric

Incorrect side—right

Incorrect term—colonoscopy (to view hepatic flexure)

CHAPTER

15

Neurology/Neurosurgery

OBJECTIVES CHECKLIST

A prepared exam candidate will know:

- ❑ Combining forms, prefixes, and suffixes related to the body system.
- ❑ Anatomical structures of the nervous system.
- ❑ Physiologic processes of the nervous system.
- ❑ Role of the nervous system as the communication network for the body.
- ❑ Imaging studies used in the identification and diagnosis of neurologic and neurosurgical diseases.
- ❑ Laboratory studies used in the diagnosis and treatment of neurologic symptoms, disorders, and diseases.
- ❑ Common medications prescribed for neurologic symptoms, disorders, and diseases.
- ❑ Transcription standards related to EEGs.

RESOURCES FOR STUDY

1. *The Language of Medicine*
   Chapter 10: Nervous System, pp. 333–382.
2. *H&P: A Nonphysician's Guide to the Medical History and Physical Examination*
   Chapter 12: Review of Systems: Neuromuscular, pp. 107–116.
   Chapter 27: The Neurologic Examination, pp. 261–272.
   Chapter 28: The Formal Mental Status Examination, pp. 261–272.
3. *Human Diseases*
   Chapter 19: Diseases of the Nervous System, pp. 291–314.
4. *Laboratory Tests & Diagnostic Procedures in Medicine*
   Chapter 5: Electroencephalography, Electromyography, and Related Tests, pp. 61–62.
5. *Understanding Pharmacology for Health Professionals*
   Chapter 24: Neurological Drugs, pp. 262–278.
6. *The AAMT Book of Style for Medical Transcription*
   Electroencephalographic Terms, pp. 159–160.

SAMPLE REPORTS

The following five reports are examples of reports you might encounter while transcribing neurology and neurosurgery.

ELECTROENCEPHALOGRAM

HISTORY
The patient is an 82-year-old gentleman with a history of possible subclinical status epilepticus, given the persistent depressed neurological status.

DESCRIPTION OF PROCEDURE
Cerebral activity was grossly disorganized, with asynchrony between the two cerebral hemispheres. Cerebral activity over the left side consisted of medium- to high-amplitude, poorly sustained, 4-Hz to 5-Hz waveforms. Cerebral activity on the right hemisphere consisted of high-amplitude slow waves, often interspersed with spike and spike-and-wave complexes. Periods of attenuation of cerebral activity were noted to occur in the right cerebral hemisphere. At times, the spike and spike-and-wave complexes occurred in a periodic fashion. Superimposed low-amplitude beta activity was noted to occur over the left cerebral hemisphere.

The patient was reported to be obtunded throughout the tracing.

Simultaneous electrocardiogram recording revealed no cardiac arrhythmias.

Activation hyperventilation could not be performed; photic stimulation was not performed.

IMPRESSION
1. Periodic lateralizing epileptiform discharges over the right cerebral hemisphere, as may be seen following an ischemic insult.
2. Global disorganization and slowing of the cerebral activity signifying generalized encephalopathy.

ELECTROMYOGRAM

HISTORY
This is a 76-year-old, right-handed gentleman who presents with a history of many months of worsening intermittent burning, numbness, and tingling involving the hands, predominantly involving the thumb, index, and middle fingers, somewhat more on the left than the right side. The symptoms lead to awakening around 4 a.m. He reports no significant weakness of the hands or tendency to drop objects, etc. There is no significant cervical pain. There is no history of pain involving the feet. There is a strong family history of carpal tunnel syndrome. There is no family history of diabetes.

EXAMINATION
Pertinent neurological examination shows weakness of the thenar muscles with slight atrophy, more on the left than the right side. There are sensory disturbances involving the palmar aspect of the hands. Positive Tinel sign. Negative median compression. Negative Phalen test bilaterally. Range of motion of the neck is painless though globally limited.

INTERPRETATION
1. Severe prolongation of the distal motor latencies, negligible compartment selection potentials, and reduction of motor conduction velocity in the right median nerve.
2. Marked prolongation of the resting motor latencies, reduction of compartment selection potentials, and normal conduction velocity in the left median nerve.
3. Prolongation of the distal motor latencies, reduction of the compartment selection potentials, and reduction of motor conduction velocities in both ulnar nerves.
4. Unobtainable F-wave latency of the right median nerve.
5. Prolongation of the F-wave latency in the left median nerve.
6. Marked prolongation of the distal motor latencies in both ulnar nerves.
7. Unobtainable NAP and SNAP amplitudes on the right median nerve.
8. Severe reduction of the NAP and SNAP amplitudes and moderate to severe reduction in sensory conduction velocity in the left median nerve.
9. Normal NAP and SNAP amplitudes and marked slowing of the sensory conduction velocity in both ulnar nerves.
10. Needle EMG of the muscles of the upper extremities reveals mild to moderate denervation changes involving the median-innervated hand muscles.

IMPRESSION
This study is consistent with bilateral sensorimotor median neuropathy at the wrists, as seen in association with carpal tunnel syndrome. This is of a severe degree on the right side and a moderate to severe degree on the left side. Surgical release is warranted to prevent ongoing axonal loss.

This study also reveals evidence of a mild bilateral sensory neuropathy. There is no evidence of lower cervical radiculopathy involving the upper extremities.

(continued)

RECOMMENDATIONS

1. Staged surgical release of the carpal tunnels, right followed by the left.
2. Staged steroid injections in the carpal tunnels while waiting for surgical release.
3. Cock-up wrist splints can be placed, properly fitting.
4. Avoidance of repetitive wrist movements and weight lifting.
5. Two-hour glucose tolerance test, CBC, Chem-25, ESR, ANA, RA, and TSH, if not already done.

OPERATIVE NOTE

DATE OF OPERATION
05/15/2004

ATTENDING SURGEON
John Smith, MD.

PREOPERATIVE DIAGNOSIS
Acquired cranial defect.

POSTOPERATIVE DIAGNOSIS
Acquired cranial defect.

PROCEDURE PERFORMED
Titanium bar and methyl methacrylate cranioplasty, left frontal, greater than 5 cm.

ANESTHESIA
General endotracheal.

INDICATIONS FOR PROCEDURE
The patient is a 33-year-old white male status post gunshot wound to the left frontal region. He has recovered well and presents now for replacement of the bone flap with a cranioplasty.

DESCRIPTION OF PROCEDURE
The patient was brought to the operating room and placed on the table in the supine position, intubated, and given general endotracheal anesthesia. The head was turned to the right side. The frontal portion of the skull was shaved and prepped with Betadine scrub and Betadine solution. The previous biparietal flap was identified, but it was opted to include our incision within the boundaries of the flap in order to minimize the amount of dissection.

A frontotemporal flap was then traced out and infiltrated with 0.5% lidocaine with 1:200,000 epinephrine, and a skin incision was made with a #10 blade. This incision was carried down through the pericranium. Raney clips were placed on the edges for hemostasis. The temporal muscle was left intact, and the flap was rotated anteriorly and held in place with towel clips. Using sharp dissection, we lifted the flap off the underlying dura. We revised the edges of the bone and then we placed several KLS Martin plates across the defect holding them in place with 5-mm screws.

With this being done, we mixed the methyl methacrylate and placed it over the cranial defect in order to approximate the shape and size of the defect. Once the plastic had cured adequately, and after copious amounts of antibiotic irrigation, we closed the galea with 2-0 Vicryl. The skin was closed with 3-0 Prolene, and we placed a sterile dressing over the area.

The patient was subsequently transferred to the recovery room in stable condition.

ESTIMATED BLOOD LOSS
Approximately 150 mL.

COMPLICATIONS
None.

OPERATIVE REPORT

OPERATIVE DATE
05/15/2004

ATTENDING SURGEON
John Smith, MD.

PREOPERATIVE DIAGNOSES
1. Open bitable frontal sinus fracture.
2. Cerebrospinal fluid leak.

POSTOPERATIVE DIAGNOSES
1. Open bitable frontal sinus fracture.
2. Cerebrospinal fluid leak.

PROCEDURES PERFORMED
1. Bifrontal craniotomy.
2. Exenteration of frontal sinuses.
3. Primary repair of dural tear and closure with pericranium of frontobasal dural tear.
4. Placement of lumbar drain.

ANESTHESIA
General endotracheal anesthesia.

COMPLICATIONS
None.

ESTIMATED BLOOD LOSS
Approximately 250 mL.

INDICATIONS FOR PROCEDURE
The patient is a 19-year-old female status post blunt head trauma to the right forehead and frontal region after she hit a tree during a boating accident. She lost consciousness but was initially a Glasgow coma score of 14 upon initial evaluation. She was subsequently intubated on the scene and transported to our facility for further management.

Her CT scan revealed a bitable frontal sinus fracture carrying down to the level of the cribriform plate and near the sella turcica. She also had cerebrospinal fluid emanating from the frontal skull fracture. She was awake and following commands at that time, although she was still intubated.

PROCEDURE IN DETAIL
After the patient was taken to the operating room and placed in the supine position, adequate general endotracheal anesthesia was induced. Her right bifrontal region was shaved and prepped in the usual sterile fashion.

(continued)

At this time, she was placed in the reflex position with the head up. The bifrontal skin flap was connected utilizing the existing laceration and carried down to approximately 1 cm above the zygoma bilaterally. The coronal skin flap was reflected anteriorly and, with the aid of the Bovie electrocautery, we carried the flap forward and undermined the temporalis muscle at the pericranium. This dissection was carried down to the level of the supraorbital ridge and also to the keyholes laterally.

Next, 1 bur hole each was placed on the keyhole sites as well as 2 parasagittal bur holes posteriorly, along with 1 midline bur hole near the midline over the sinus. After the underlying dura was dissected free with a #3 Penfield dissector, the craniotome was used to connect the bur holes. No dural tear was evident and the bone flap was elevated.

At this time, the exenteration of the frontal sinus was completed with the use of rongeurs as well as curettes. The posterior walls of the frontal sinus were bitten off with Leksell rongeurs. At this time, attention was turned to the frontal basilar dural tear, and the brain retractor was used to retract the frontal lobe backwards. The #1 Penfield dissector was used to dissect the dura away from the crista galli. A linear, anteroposterior, long dural tear, approximately 3 cm in length, was noted along the left basal frontal region over the cribriform plate. The area was irrigated and the anterior portion of the tear was closed primarily with a 5-0 Prolene suture.

Because of the depth of the injury and the possible injury that could be caused by further retraction and dissection, it was decided that a piece of pericranium would be used to cover the dural tear and a lumbar drain would be placed at the end of the procedure. The remainder of the dura was carefully inspected and no other dural tears were encountered. Dural tack-ups with 4-0 Prolene were next performed. Surgicel was placed over the bony edges as well as over the superior sagittal sinus. Adequate hemostasis was obtained with the above as well as with Gelfoam and bipolar electrocautery.

At this time, the procedure was turned over to the oral-maxillofacial surgery service for reconstruction of the frontal bone as well as the left orbital roof defect. A lumbar drain was placed at the end of this procedure.

Sponge, laparotomy pad, instrument, and needle counts were correct x2 at the end of our procedure. The patient tolerated this portion of the procedure well, remaining hemodynamically stable. She was given intravenous antibiotics as well as Dilantin.

HISTORY & PHYSICAL

This is a 23-year-old adult white male who was seen in neurological evaluation for a history of recurrent syncope. He reports his first episode took place in 1997, the second one in 2000, and the third one was in 2001. Each of these episodes was connected with drawing of blood, and right after that he passed out for a few seconds. There was no reported history of convulsant movements and no reported history of confusion following the episodes.

PAST MEDICAL HISTORY
He denies any injuries to his head. He has had some broken bones in his arms in the past. He denies any trouble seeing, hearing, or swallowing and has had no weakness, no numbness, no sphincter disturbances. He denies any chest pain, cough, nausea, vomiting, or urinary symptoms on review of systems.

SOCIAL HISTORY
He states that he is the only child in his family. His father used to have similar problems of passing out when blood was drawn in an office situation, but he does not pass out when blood is drawn in the home situation.

ALLERGIES
No known drug allergies.

PAST SURGICAL HISTORY
Positive for a tonsillectomy in the past.

PHYSICAL EXAMINATION
GENERAL: This is a well-built, tall-looking male who appears to be in no acute distress.
HEAD: Normocephalic.
EENT: Extraocular movements are full, pupils are reactive to light, and disks are sharp. No apparent facial asymmetry seen. Facial sensations are preserved. Hearing is intact. Swallowing is intact. Tongue is midline on protrusion.
NECK: Supple, no bruit heard.
CHEST: Clear.
HEART: Normal sinus rhythm.
ABDOMEN: Soft, nontender with no organomegaly.
EXTREMITIES: Moves all four extremities.
NEUROLOGICAL EXAMINATION: Alert, mental status intact, cranial nerves intact, motor system intact for strength, tone, and bulk. Sensory examination intact to all modalities. Cerebellar functions are intact. Reflexes are 2+ to 3+ and symmetrical. Bilateral plantars are downgoing. Neurovascular examination is unremarkable.

IMPRESSION
Vasovagal syncope. Neurologically, no other significant abnormalities are noted. As he has never had an EEG, an EEG might be needed to exclude any possible seizure discharges. I doubt this, as his history does not indicate any evidence suggestive of seizures at this time.

REVIEW QUESTIONS

The goal of these questions is to test your knowledge in the areas of neurology and neurosurgery.

Directions: Select the correct answer for each of the multiple-choice questions provided below. *Answers are provided at the end of this chapter.*

1. The trigeminal (cranial) nerve is number:
   - A. I
   - B. II
   - C. V
   - D. VII
2. An inflammation of the membrane covering of the brain and spinal cord is called:
   - A. Myelitis
   - B. Meningitis
   - C. Neuritis
   - D. Radiculitis
3. The term somnambulism means:
   - A. Sleepwalking
   - B. Excessive dreaming
   - C. REM sleep
   - D. Chronic insomnia
4. Paralysis on only one side of the body is termed:
   - A. Paraplegia
   - B. Hemiplegia
   - C. Quadriplegia
   - D. Diplegia
5. The suffix meaning seizure is:
   - A. -plegia
   - B. -phasia
   - C. -lepsy
   - D. -lexia
6. Cephalgia means:
   - A. Head pain
   - B. Perineal pain
   - C. Sinus pain
   - D. Brain swelling
7. Loss of the power of expression by speech is called:
   - A. Aphakia
   - B. Dyslexia
   - C. Coprolalia
   - D. Aphasia
8. A glioma is a tumor consisting of:
   - A. Myelin
   - B. Neuroglial cells
   - C. Meningeal cells
   - D. Ganglion cells
9. The root word meaning "root of a spinal nerve" is:
   - A. Myel/o
   - B. Radicul/o
   - C. Mening/o
   - D. Gangli/o
10. Encephalomalacia literally means:
    - A. Brain tumor
    - B. Absence of brain matter
    - C. Headache
    - D. Softening of brain
11. Which of the following terms would be used in an electroencephalogram?
    - A. ST-T waves
    - B. Hypoechoic
    - C. Mu pattern
    - D. QRS axis
12. Under which heading in the physical examination would you find mention of "dysdiadochokinesia"?
    - A. HEENT examination
    - B. Abdominal examination
    - C. Neurological examination
    - D. Musculoskeletal examination

13. A ventriculoperitoneal shunt is placed to relieve:
    A. Spina bifida
    B. Hydrocephalus
    C. Hirschsprung disease
    D. Strabismus.

14. An incomplete closure of the vertebrae in newborns is:
    A. Cerebral palsy
    B. Muscular dystrophy
    C. Spina bifida
    D. Myasthenia gravis

15. One type of brain cancer is:
    A. Astrocytoma
    B. Retinoblastoma
    C. Osteosarcoma
    D. Epithelioma

16. The central nervous system is made up of the:
    A. Brain and ventricles
    B. Spinal cord and cerebrospinal fluid
    C. Brain and spinal cord
    D. Peripheral nervous system and CSF

17. A cerebral concussion is usually caused by:
    A. Blunt trauma
    B. Cerebral aneurysm
    C. Loss of consciousness
    D. Aspirin overdose

18. Damage to the right side of the brain may cause:
    A. Right sided paralysis
    B. Quadriplegia
    C. Left sided paralysis
    D. Paraplegia

19. Cerebral aneurysm is sometimes treated with:
    A. Craniectomy
    B. Clipping
    C. Biopsy
    D. Coumadin therapy

20. Acute bacterial meningitis may occur as a sequela to:
    A. Claudication
    B. Otitis media
    C. Viral encephalitis
    D. Fibroadenoma

21. Encephalitis may result following:
    A. Rubella
    B. Seizure activity
    C. Decubitus ulcers
    D. Parkinson disease

22. Which of these is a type of epileptic seizure?
    A. Apraxic
    B. Absence
    C. Kyphotic
    D. Lordotic

23. If a patient with a migraine took Imitrex with relief of her headache, her symptoms can said to have been:
    A. Elevated
    B. Alleviated
    C. Aggravated
    D. Allocated

24. Diazepam is a benzodiazepine that is used to treat anxiety and acute muscle spasms. One other use of diazepam is for the treatment of:
    A. Status epilepticus
    B. Migraine headaches
    C. Cocaine overdose
    D. Multiple sclerosis

25. Which test would be used to assess the brain?
    A. Meckel scan
    B. Doppler
    C. MRI
    D. VQ scan

26. The electrical activity of the brain is recorded via:
    A. Electrocardiogram
    B. Thermogram
    C. Electroencephalogram
    D. Sonogram

27. Involuntary reflexes are termed:
    A. Somatic
    B. Autonomic
    C. Proprioceptive
    D. Polarized

28. An ICP monitor may be placed by the neurosurgeon by drilling into the:
    A. Skull
    B. Auricular canal
    C. Olecranon
    D. Mandible

29. The number of cranial nerve pairs:
    A. 6
    B. 10
    C. 12
    D. 24

30. A lumbar puncture is done to test the:
    A. Cerebrospinal fluid
    B. Cauda equina
    C. Dura mater
    D. Grey and white matter

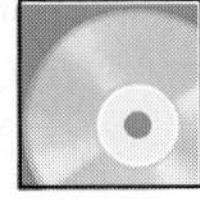

Please see the accompanying CD for additional review materials for this section.

PROOFREADING EXERCISES

These three proofreading exercises are provided to improve your skills in the areas of editing and effective identification and correction of errors in the medical record.

Directions: Identify and correct the transcription errors found in the exercises below. *Answers are provided at the end of this chapter.*

PROOFREADING EXERCISE #1

This is a standard digital ECG on a 72-year-old female, done for altered dental status, lethargy, and confusion.

The general cerebral background activity consists of symmetrical, fairly regular, 6–7 Hz dominant rhythm with bay activity symmetrically on both sides. The tracing also shows drowsy and light sleep stages.

Phobic stimulation and hyperventilation were not performed.

IMPRESSION: Slightly slow, but fairly regular, sustained basic cerebral rhythm.

There are no excessive slow waves. There are no abnormal discharges and no vocal abnormalities.

PROOFREADING EXERCISE #2

HISTORY OF PRESENT ILLNESS
This is a 17-year-old girl who was admitted here following 2 seizure episodes. She says that she has been having seizures since the age of 5 and she has frequent seizures. She feels dizzy prior to the onset of a seizure, looses consciousness, and has a major motor seizure. She denies any headache or visual difficulties, weakness, numbness, or sphincter disturbances. She states she had no history of injury or central nervous system infections.

ALLERGIES
No known drug allergies.

PAST SURGICAL HISTORY
None.

MEDICATIONS
Her Diflucan level of 17.

FAMILY HISTORY
Her father has seizures as does a cousin on the maternal side. She has 3 siblings and they have no history of seizures.

PHYSICAL EXAMINATION
GENERAL: On examination, this is an average-built young woman who appears to be in no acute distress.
HEENT: Normocephalic and atraumatic. Extra ocular movements intact. Pupils are equal, round, regular, and reactive to light and accommodation. Discs are sharp with no apparent facial asymmetry seen. Fascial sensations are preserved. Hearing is intact. Swallowing is intact. Tongue is midline on protrusion.
NECK: Supple, no jugular venous distension, and no bruit.
CHEST: Clear.
HEART: Normal sinus rhythm.
ABDOMEN: Soft and nontender with no organomegaly or hepatosplenomegaly.
EXTREMITIES: She moves all 4 extremities well.

(continued)

NEUROLOGIC: Alert. Mental status is intact. Cranial nerves intact. Motor system intact for strength, tone, and bulk. Century examination is intact to all modalities. Lamellar functions are intact. Reflexes are 2+ to 3+ and symmetrical. Plantars are downgoing bilaterally. Neuro vascular status is unremarkable.

IMPRESSION
Seizure disorder.

RECOMMENDATIONS
An electrocardiogram is being done but, neurologically, there are no focal deferents. We will see her again in followup on an as needed basis.

PROOFREADING EXERCISE #3

DATE OF SURGERY
05/15/2004

ATTENDING SURGEON
John Smith, MD.

FIRST ASSISTANT SURGEON
Mary Jones, MD.

PREOPERATIVE DIAGNOSIS
Left central parietal occipital oppressed skull fracture.

POSTOPERATIVE DIAGNOSIS
Same.

PROCEDURES PERFORMED
1. Elevation of oppressed fracture.
2. Craniectomy.
3. Irrigation and debridement of bone fragments.

ANESTHESIA
General endotracheal.

INTRAVENOUS FLUIDS
Crystalloid.

ESTIMATED BLOOD LOSS
Approximately 200 mL.

INDICATIONS FOR PROCEDURE
The patient is a 23-year-old male status post motor vehicle accident while driving a speedboat. The patient crashed into a bridge. The patient came in with a Glasgow coma score of 115 and was intubated. He had a right temporal confusion and a left open parietooccipital depressed fracture with evidence of new Mohs acephalus. The patient also had a C7 burst fracture with about 10% compromise of the ventral canal. The patient was taken immediately to the operating room to irritate and débride the dirty wound as well as to elevate the depressed fragment.

(continued)

DESCRIPTION OF PROCEDURE

The patient was transferred to the operating room table and placed in 3-point fixation on a Mayfield head holder. Close attention was paid to the patient's unstable cervical fracture. There was no misalignment. The patient was taken off the bored after being log-rolled very carefully, maintaining the head in traction.

The hair was removed using a racer blade and the stapled, jagged, 15-cm incision was prepped using sterile standard technique, at which time the wound was irrigated with approximately 2 liters of antibiotic-impregnated phthalein. After prepping and setting up the standard craniotomy operative site, the incision was extended in a lazy-S fashion, both in a vertical direction as well as in a slight horizontal fashion.

The incision edges were tamponaded using Raney clips after which towel clips were used to expose the depressed skull fracture. A bur hole was placed at the base of the decision away from the depressed fragment, after which a rongeur and a Kerrison were used to craniectomize the depressed fragment.

There was no evidence of mural tears or cerebrospinal fluid leakage. All of the depressed bone fragments were débrided. The wound itself was also débrided. The incision edges were débrided as well as the jagged incisions. The entire wound was then irrigated with approximately 4 liters of antibiotic-impregnated normal saline, after which the Raney clips were removed. All scalp leaders were coagulated, and the wound was closed using 2-0 Prolene in interrupted dress sutures.

The patient tolerated the procedure well and his vital signs remained stable. After covering the incision, the patient was placed in tong traction. He was subsequently placed on a Roto-Rest bed, paying close attention to his surgical spine. The patient remained intubated and was transferred to the neurosurgical intensive care unit.

ANSWER KEYS

REVIEW QUESTIONS ANSWER KEY

1. C
2. B
3. A
4. B
5. C
6. A
7. D
8. B
9. B
10. D
11. C
12. C
13. B
14. C
15. A
16. C
17. A
18. C
19. B
20. B
21. A
22. B
23. B
24. A
25. C
26. C
27. B
28. A
29. C
30. A

PROOFREADING EXERCISE #1 KEY

This is a standard digital ECG on a 72-year-old female, done for altered dental status, lethargy, and confusion.

The general cerebral background activity consists of symmetrical, fairly regular, 6–7 Hz dominant rhythm with bay activity symmetrically on both sides. The tracing also shows drowsy and light sleep stages.

Phobic stimulation and hyperventilation were not performed.

IMPRESSION: Slightly slow, but fairly regular, sustained basic cerebral rhythm.

There are no excessive slow waves. There are no abnormal discharges and no vocal abnormalities.

Incorrect abbreviation—EEG

Incorrect term—mental

Incorrect term—beta

Incorrect term—photic

Incorrect term—focal

PROOFREADING EXERCISE #2 KEY

Incorrect word—loses

Incorrect term—infarctions

Incorrect drug—Dilantin

Use combined form—extraocular

Incorrect spelling—facial

HISTORY OF PRESENT ILLNESS
This is a 17-year-old girl who was admitted here following 2 seizure episodes. She says that she has been having seizures since the age of 5 and she has frequent seizures. She feels dizzy prior to the onset of a seizure, looses consciousness, and has a major motor seizure. She denies any headache or visual difficulties, weakness, numbness, or sphincter disturbances. She states she had no history of injury or central nervous system infections.

ALLERGIES
No known drug allergies.

PAST SURGICAL HISTORY
None.

MEDICATIONS
Her Diflucan level is 17.

FAMILY HISTORY
Her father has seizures as does a cousin on the maternal side. She has 3 siblings and they have no history of seizures.

PHYSICAL EXAMINATION
GENERAL: On examination, this is an average-built young woman who appears to be in no acute distress.
HEENT: Normocephalic and atraumatic. Extra ocular movements intact. Pupils are equal, round, regular, and reactive to light and accommodation. Discs are sharp with no apparent facial asymmetry seen. Fascial sensations are preserved. Hearing is intact. Swallowing is intact. Tongue is midline on protrusion.

NECK: Supple, no jugular venous distension, and no bruit.
CHEST: Clear.
HEART: Normal sinus rhythm.
ABDOMEN: Soft and nontender with no organomegaly or hepatosplenomegaly.
EXTREMITIES: She moves all 4 extremities well.
NEUROLOGIC: Alert. Mental status is intact. Cranial nerves intact. Motor system intact for strength, tone, and bulk. Century examination is intact to all modalities. Lamellar functions are intact. Reflexes are 2+ to 3+ and symmetrical. Plantars are downgoing bilaterally. Neuro vascular status is unremarkable.

Incorrect term—sensory

Incorrect term—cerebellar

IMPRESSION
Seizure disorder.

RECOMMENDATIONS
An electrocardiogram is being done but, neurologically, there are no focal deferents. We will see her again in followup on an as needed basis.

Incorrect test—electroenceph-alogram

Incorrect term—deficits

PROOFREADING EXERCISE #3 KEY

Use combined form—parieto-occipital

Repeat full text, do not use "same"

Flag—invalid number for Glasgow scale

Incorrect word—depressed

Incorrect term—contusion

DATE OF SURGERY
05/15/2004

ATTENDING SURGEON
John Smith, MD.

FIRST ASSISTANT SURGEON
Mary Jones, MD.

PREOPERATIVE DIAGNOSIS
Left central parietal occipital oppressed skull fracture.

POSTOPERATIVE DIAGNOSIS
Same.

PROCEDURES PERFORMED

1. Elevation of oppressed fracture.
2. Craniectomy.
3. Irrigation and debridement of bone fragments.

ANESTHESIA
General endotracheal.

INTRAVENOUS FLUIDS
Crystalloid.

ESTIMATED BLOOD LOSS
Approximately 200 mL.

INDICATIONS FOR PROCEDURE
The patient is a 23-year-old male status post motor vehicle accident while driving a speedboat. The patient crashed into a bridge. The patient came in with a Glasgow coma score of 115 and was intubated. He had a right temporal confusion and a left open parietooccipital depressed fracture with

evidence of new Mohs acephalus. The patient also had a C7 burst fracture with about 10% compromise of the ventral canal. The patient was taken immediately to the operating room to irritate and débride the dirty wound as well as to elevate the depressed fragment.

Incorrect terms—pneumocephalus

Incorrect term—central

Incorrect word—irrigate

DESCRIPTION OF PROCEDURE

The patient was transferred to the operating room table and placed in 3-point fixation on a Mayfield head holder. Close attention was paid to the patient's unstable cervical fracture. There was no misalignment. The patient was taken off the bored after being log-rolled very carefully, maintaining the head in traction.

Incorrect spelling—board

The hair was removed using a racer blade and the stapled, jagged, 15-cm incision was prepped using sterile standard technique, at which time the wound was irrigated with approximately 2 liters of antibiotic-impregnated phthalein. After prepping and setting up the standard craniotomy operative site, the incision was extended in a lazy-S fashion, both in a vertical direction as well as in a slight horizontal fashion.

Incorrect term—saline

Incorrect word—razor

The incision edges were tamponaded using Raney clips after which towel clips were used to expose the depressed skull fracture. A bur hole was placed at the base of the decision away from the depressed fragment, after which a rongeur and a Kerrison were used to craniectomize the depressed fragment.

Incorrect term—incision

There was no evidence of mural tears or cerebrospinal fluid leakage. All of the depressed bone fragments were débrided. The wound itself was also débrided. The incision edges were débrided as well as the jagged incisions. The entire wound was then irrigated with approximately

Incorrect term—dural

4 liters of antibiotic-impregnated normal saline, after which the Raney clips were removed. All scalp leaders were coagulated, and the wound was closed using 2-0 Prolene in interrupted dress sutures.

The patient tolerated the procedure well and his vital signs remained stable. After covering the incision, the patient was placed in tong traction. He was subsequently placed on a Roto-Rest bed, paying close attention to his surgical spine. The patient remained intubated and was transferred to the neurosurgical intensive care unit.

Incorrect word—bleeders

Incorrect word—mattress

Incorrect term—cervical

CHAPTER

16

Obstetrics & Gynecology/ Genetics/Pediatrics

OBJECTIVES CHECKLIST

A prepared exam candidate will know:

- ❑ Combining forms, prefixes, and suffixes related to the body system.
- ❑ Anatomy and structures of the reproductive system.
- ❑ Physiology and function of the organs of the reproductive system.
- ❑ Role of hormones in the reproductive process and reproductive health.
- ❑ Terminology related to gestation, labor, delivery, and neonatal care.
- ❑ Role of genetic testing in diagnosing and treating developmental disorders.
- ❑ Common imaging and diagnostic studies used in the treatment of obstetric and gynecologic diseases.
- ❑ Common imaging and diagnostic studies used in the treatment of diseases unique to pediatrics.
- ❑ Laboratory tests ordered to diagnose and monitor the symptoms and diseases related to reproductive medicine.
- ❑ Laboratory tests ordered to diagnose and monitor the symptoms and diseases related to genetics and pediatrics.
- ❑ Transcription standards pertaining to gestational terminology, labor and delivery, and chromosomal delineation.

RESOURCES FOR STUDY

1. *The Language of Medicine*
   Chapter 8: Female Reproductive System, pp. 253–304.
2. *H&P: A Nonphysician's Guide to the Medical History and Physical Examination*
   Chapter 11: Review of Systems: Genitourinary, pp. 97–106.
   Chapter 25: Examination of the Abdomen, Groins, Rectum, Anus, and Genitalia, pp. 235–248.
   Chapter 29: The Pediatric History and Physical Examination, pp. 281–290.
3. *Human Diseases*
   Chapter 2: Genetic Disorders, pp. 15–26.
   Chapter 13: Diseases of the Female Reproductive System, pp. 189–204.
   Chapter 14: Pregnancy and Childbirth, pp. 205–222.
4. *Laboratory Tests & Diagnostic Procedures in Medicine*
   Chapter 8: Examination of the Digestive Tract and Genitourinary System, pp. 107–118.
   Chapter 20: Chemical Examination of the Blood (Hormones), pp. 366–367.
   Chapter 23: Molecular Biology (Medical Genetics, Genetic Abnormalities, and Genetic Testing), pp. 423–436
5. *Understanding Pharmacology for Health Professionals*
   Chapter 23: Obstetric/Gynecologic Drugs, pp. 243–261.
6. *The AAMT Book of Style for Medical Transcription*
   Obstetrics, pp. 289–291.
   Genetics, pp. 183–186.
   Genes, pp. 186–188.

SAMPLE REPORTS

The following six reports are examples of reports you might encounter while transcribing obstetrics and gynecology, genetics, and pediatrics.

OPERATIVE REPORT

SURGEON OF RECORD
John Smith, MD.

RESIDENT SURGEON
Mary Jones, MD.

PREOPERATIVE DIAGNOSIS
Oligohydramnios with breech presentation at 35 weeks estimated gestational age.

POSTOPERATIVE DIAGNOSIS
Oligohydramnios with breech presentation at 35 weeks estimated gestational age.

PROCEDURE
Primary low transverse cesarean section via Pfannenstiel skin incision.

ANESTHESIA
Spinal.

ESTIMATED BLOOD LOSS
Approximately 500 mL.

FINDINGS
A viable male infant in the breech presentation, right sacrum anterior. Normal tubes and ovaries bilaterally. Two small fibroids are noted in the uterus. The infant weighed 5 pounds 12 ounces and Apgar scores were 9 and 9.

PROCEDURE
The patient was taken to the operating room and placed in the dorsal lithotomy position after being given a spinal anesthesia without difficulty. She was then prepped and draped in the usual sterile fashion. A Pfannenstiel skin incision was made with a scalpel and carried through the underlying layer of fascia with the use of electrocautery. The fascial incision was extended laterally, and the superior aspect of the fascial incision was grasped with Kocher clamps, elevated upward, and the rectus muscle was dissected off with the use of cautery. In a similar fashion, this was done at the inferior aspect of the fascial incision.

The muscles were separated. The peritoneum was entered and the incision was extended with the use of a gentle tug. A bladder blade was inserted, and the vesicouterine peritoneum was identified, held with pickups, and entered with Metzenbaum scissors. The incision was extended laterally and a bladder flap was created digitally. The bladder blade was then inserted.

(continued)

The lower uterine segment was incised in transverse fashion, and the incision was extended laterally with the use of bandage scissors. The baby was delivered from a frank breech presentation. The mouth and nose were suctioned and the cord was clamped and cut. Cord blood was sent to pathology, and the infant was then handed off to the awaiting neonatologist.

The placenta was removed manually. The uterus was exteriorized and cleared of all clots and debris. The incision was repaired with #0 Vicryl in running, locked fashion. The uterus was then returned to the pelvis. The gutters were cleared of clots and debris. Hemostasis was assured. The fascia was reapproximated with #0 Vicryl in running fashion. The subcutaneous fat was irrigated, and any bleeders were cauterized and hemostasis was assured. The skin was reapproximated in a subcuticular fashion with the use of 4-0 Vicryl.

The patient tolerated the procedure well. Sponge, instrument, and needle counts were correct x2. The patient was taken to the recovery room in stable condition.

OPERATIVE REPORT

SURGEON
John Smith, MD.

PREOPERATIVE DIAGNOSES
1. Ovarian cyst.
2. Pelvic fluid.

POSTOPERATIVE DIAGNOSES
1. Ovarian cyst.
2. Pelvic fluid.

PROCEDURE
Diagnostic laparoscopy with suction of pelvic fluid for cytology as well as culture and sensitivity.

ANESTHESIA
General endotracheal.

PROCEDURE IN DETAIL
Under satisfactory general anesthesia, the patient was placed in the dorsal lithotomy position, and a tenaculum and cannula were applied to the cervix in the usual manner. The bladder was emptied by simple catheterization. The entire abdomen was then prepped and painted with Betadine soap and solution, cleansed with alcohol solution, and then draped with sterile sheets in the usual manner.

A small subumbilical vertical incision was made at the previous scar line. This incision was deepened through the skin. The primary trocar and cannula were inserted into the abdominal cavity and the primary trocar was removed. Through the primary cannula, the laparoscope was introduced, and the pelvic cavity was well visualized. Meanwhile, carbon dioxide gas was insufflated, and we obtained an adequate pneumoperitoneum. A second puncture was made at McBurney point in the usual manner, and through the second puncture, the retractor was introduced and the abdominal and pelvic cavities were explored.

We found the uterus to be slightly enlarged, with a few leiomyomata noted which appeared to be more of the intramural type. These were located at the top of the uterine fundus. No other abnormalities were noted. Both tubes revealed evidence of an old tubal ligation. Both ovaries were small and cystic, with no evidence of operation noted. No adhesions were noted. The cul-de-sac was inspected and showed a moderate amount of pelvic fluid which was clear. This fluid was subsequently suctioned in the usual manner and sent for cytology and culture and sensitivity. At this point, the procedure was completed.

The laparoscope and retractors were removed from the abdominal cavity. All carbon dioxide gas was also removed, and both primary and secondary cannulas were removed. The deep fascia of the subumbilical wound was suture ligated with #0 Vicryl using interrupted sutures. The subcutaneous tissue of the wound was suture ligated with 2-0 plain using multiple interrupted simple sutures. The skin was approximated with 3-0 plain using continuous subcuticular stitches. The wound of the second puncture was also approximated with 3-0 plain using single simple sutures. A sterile dressing was placed. The tenaculum and cannulas were removed from the vagina and bleeders were checked.

The patient tolerated the procedure well and was sent to the recovery room in stable condition.

ESTIMATED BLOOD LOSS
Less than 10 mL.

HISTORY & PHYSICAL

CHIEF COMPLAINT/HISTORY OF PRESENT ILLNESS
The patient is a 4-year-old African-American female who presented to the office today with a history of a cold for approximately 1 week. She began complaining of right ear pain last evening, and this continued throughout the night, with the patient waking up multiple times throughout the night complaining of pain. She has had a runny nose, but the nasal discharge was clear and this has been improving. She has also had a cough, which has been nonproductive but is worse at nighttime. She has had no vomiting or diarrhea and no rashes have been noted.

PAST MEDICAL HISTORY
Unremarkable with no history of asthma.

IMMUNIZATIONS
Up to date.

ALLERGIES
No known drug allergies.

CURRENT MEDICATIONS
Tylenol, with the last dose at 0400 today.

PHYSICAL EXAMINATION
VITAL SIGNS: Temperature is 97, pulse 105, respirations 24, blood pressure 110/83, and weight is 19.5 kg.
GENERAL: The patient is awake, alert, and cooperative for the examination. She answers appropriately and is nontoxic-appearing.
SKIN: Warm, dry, and intact with no rashes.
HEENT: Head is normocephalic and atraumatic. Pupils are equal, round, and reactive to light, extraocular muscle movements are intact, and she has a normal red reflex bilaterally. The conjunctivae are clear. The left tympanic membrane is normal. The right tympanic membrane is pulsing and erythematous with poor landmarks and decreased mobility. The nose is remarkable for mild mucosal congestion and clear nasal discharge. Oropharynx is clear without erythema or exudates. Mucous membranes are moist.
NECK: Full range of motion with no meningismus. There is mild anterior cervical lymphadenopathy which is nontender and mobile.
CHEST: She has slightly diffuse wheezes on expiration. Aeration is good, there is no respiratory distress, and no retractions are noted.
HEART: Regular rate and rhythm with normal S1 and S2; no murmurs appreciated.
ABDOMEN: Benign.
EXTREMITIES: Peripheral pulses of 2+ were noted, and capillary refill is less than 2 seconds. Extremities are normal.

OFFICE PROCEDURES
During her stay in the office, she was given 2 puffs of albuterol along with a metered-dose inhaler. Subsequently re-evaluation revealed resolution of wheezing with only slightly coarse breath sounds bilaterally and no respiratory distress. The patient was sent home with diagnoses of:

(continued)

DIAGNOSES

1. Right otitis media.
2. Wheezing.
3. Upper respiratory infection.

DISCHARGE INSTRUCTIONS

Amoxicillin 2 teaspoons (250/5 mL) to be given q.12 h. for 10 days, and albuterol 2 puffs with spacer q.i.d. Mother is to encourage fluid intake, avoid contact with cigarette smoke, run a vaporizer in the patient's room with daily water changes, and follow up with my office in 1 week for a repeat evaluation of the wheezing. She is to contact me if the child's symptoms do not improve 24 to 48 hours after starting antibiotics, if symptoms worsen, or if mother has further questions or concerns.

OPERATIVE REPORT

PREOPERATIVE DIAGNOSIS
Fetal malposition, double footling breech.

POSTOPERATIVE DIAGNOSES
1. Fetal malposition, double footling breech.
2. Spigelian hernia.

SURGERY PERFORMED
1. Primary cesarean section, low segment transverse.
2. Spigelian hernia repair.

SURGEON OF RECORD
John Smith, MD.

PROCEDURE IN DETAIL
The patient was taken to the operating theater and given anesthesia without difficulty. She was then sterilely prepped and draped in the usual fashion. A Pfannenstiel skin incision was made transversely, and this was taken down through the anatomical layers. The abdomen was opened atraumatically. A low segment, transverse uterine incision was initiated with the scalpel and bluntly separated with the surgeon's fingers. A breech baby (male) was found in a double footling presentation. Apgar scores were 9 and 9, and the baby weighed 8 pounds 8 ounces. The placenta was delivered spontaneously.

The uterine incision was repaired using #1 Monocryl in a single, running fashion. The peritoneum was well irrigated, and no evidence of active bleeding was noted. The uterus, tubes, and ovaries were found to be within normal limits. The peritoneum was then closed with 2-0 Monocryl in a single, running fashion. The rectus sheath, posterior leaf, was reapproximated at the midline with interrupted #1 sutures of Monocryl for correction of the spigelian hernia. The aponeurosis of the externus and internus were reapproximated using #0 Monocryl in single, running fashion.

The patient tolerated the procedure well without any complications, and she was transferred to the recovery room in stable condition. Skin staples had been applied to the incision site, and these are to be removed 3 days post surgery.

OFFICE NOTE

The patient is a 2½-year-old, here to recheck his eye. Mom reports that overall he did better yesterday but then last night was up screaming and crying and ended up having to go to the emergency room to have it looked at. The emergency room gave him some Tylenol with codeine, and that seemed to provide him relief. They are back this morning for a recheck.

EXAM
He is a very well-appearing 2-year-old, smiling and playful, in no acute distress. He is afebrile. Eye, however, is still very erythematous and swollen, especially inferior to the orbit, but it seems to be nontender. There is now some thick yellow discharge out of the eye.

ASSESSMENT
Conjunctivitis with cellulitis, improving.

PLAN
We will give him one more injection of Rocephin 750 mg IM today in clinic. We'll see him back again first thing tomorrow morning. Same precautions as yesterday, that if he worsens, fever reappears, or if he appears lethargic at all, to call immediately.

OFFICE NOTE

This is an 8-year-old with a deep cough for 4 days and low-grade fever, congestion. Mom says she has a history of bronchial asthma that requires breathing treatments each winter and was originally diagnosed at age 3. She has an SVN machine at home that they have been using intermittently.

PHYSICAL EXAM
She is a well-appearing 8-year-old. She is alert and afebrile. Posterior pharynx is mildly erythematous. Cervical lymphadenopathy. Tympanic membranes are also mildly erythematous but thin. Chest shows decreased aeration, and she coughs frequently with deep breaths. SVN given with 25 mL albuterol and normal saline with good response.

ASSESSMENT
1. Bronchitis.
2. Reactive airway disease.

PLAN
Zithromax 200 mg/5 mL 1¾ teaspoon p.o. today and 1 teaspoon p.o. days 2 through 5. Increase SVNs q.4–6 h. until patient improves.

REVIEW QUESTIONS

The goal of these questions is to test your knowledge in the areas of obstetrics and gynecology, genetics, and pediatrics.

Directions: Select the correct answer for each of the multiple-choice questions provided below. *Answers are provided at the end of this chapter.*

1. The medical term for sexual intercourse is:
   A. Cohabitation
   B. Conjugation
   C. Coitus
   D. Procreation

2. The root word meaning ovary is:
   A. Oophor/o
   B. Vulv/o
   C. Uter/o
   D. Salping/o

3. The neck of the uterus is called the:
   A. Vagina
   B. Adnexa
   C. Cervix
   D. Vulva

4. Clomid is an example of:
   A. A labor-inducing drug
   B. A birth control pill
   C. Hormone replacement therapy
   D. An ovulation-stimulating drug

5. The patient is a 31-year-old gravida 2, para 1, abortus 1. How many living children does she have?
   A. One
   B. Two
   C. None
   D. Three

6. To produce milk following birth is to:
   A. Lacrimate
   B. Lactate
   C. Micturate
   D. Procreate

7. Surgical removal of the fallopian tubes is called:
   A. Salpingogram
   B. Salpingectomy
   C. Oophorectomy
   D. Hysterectomy

8. The membrane enveloping the fetus is called the:
   A. Chorion
   B. Uterus
   C. Oviduct
   D. Amnion

9. An episiotomy is performed to aid in:
   A. Bladder reconstruction
   B. Hemorrhoidectomy
   C. Childbirth
   D. Menstruation

10. Gravida 1, para 2, abortus 0 would mean:
    A. Twins
    B. Triplets
    C. Singleton
    D. Three miscarriages

11. The first feces of the newborn is called:
    A. Meconium
    B. Mentation
    C. Mercurochrome
    D. Melena

12. The pituitary hormone which stimulates uterine contractions is:
    A. Pitocin
    B. Oxytocin
    C. Estrogen
    D. FSH

13. Why is it dangerous for a newborn to have a bowel movement in utero?
    A. Malrotation can develop.
    B. Feces could be aspirated.
    C. Intussusception is possible.
    D. Volvulus can result.

14. A 24-year-old woman comes into the ER with abdominal pain, and a tentative diagnosis of ectopic pregnancy is made. What lab test must be ordered?
    A. AFP
    B. PSA level
    C. beta HCG level
    D. Free P2 and P4 levels

15. A pelvic sonogram in a woman with menometrorrhagia and chronic hypogastric pain might help diagnose:
    A. Vena cava syndrome
    B. Hiatal hernia
    C. Vaginal atrophy
    D. Leiomyoma uteri

16. You are given this information: The woman is gravida 2, para 3-0-0-3. What could this mean?
    A. She had two pregnancies, 3 live births, 3 miscarriages
    B. She had two pregnancies, 0 live births, 3 abortions
    C. She had 1 singleton pregnancy, 1 twin pregnancy, has 3 living children
    D. She had 2 live births, 3 vaginal deliveries (one stillborn), 3 abortions

17. PMDD is the abbreviation for:
    A. Premenstrual dysphoric disorder
    B. Post menopausal dysphoric disorder
    C. Para-mercuribenzoate dinitrate
    D. Premenstrual dysmenorrhea and dysphoria

18. A benign tumor of breast tissue is called a:
    A. Neoplasia
    B. Fibroadenoma
    C. Astrocytoma
    D. Teratoma

19. Why is silver nitrate or erythromycin placed in the newborn infant's eyes?
    A. To prevent blindness
    B. To prevent infection in the newborn after passing through the birth canal
    C. To prevent infection passed between babies in the newborn nursery
    D. To treat the yellowness caused by elevated bilirubin

20. Malabsorption syndrome in children is also called:
    A. Short gut syndrome
    B. Failure to thrive
    C. GERD
    D. Pyloric stenosis

21. In a gravid female, the abbreviation PROM stands for:
    A. Partial range of motion
    B. Pregnancy related osteomyelitis
    C. Premature rupture of membranes
    D. Passive range of motion

22. A cesarean section performed due to CPD indicates:
    A. Cephalopelvic disproportion
    B. Calcium pyrophosphate deposition
    C. Contagious pustular dermatitis
    D. The mother has an STD

23. The term effacement refers to:
    A. Placental abruption
    B. Dilation of the cervix
    C. Rupture of membranes
    D. Crescendo of labor

24. Dyspareunia means:
    A. Lack of menstruation
    B. Inability to use tampons
    C. Pain with sexual intercourse
    D. Transient headaches during menses

25. The teacher reports that nits were found in your child's hair. The child likely has:
    A. Scabies
    B. Lice
    C. Varicella
    D. Roseola

26. A child with bulging tympanic membranes, fever, and irritability would have a differential diagnosis of:
    A. Group B strep
    B. Pharyngitis
    C. Bilateral otitis media
    D. Bilateral otitis externa

27. Chlamydia infections are treated with:
    A. Antibiotics
    B. Antiviral medications
    C. Nothing, there is no treatment
    D. Silvadene

28. The occurrence of cerebral palsy is highest in:
    A. Males
    B. Females
    C. Post-term infants
    D. Premature infants

29. Projectile vomiting in a newborn may signify:
    A. Cerebral palsy
    B. Pyloric stenosis
    C. Hirschsprung disease
    D. Spina bifida

30. Which of the following methods is not used to assess chromosomal disorders?
    A. Karyotyping
    B. Meiosis
    C. Polymerase chain reaction (PCR)
    D. DNA probe

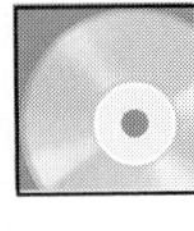

Please see the accompanying CD for additional review materials for this section.

PROOFREADING EXERCISES

These five proofreading exercises are provided to improve your skills in the areas of editing and effective identification and correction of errors in the medical record.

Directions: Identify and correct the transcription errors found in the exercises below. *Answers are provided at the end of this chapter.*

PROOFREADING EXERCISE #1

PREOPERATIVE DIAGNOSIS
Lesion of the right breast, ideology undetermined.

POSTOPERATIVE DIAGNOSIS
Lesion of the right breast, pending permanent session for final diagnosis.

OPERATION
1. Right breast needle localization.
2. Incisional biopsy of the right breast lesion.

ANESTHESIA
General.

PROCEDURE IN DETAIL
With the patient in the sublime position, satisfactory general anesthesia was given. The left crest was prepped with Betadine and draped as usual. The patient received 1 g of Ancef prior to surgery.

A skin incision was made and bleeders were controlled with electric chorea utilizing the needle-tip Bovie. Exposure was obtained, and then the tip of the vocalizing wire was identified. It was grasped with an Alice clamp and the tissue was pulled upward. Using the scalpel, the lesion was excised en toto. The wire was transected at the outer portion of the skin, and the specimen was sent to the pathologist in a container with saline as requested.

(continued)

The wound was inspected, and a couple of bleeders were controlled with suture ligatures of 3-0 chromic catgut; the rest were controlled with the electrocautery using the needle-tip boogie. The wound was irrigated with saline and then aspirated. The wound was then approximated in the deep potion and the midportion with 3-0 and 4-0 chromic catgut.

Following this, the subcutaneous tissue was approximated with 40 chromic catgut, and then the subcuticular tissue was approximated in a stunning fashion with 5-0 Monocryl on a P3 needle. The skin was further protected with Steri-Strips and a sterile dressing. Sponge, needle, and instrument counts were reported as correct by the nurse. The patient was then transferred to the recovery room in satisfactory condition.

PROOFREADING EXERCISE #2

PREOPERATIVE DIAGNOSIS
Multiple uterine stomata.

POSTOPERATIVE DIAGNOSIS
Multiple uterine stomata.

PROCEDURE
Total abdominal hysterectomy.

ANESTHESIA
General.

PROCEDURE IN DETAIL
The patient was placed in the supine position on the operating table and, after the induction of adequate general anesthesia, the operative area was prepped and draped in the usual manner. A Foley catheter was inserted for independent drainage. A midlung vertical skin incision was made and carried down to the fascia. All bleeders were electrocoagulated and the fascia was incised longitudinally. The perineum was entered without difficulty.

Upon entry into the pelvic cavity, the uterus was noted to be irregularly enlarged due to multiple fibroids. There was also a simple ovarian cyst on the left ovary measuring 4 to 5 cm in diameter. The right adnexal was normal.

A total abdominal hysterectomy was carried out as follows: First, both sound ligaments were clamped, cut, and suture ligated with #0 Vicryl, and both infundibulopelvic ligaments were clamped, cut, and suture ligated with Vicryl bilaterally. Then, a bladder flap was made and separated from the uterus. Both uterine vessels were clamped, cut, and suture ligated with #0 Vicryl and both carinal ligaments were likewise clamped, cut, and suture ligated with the same suture material. Then, both uterosacral liniments were severed and the vaginal canal was entered posteriorly. The entire uterine specimen was removed. The vaginal puff was closed using a continuous, interlocking suture of #0 Vicryl and each corner of the vaginal cuff was transfixed to each cardinal ligament.

(continued)

Following this, complete hemostasis was obtained from the virginal cuff, and then retroperitonealization was carried out with continuous 2-0 chromic catgut suture material. Complete hemostasis was obtained from the pelvic floor, and then the posterior peritoneum was closed with continuous 2-0 chromic catgut suture. The fascia was closed with continuous, running #1 PDS with additional interrupted #1 PDS, and then the skin edges were reapproximated with skin staples.

The patient tolerated the procedure well.

ESTIMATED BLOOD LOSS
Approximately 200 mL.

PROOFREADING EXERCISE #3

PREOPERATIVE DIAGNOSIS
Mist abortion at 5½ weeks.

POSTOPERATIVE DIAGNOSIS
Mist abortion at 5½ weeks.

PROCEDURE
Suction dilatation and carriage.

ANESTHESIA
Intravenous sedation with Femoral and Versed.

COMPLICATIONS
None.

INTRAVENOUS FLUIDS
Lactated Ringer solution, 500 mL.

INDICATIONS FOR PROCEDURE
The patient is a 32-year-old gravida 2, para 0010 who presented to the gynecology emergency room with vaginal bleeding and was found to have a missed abortion at 5½ weeks by ultrasound. The patient presents today for an elective digitation and curettage.

FINDINGS DURING SURGERY
Ate, weak-sized uterus and a moderate amount of products of contraception.

(continued)

PROCEDURE IN DETAIL

The patient was taken to the operating room where her intravenous sedation was found to be adequate. She was then prepped and draped in the normal sterile fashion and placed in the dorsal lithography position. A sterile speculate was placed into the vagina, and the anterior lip of the cervix was grasped with a retinaculum and the uterus rounded to 8 cm. The cervix was dilated with progressive dilators to accommodate a 7-mm suction curette. Suction curettage was performed, with a moderate amount of tissue obtained. A sharp burette was then used to ensure that all tissue had been removed. Excellent hemostasis was achieved and all instruments were removed from the vagina.

The patient tolerated the procedure well. Sponge, instrument, and needle counts were correct at the end of the procedure, and the patient was transferred to the recovery room in stable condition.

PROOFREADING EXERCISE #4

SURGEON OF RECORD
John Smith, MD.

RESIDENT SURGEON
Mary Jones, MD.

PREOPERATIVE DIAGNOSIS
Multiplayer; desires permanent sterilization.

POSTOPERATIVE DIAGNOSIS
Multiplayer; desires permanent sterilization.

PROCEDURE
Postpartum bilateral double ligation via the modified Pomeroy method.

ANESTHESIA
Epidermal.

COMPLICATIONS
None.

INTRAVENOUS FLUIDS
Lactated Ringers, 500 mL.

INDICATIONS FOR PROCEDURE
The patient is a 22-year-old female, para 2-0-0-2, who is status post normal spontaneous vaginal delivery and who desires permanent sterilization. The risks and benefits of the procedure were discussed with the patient, including the risk of failure of 1 in 300 and the increased risk of an atopic gestation should pregnancy occur.

FINDINGS DURING SURGERY
A normal post partum uterus, normal tubes and ovaries bilaterally.

(continued)

PROCEDURE IN DETAIL

The patient was taken to the operating room where her epidural anesthesia was found to be adequate. A small transverse infraumbilical incision was made with a scalpel. The incision was carried down through the underlying layer of fascia until the peritoneum was identified and entered. The peritoneum was noted to be free of any adhesins and the incision was extended with blunt direction. The patient's left fallopian tube was then identified, brought through the incision, and grasped with a Bab cock clamp. The tube was then followed to the fimbria. The Babcock clamp was used to grasp the tube approximately 4 cm from the corneal region. A 3-cm segment of tube was then ligated with 2 free-ties of plane catgut and excised. Good hemostasis was noted and the tube was returned to the abdomen. The right fallopian tube was then ligated with 2 free-ties of plane catgut and a 3-cm segment exercised in a similar fashion. Excellent hemostasis was noted and the tube was returned to the abdomen.

The fascia and peritoneum were closed in a single layer using #0 Velcro. The skin was closed in a subcuticular fashion using 3-0 Vicryl on a Keith needle.

The patient tolerated the procedure well. Sponge, instrument, and needle counts were correct times two. The patient was transferred to the recovery room in stable condition.

PROOFREADING EXERCISE #5

The patient is a 25-year-old gravida 1, para 0 at 28 weeks 2 days by ultrasound performed at 10 weeks. She is here today for a repeat ultrasound. She has had no spotting, contractions, or other problems. She reports the baby is active with ticking and hiccups.

OBJECTIVE
Weight 160 pounds, up 5 pounds since last visit. Dip stick is negative, specifically for sucrose and protein.

A trans abdominal ultrasound was performed. A singleton fetus is in the vortex presentation. Good movements were visualized including breathing, arms, and legs. Cardiac activity was also visualized. The placenta is posterior and high. Atomically, the fetus is normal, including intracranial anatomy, spine, all 4 chambers of the heart, kidneys, stomach, bladder, cor, and extremities. Fatal heart rate is 166 bpm. Fetal biometry indicates average fetal age to be 28 weeks 4 days. The estimated fetal wait is appropriate at 5101 g. Estimated date of confinement is April 1, 2004.

ASSESSMENT
Abnormal anatomical ultrasound.

PLAN
The patient will follow up in 4 weeks for her routine appointment.

ANSWER KEYS

REVIEW QUESTIONS ANSWER KEY

1. C
2. A
3. C
4. D
5. A
6. B
7. B
8. D
9. C
10. A
11. A
12. B
13. B
14. C
15. D
16. C
17. A
18. B
19. B
20. B
21. C
22. A
23. B
24. C
25. B
26. C
27. A
28. D
29. B
30. B

PROOFREADING EXERCISE #1 KEY

PREOPERATIVE DIAGNOSIS
Lesion of the right breast, ideology undetermined.

POSTOPERATIVE DIAGNOSIS
Lesion of the right breast, pending permanent session for final diagnosis.

OPERATION
1. Right breast needle localization.
2. Incisional biopsy of the right breast lesion.

ANESTHESIA
General.

PROCEDURE IN DETAIL
With the patient in the sublime position, satisfactory general anesthesia was given. The left crest was prepped with Betadine and draped as usual. The patient received 1 g of Ancef prior to surgery.

A skin incision was made and bleeders were controlled with electric chorea utilizing the needle-tip Bovie. Exposure was obtained, and then the tip of the vocalizing wire was identified. It was grasped with an Alice clamp and the tissue was pulled upward. Using the scalpel, the lesion was excised en toto. The wire was transected at the outer portion of the skin, and the specimen was sent to the pathologist in a container with saline as requested.

Incorrect term—etiology

Incorrect term—section

Incorrect term—excisional

Incorrect term—supine

Incorrect side—right

Incorrect word—breast

Incorrect term—electrocautery

Incorrect word—localizing

Incorrect spelling—Allis

The wound was inspected, and a couple of bleeders were controlled with suture ligatures of 3-0 chromic catgut; the rest were controlled with the electrocautery using the needle-tip ~~boogie.~~ The wound was irrigated with saline and then aspirated. The wound was then approximated in the deep ~~potion~~ and the midportion with 3-0 and 4-0 chromic catgut.

Incorrect term—Bovie

Incorrect word—portion

Following this, the subcutaneous tissue was approximated with ~~40~~ chromic catgut, and then the subcuticular tissue was approximated in a ~~stunning~~ fashion with 5-0 Monocryl on a P3 needle. The skin was further protected with Steri-Strips and a sterile dressing. Sponge, needle, and instrument counts were reported as correct by the nurse. The patient was then transferred to the recovery room in satisfactory condition.

Incorrect format—4-0

Incorrect word—running

PROOFREADING EXERCISE #2 KEY

PREOPERATIVE DIAGNOSIS
Multiple uterine stomata.

POSTOPERATIVE DIAGNOSIS
Multiple uterine stomata.

PROCEDURE
Total abdominal hysterectomy.

ANESTHESIA
General.

PROCEDURE IN DETAIL
The patient was placed in the supine position on the operating table and, after the induction of adequate general anesthesia, the operative area was prepped and draped in the usual manner. A Foley catheter was inserted for independent drainage. A midlung vertical skin incision was made and carried down to the fascia. All bleeders were electrocoagulated and the fascia was incised longitudinally. The perineum was entered without difficulty.

Upon entry into the pelvic cavity, the uterus was noted to be irregularly enlarged due to multiple fibroids. There was also a simple ovarian cyst on the left ovary measuring 4 to 5 cm in diameter. The right adnexal was normal.

A total abdominal hysterectomy was carried out as follows: First, both sound ligaments were clamped, cut, and suture ligated with #0 Vicryl, and both infundibulopelvic ligaments were clamped, cut, and suture ligated with Vicryl bilaterally. Then, a bladder flap was made and separated from the uterus. Both uterine vessels were clamped, cut, and suture ligated with #0 Vicryl and both carinal

Incorrect term—myomata

Incorrect word—dependent

Incorrect word—midline

Incorrect term—peritoneum

Incorrect term—adnexa

Incorrect word—round

Incorrect word—cardinal

Incorrect term—ligaments

ligaments were likewise clamped, cut, and suture ligated with the same suture material. Then, both uterosacral liniments were severed and the vaginal canal was entered posteriorly. The entire uterine specimen was removed. The vaginal puff was closed using a continuous, interlocking suture of #0 Vicryl and each corner of the vaginal cuff was transfixed to each cardinal ligament.

Incorrect word—cuff

Incorrect term—vaginal

Following this, complete hemostasis was obtained from the virginal cuff, and then retroperitonealization was carried out with continuous 2-0 chromic catgut suture material. Complete hemostasis was obtained from the pelvic floor, and then the posterior peritoneum was closed with continuous 2-0 chromic catgut suture. The fascia was closed with continuous, running #1 PDS with additional interrupted #1 PDS, and then the skin edges were reapproximated with skin staples.

Incorrect term—anterior

The patient tolerated the procedure well.

ESTIMATED BLOOD LOSS
Approximately 200 mL.

PROOFREADING EXERCISE #3 KEY

PREOPERATIVE DIAGNOSIS
Mist abortion at 5½ weeks.

Incorrect word—missed

POSTOPERATIVE DIAGNOSIS
Mist abortion at 5½ weeks.

PROCEDURE
Suction dilatation and carriage.

Incorrect term—curettage

ANESTHESIA
Intravenous sedation with Femoral and Versed.

Incorrect drug—Demerol

COMPLICATIONS
None.

INTRAVENOUS FLUIDS
Lactated Ringer solution, 500 mL.

INDICATIONS FOR PROCEDURE
The patient is a 32-year-old gravida 2, para 0010 who presented to the emergency room with vaginal bleeding and was found to have a missed abortion at 5½ weeks by ultrasound. The patient presents today for an elective digitation and curettage.

Incorrect format—0-0-1-0

Incorrect term—dilatation

FINDINGS DURING SURGERY
Ate, weak-sized uterus and a moderate amount of products of contraception.

Incorrect phrase—eight-week-sized

Incorrect term—conception

PROCEDURE IN DETAIL
The patient was taken to the operating room where her intravenous sedation was found to be adequate. She was then prepped and draped in the normal sterile fashion and placed in the dorsal lithography position. A sterile speculate was placed into the vagina, and the anterior lip of the cervix

Incorrect term—lithotomy

Incorrect term—speculum

was grasped with a retinaculum and the uterus rounded to 8 cm. The cervix was dilated with progressive dilators to accommodate a 7-mm suction curette. Suction curettage was performed, with a moderate amount of tissue obtained. A sharp burette was then used to ensure that all tissue had been removed. Excellent hemostasis was achieved and all instruments were removed from the vagina.

The patient tolerated the procedure well. Sponge, instrument, and needle counts were correct at the end of the procedure, and the patient was transferred to the recovery room in stable condition.

Incorrect term—sounded

Incorrect term—curettage

Incorrect term—tenaculum

PROOFREADING EXERCISE #4 KEY

SURGEON OF RECORD
John Smith, MD.

RESIDENT SURGEON
Mary Jones, MD.

PREOPERATIVE DIAGNOSIS
Multiplayer, desires permanent sterilization.

Incorrect term—multiparity

POSTOPERATIVE DIAGNOSIS
Multiplayer; desires permanent sterilization.

PROCEDURE
Postpartum bilateral double ~~ligation~~ ligation via the modified Pomeroy method.

Incorrect term—tubal

ANESTHESIA
Epidermal.

Incorrect term—epidural

COMPLICATIONS
None.

INTRAVENOUS FLUIDS
Lactated Ringers, 500 mL.

INDICATIONS FOR PROCEDURE
The patient is a 22-year-old female, para 2-0-0-2, who is status post normal spontaneous vaginal delivery and who desires permanent sterilization. The risks and benefits of the procedure were discussed with the patient, including the risk of failure of 1 in 300 and the increased risk of an atopic gestation should pregnancy occur.

Incorrect term—ectopic

FINDINGS DURING SURGERY
A ~~normal~~ post partum uterus, normal tubes and ovaries bilaterally.

Use combined form—postpartum

PROCEDURE IN DETAIL

The patient was taken to the operating room where her epidural anesthesia was found to be adequate. A small transverse infraumbilical incision was made with a scalpel. The incision was carried down through the underlying layer of fascia until the peritoneum was identified and entered. The peritoneum was noted to be free of any adhesins and the incision was extended with blunt direction. The patient's left fallopian tube was then identified, brought through the incision, and grasped with a Bab cock clamp. The tube was then followed to the fimbria. The Babcock clamp was used to grasp the tube approximately 4 cm from the corneal region. A 3-cm segment of tube was then ligated with 2 free-ties of plane catgut and excised. Good hemostasis was noted and the tube was returned to the abdomen. The right fallopian tube was then ligated with 2 free-ties of plane catgut and a 3-cm segment exercised in a similar fashion. Excellent hemostasis was noted and the tube was returned to the abdomen.

The fascia and peritoneum were closed in a single layer using #0 Velcro. The skin was closed in a subcuticular fashion using 3-0 Vicryl on a Keith needle.

The patient tolerated the procedure well. Sponge, instrument, and needle counts were correct times two. The patient was transferred to the recovery room in stable condition.

Incorrect term—adhesions

Incorrect word—dissection

Incorrect term—Babcock

Incorrect spelling—plain

Incorrect term—cornual

Incorrect spelling—plain

Incorrect term—excised

Incorrect term—Vicryl

Incorrect format—x2

PROOFREADING EXERCISE #5 KEY

The patient is a 25-year-old gravida 1, para 0 at 28 weeks 2 days by ultrasound performed at 10 weeks. She is here today for a repeat ultrasound. She has had no spotting, contractions, or other problems. She reports the baby is active with ticking and hiccups.

Incorrect word—kicking

OBJECTIVE

Weight 160 pounds, up 5 pounds since last visit. Dip stick is negative, specifically for sucrose ~~and~~ protein.

Use combined form—dipstick

Incorrect term—glucose

~~A~~ trans abdominal ultrasound was performed. A singleton fetus is in the vortex ~~presentation~~. Good movements were visualized including breathing, arms, and legs. Cardiac activity was also visualized. The placenta is posterior and high. Atomically, ~~the~~ fetus is normal, including intracranial anatomy, spine, all 4 chambers of the heart, kidneys, stomach, ~~bladder~~, cor, and extremities. Fatal ~~heart~~ rate is 166 bpm. Fetal biometry indicates average fetal age to be 28 weeks 4 days. The estimated ~~fetal~~ wait is appropriate at 5101 g. Estimated date of confinement is April 1, 2004.

Use combined form—transabdom-inal

Incorrect term—vertex

Incorrect term—anatomically

Incorrect term—cord

Incorrect word—fetal

Incorrect word—weight

ASSESSMENT

Abnormal anatomical ultrasound.

"normal"—no abnormal results reported

PLAN

The patient will followup ~~in 4~~ weeks for her routine appointment.

Verb form—follow up

CHAPTER

17

Ophthalmology

OBJECTIVES CHECKLIST

A prepared exam candidate will know:

- ❑ Combining forms, prefixes, and suffixes related to the body system.
- ❑ Anatomy and physiology of the eye, both internal and external.
- ❑ Visual pathway of light from the cornea to the cerebral cortex.
- ❑ Errors of refraction related to visual acuity.
- ❑ Common pathologic conditions of the eye.
- ❑ Clinical and diagnostic procedures used in the identification of diseases and disorders of the eye.
- ❑ Medications commonly prescribed for symptoms, disorders, and diseases of the eye.

RESOURCES FOR STUDY

1. *The Language of Medicine*
   Chapter 17: Sense Organs: The Eye and the Ear, pp. 669–689.
2. *H&P: A Nonphysician's Guide to the Medical History and Physical Examination*
   Chapter 7: Review of Systems: Head, Eyes, Ears, Nose, Throat, Mouth, Teeth, pp. 59–70.
   Chapter 19: Examination of the Eyes, pp. 179–188.
3. *Human Diseases*
   Chapter 18: Diseases of the Eye, pp. 291–314.
4. *Laboratory Tests & Diagnostic Procedures in Medicine*
   Chapter 3: Measurement of Vision and Hearing, pp. 29–38.
   Chapter 7: Endoscopy: Visual Examination of the Eyes, Ears, Nose, and Respiratory Tract, pp. 95–106.
5. *Understanding Pharmacology for Health Professionals*
   Chapter 20: Ophthalmic Drugs, pp. 217–227.

SAMPLE REPORTS

The following five reports are examples of reports you might encounter while transcribing ophthalmology.

OPERATIVE NOTE

PREOPERATIVE DIAGNOSIS
Medically uncontrolled glaucoma, right eye.

POSTOPERATIVE DIAGNOSIS
Medically uncontrolled glaucoma, right eye.

OPERATION
Trabeculectomy, right eye.

SURGEON
John Smith, MD.

ANESTHESIA
Local with standby.

PROCEDURE
Peribulbar anesthesia of the right eyelids and globe was obtained by injecting 2% Xylocaine into the right eye, and the right eye was sterilely prepped and draped. A lid speculum was inserted, and a 4-0 black silk superior rectus traction suture was placed and additional anesthesia obtained with 2% Xylocaine subconjunctivally. A large limbal-based conjunctival flap was fashioned with scissors. The Tenon capsule was excised. Bleeding areas were meticulously cauterized, and a 4 x 4 half-thickness scleral flap was created with a #69 blade.

Mitomycin 0.5 mg/mL was applied to the underside of the flap in the bare sclera for 2 minutes and then copiously irrigated off the eye. The anterior chamber was entered with a #75 blade. A trabeculectomy punch was used to double punch a hole in the trabecular meshwork, and a peripheral iridectomy was performed. The scleral flap was positioned posteriorly with two 10-0 nylon sutures. Irrigation through a side port showed easy flow underneath the flap. The conjunctiva was then closed with running, locked 8-0 Vicryl suture, giving a watertight closure.

At the close of the procedure the chamber was deep and the eye was soft. Ancef and Celestone were injected subconjunctivally. Maxitrol was instilled in the eye. The eye was patched, and the patient tolerated the procedure well.

OPERATIVE NOTE

PREOPERATIVE DIAGNOSIS
Esotropia, both eyes.

POSTOPERATIVE DIAGNOSIS
Esotropia, both eyes.

OPERATION
A 3.5-mm bimedial recession.

SURGEON
John Smith, MD.

ANESTHESIA
General.

PROCEDURE
After successful induction of general anesthesia, both eyes were sterilely prepped and draped in the usual manner for strabismus surgery. Attention was first turned to the right eye.

A lid speculum was inserted, a 5-0 Mersilene limbal traction suture placed, and the eye placed in an abducted position. A limbal peritomy was performed with scissors. The medial rectus was isolated on a muscle hook and attachments to the Tenon capsule cut. At this point, 6-0 Vicryl was threaded through the insertion. The muscle was disinserted and reinserted 3.5 mm from the original point of insertion. The conjunctiva was then closed with a 6-0 plain suture. Maxitrol was instilled into the eye, and the eye was not patched.

Attention was then turned to the left eye where a similar operation was performed by isolating the medial rectus on a muscle hook, recessing it 3.5 mm and closing the conjunctiva with 6-0 plain. Maxitrol was instilled into the eye and the eye was again not patched.

The patient tolerated both procedures well and was taken to the recovery room and then discharged home in excellent condition.

OPERATIVE NOTE

PREOPERATIVE DIAGNOSIS
Pseudophakic bullous keratopathy, right eye.

POSTOPERATIVE DIAGNOSIS
Pseudophakic bullous keratopathy, right eye.

OPERATION
An 8-mm penetrating keratoplasty, right eye.

SURGEON
John Smith, MD.

ANESTHESIA
Local with standby.

PROCEDURE
Peribulbar anesthesia of the right eyelids and globe was obtained by injection of 2% Xylocaine. The right eye was sterilely prepped and draped. A lid speculum was inserted and attention was turned to the donor eye.

The donor was a 47-year-old intracerebral bleed patient who died on 1/05, and the cornea was preserved on the same day and used today. It was removed from the transport medium and placed on the Teflon chopping block epithelial side up. An 8.25-mm button was punched through from the posterior surface. This was flooded with transport media and brought to the operative field.

Attention was returned to the patient, where an 8-mm trephine was placed on the cornea and used to trephine into the anterior chamber. The cornea was cut through with right and left corneal scissors. Healon was used to deepen the fornices in the anterior chamber. The donor button was placed into the recipient bed and sutured in place with four 10-0 nylon cardinal sutures, an additional four 10-0 nylon interrupted sutures and, finally, a 16-bite 10-0 nylon, pulled up once and tied in the wound. The wound was felt to be watertight.

Celestone and Garamycin were injected subconjunctivally, TobraDex instilled in the eye, and the eye patched and shielded. The patient tolerated the procedure well.

DISCHARGE SUMMARY

FINAL DIAGNOSIS
Cataract, right eye.

OPERATION PERFORMED
Kelman phacoemulsification, right eye, with insertion of an AcrySof 19-diopter posterior chamber intraocular lens under local and general anesthesia with microscopic control.

SUMMARY
This is the second outpatient admission for this 65-year-old female who has had decreased vision in both eyes for the last several years. The patient had cataract surgery in the left eye with good visual results. She is now admitted for cataract surgery of the right eye. Her best-corrected vision is 20/80 in the right and 20/40 in the left. Pressures are normal and slit-lamp examination is normal except for corneal scarring. The lens revealed 3+ nuclear sclerosis, and the fundus examination was normal.

DIAGNOSIS
Cataract, right eye.

DISPOSITION
The patient was advised of the above and desired to have cataract surgery. She was seen by a medical doctor and cleared for surgery. She underwent an uncomplicated cataract extraction, right eye, with implant. She tolerated the procedure well and was discharged postoperatively.

She was discharged on Pred Forte drops, Maxitrol drops, patch and shield. She was given postoperative care instructions, and she is to see us for followup in the office in the morning.

OPERATIVE REPORT

PREOPERATIVE DIAGNOSIS
Chronic blepharitis and severe ectropion, left lower lid.

POSTOPERATIVE DIAGNOSIS
Chronic blepharitis and severe ectropion, left lower lid.

OPERATION
Repair of ectropion, left lower lid with excisional biopsy, left lower lid.

SURGEON
John Smith, MD.

ANESTHESIA
Local with standby.

PROCEDURE
Anesthesia of the left lower lid was obtained by injection of 2% Xylocaine in the distribution of the infraorbital nerve and subcutaneously. The left eye was sterilely prepped and draped in the usual manner for major eyelid surgery. An incision was made along the inferior lash line to the lateral canthus, angled out at 15 degrees. A skin and muscle flap was created with Westcott scissors. A 10-mm section of the left lower lid was excised temporally and sent to pathology for permanent section.

The lid was then closed with a 4-0 silk to the grey line, 6-0 silk to the anterior and posterior lid margins, 5-0 chromic to the deep muscle tissues and 6-0 silk to the skin, leaving a good closure. The lid sutures were left long and taped to the face. Maxitrol was applied to the wound and the eye was patched. The patient tolerated the procedure well.

REVIEW QUESTIONS

The goal of these questions is to test your knowledge in the area of ophthalmology.

Directions: Select the correct answer for each of the multiple-choice questions provided below. *Answers are provided at the end of this chapter.*

1. The cranial nerve pertaining to the eye is:
   A. One
   B. Two
   C. Four
   D. Five
2. A doctor who prescribes glasses but is not an M.D. is an:
   A. Optometrist
   B. Orthoptist
   C. Ophthalmologist
   D. Optician
3. An inflammation of the eyelids is called:
   A. Blepharitis
   B. Scleritis
   C. Conjunctivitis
   D. Dacryocystitis
4. The white part of the eye is called the:
   A. Sclera
   B. Cornea
   C. Iris
   D. Conjunctiva
5. To cry is to:
   A. Lactate
   B. Lacrimate
   C. Acelomate
   D. Lamellate
6. Removal of part of the iris is termed:
   A. Iridectomy
   B. Iridotomy
   C. Iridoplasty
   D. Iridesis
7. A disease process of the retina is called:
   A. Retinopathy
   B. Cataract
   C. Strabismus
   D. Amblyopia
8. That which is removed in a cataract operation is the:
   A. Fovea
   B. Retina
   C. Lens
   D. Pupil
9. Ptosis of the eyelids means:
   A. Prolapse
   B. Drooping
   C. An inability to close
   D. Paralysis
10. The ophthalmologic abbreviation RLF stands for:
    A. Right lateral fovea
    B. Ruptured lateral fovea
    C. Retrolental fibroplasia
    D. Radiographic lens fibrosis
11. Diabetic eye problems usually involve both:
    A. Retinas
    B. Retinaculum
    C. Retinacula
    D. Retinae
12. The muscle which surrounds the eye is the:
    A. Zygomaticus
    B. Buccinator
    C. Aponeurosis
    D. Orbicularis oculi
13. The part of the eye that opens and closes to control light input is the:
    A. Retina
    B. Iris
    C. Cornea
    D. Pupil

14. "Amaurosis fugax" would be placed under which category in the review of systems?
    A. Neurologic
    B. HEENT
    C. OB/GYN
    D. Endocrine

15. Which of the following transplanted organs is the least likely to be rejected?
    A. Cornea
    B. Kidney
    C. Liver
    D. Heart

16. The instrument used to view the inside of the eye is the:
    A. Proctoscope
    B. Ophthalmoscope
    C. Endoscope
    D. Amblyoscope

17. Back and forth or rotatory movement of the eyes is called:
    A. Astigmatism
    B. Asterixis
    C. Strabismus
    D. Nystagmus

18. The medical term for a stye is:
    A. Pterygium
    B. Coloboma
    C. Hordeolum
    D. Conjunctivitis

19. Dilation of the pupils is called:
    A. Mydriasis
    B. Refraction
    C. Ptosis
    D. Aponeurosis

20. A V-shaped cutout is sometimes made in the iris to relieve pressure in persons with the diagnosis of:
    A. Coloboma
    B. Hyphema
    C. Iritis
    D. Glaucoma

21. Blood in the anterior chamber of the eye is called:
    A. Coloboma
    B. Hyphema
    C. Iridectomy
    D. Zonulitis

22. A slit lamp examination is done to:
    A. Observe the internal structures of the eye
    B. Closely view the lashes and dentate line
    C. Rule out Kerley B lines
    D. Check for glaucoma

23. An inflammation of the lacrimal ducts is called:
    A. Xanthelasma
    B. Pseudophakia
    C. Canaliculitis
    D. Strabismus

24. A diagnosis of pseudostrabismus can be made when an individual has:
    A. Deep epicanthal folds
    B. Pseudophakia
    C. Amblyopia
    D. Amaurosis fugax

25. Which of the following is a mydriatic drug?
    A. Atropine
    B. Proparacaine
    C. Betoptic
    D. Garamycin

26. Yellow-orange plaques on the eyelids are termed:
    A. Pterygium
    B. Blepharitis
    C. Xanthelasma
    D. Strabismus

27. An individual who has pseudophakia has:
    A. Retrolental fibroplasia
    B. Artificial lenses in place
    C. Macular degeneration
    D. Diabetic retinae

28. The fovea centralis is located:
    A. In the retinae
    B. In the irides
    C. In the lacrimal ducts
    D. In the choroid plexus

29. One method of cataract extraction is called:
    A. Ophthalmoscopy
    B. Lensectomy
    C. Phacoemulsification
    D. Balanced salt solution infusion

30. Convergent strabismus is also known as:
    A. Exotropia
    B. Esotropia
    C. A-pattern strabismus
    D. Alternating strabismus

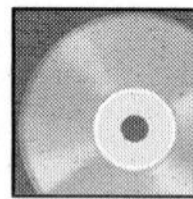

Please see the accompanying CD for additional review materials for this section.

PROOFREADING EXERCISES

These three proofreading exercises are provided to improve your skills in the areas of editing and effective identification and correction of errors in the medical record.

Directions: Identify and correct the transcription errors found in the exercises below. *Answers are provided at the end of this chapter.*

PROOFREADING EXERCISE #1

HISTORY OF PRESENT ILLNESS
This 26-year-old male was seen in consultation on 12/02 on referral by Drs. Jones and Smith. This man was said to have been beaten and robbed and was admitted from the emergency room. I was asked to see him to examine his so-called bloodshot eye and somewhat posed eye. He also complained of some loss of vision but no definite history of unconsciousness. On examination, he was alert and conscious.

PHYSICAL EXAMINATION
Vision testing revealed his right eye to be at the 20:100 level without correction. He is somewhat distressed and his eye was painful. The left eye was at the 20:40 level. Externally, he had swelling of the eyelid. The right eye was protruded about 3 mm. The left eye was within normal limits. Mobility could not be confirmed. Upward gaze was somewhat restricted. Papillary reactions, direct and consensually, were normal. Anterior chamber revealed no hyphae. The posterior pole revealed a good view with no hemorrhage and no cataract but it was somewhat more pale than the left eye. On confrontation fields, the patient was not in a comfortable position and was in distress also. Therefore, visual fields could not be done. He had some hypoesthesia in the intraorbital region, mainly in the right eye.

IMPRESSION
1. Severe contusion of right eye. Due to the protrusion, there could be a retrobulbar hemorrhage.
2. Possible sorbitol fracture.

PLAN
The patient was given some antibiotic drops and Maxalt ointment and evaluated for an orbital fracture. I reviewed the x-rays, and I will see him during his hospital course to see if anything develops.

PROOFREADING EXERCISE #2

PREOPERATIVE DIAGNOSIS
Sessile cataract, right eye.

POSTOPERATIVE DIAGNOSIS
Sessile cataract, right eye.

OPERATION
Fake emulsification and implantation of posterior chamber lens, left eye.

SURGEON
John Smith, MD.

ANESTHESIA
Local.

PROCEDURE
Peribulbar anesthesia of the right eyelids and lobe was obtained by injection of 2% Xalatan. The right eye was sterilely prepped and draped. A lid speculum was inserted, a fornix-based conjunctival flap fashioned, and bleeding areas cauterized.

The anterior chamber was entered with a #75 blade and Healon installed. Capsulotomy and hydro dissection were performed. The nucleus was then phacoemulsified. Residual cortex was removed and Healon was used to deepen the capsular bag. An Alcon SA-60-AT, 14.5 diopter lens was inspected, copiously irrigated, inserted into the capsular bag, and rotated horizontally. The Healon was removed.

The wound was closed with a single tendo nylon suture. Celestone and Garamycin were injected subconjunctivally, TobraDex instilled in the eye and the eye patched and shielded.

PROOFREADING EXERCISE #3

PREOPERATIVE DIAGNOSIS
Peridium, right eye.

POSTOPERATIVE DIAGNOSIS
Peridium, right eye.

OPERATION
Excision of pterygium, right eye with mitomycin instillation and sliding conjunctival flap closure.

SURGEON
John Smith, MD.

ANESTHESIA
Local with standby.

PROCEDURE
Perivulvar anesthesia of the right eyelids and globe was obtained by injection of 2% Xylocaine. The right eye was sterilely prepped and draped. A lead speculum was inserted and additional anesthesia was obtained by subconjunctival Xylocaine. The pterygium was grasped with a forceps and an incision was made in clear cornea and carried out in the anterior stoma to the limbus. The pterygium was then cut free with Westcott scissors. Bleeding areas were meticulously cauterized.

Mitomycin 0.5 mg/mL was applied to the vascular area for 2 minutes and then copiously irrigated off. The conjunctiva was closed by incising along the lumbus, sliding the fat into the defect and closing with multiple, interrupted 8-0 Vicryl sutures.

Zoladex instilled in the eye and the eye patched and shielded. The patient tolerated the procedure well.

ANSWER KEYS

REVIEW QUESTIONS ANSWER KEY

1. B
2. A
3. A
4. A
5. B
6. A
7. A
8. C
9. B
10. C
11. D
12. D
13. B
14. B
15. A
16. B
17. D
18. C
19. A
20. D
21. B
22. A
23. C
24. A
25. A
26. C
27. B
28. A
29. C
30. B

PROOFREADING EXERCISE #1 KEY

Incorrect term—ptosed

Incorrect format—20/100

Incorrect term—hyphema

Incorrect drug—Maxitrol

Incorrect format—20/40

Incorrect term—pupillary

Incorrect prefix—infraorbital

Incorrect term—orbital

HISTORY OF PRESENT ILLNESS

This 26-year-old male was seen in consultation on 12/02 on referral by Drs. Jones and Smith. This man was said to have been beaten and robbed and was admitted from the emergency room. I was asked to see him to examine his so-called bloodshot eye and somewhat posed eye. He also complained of some loss of vision but no definite history of unconsciousness. On examination, he was alert and conscious.

PHYSICAL EXAMINATION

Vision testing revealed his right eye to be at the 20:100 level without correction. He is somewhat distressed and his eye was painful. The left eye was at the 20:40 level. Externally, he had swelling of the eyelid. The right eye was protruded about 3 mm. The left eye was within normal limits. Mobility could not be confirmed. Upward gaze was somewhat restricted. Papillary reactions, direct and consensually, were normal. Anterior chamber revealed no hyphae. The posterior pole revealed a good view with no hemorrhage and no cataract but it was somewhat more pale than the left eye. On confrontation fields, the patient was not in a comfortable position and was in distress also. Therefore, visual fields could not be done. He had some hypoesthesia in the intraorbital region, mainly in the right eye.

IMPRESSION

1. Severe contusion of right eye. Due to the protrusion, there could be a retrobulbar hemorrhage.
2. Possible sorbitol fracture.

PLAN

The patient was given some antibiotic drops and Maxalt ointment and evaluated for an orbital fracture. I reviewed the x-rays, and I will see him during his hospital course to see if anything develops.

PROOFREADING EXERCISE #2 KEY

Incorrect term—Senile

PREOPERATIVE DIAGNOSIS
Sessile cataract, right eye.

POSTOPERATIVE DIAGNOSIS
Sessile cataract, right eye.

Incorrect term—phacoemulsification

OPERATION
Fake emulsification and implantation of posterior chamber lens, left eye.

Incorrect side—right

SURGEON
John Smith, MD.

ANESTHESIA
Local.

Incorrect term—globe

PROCEDURE
Peribulbar anesthesia of the right eyelids and lobe was obtained by injection of 2% Xalatan. The right eye was sterilely prepped and draped. A lid speculum was inserted, a fornix-based conjunctival flap fashioned, and bleeding areas cauterized.

Incorrect drug—Xylocaine

Incorrect term—instilled

The anterior chamber was entered with a #75 blade and Healon installed. Capsulotomy and hydro dissection were performed. The nucleus was then phacoemulsified. Residual cortex was removed and Healon was used to deepen the capsular bag. An Alcon SA-60-AT, 14.5 diopter lens was inspected, copiously irrigated, inserted into the capsular bag and rotated horizontally. The Healon was removed.

Use combining form—hydrodissection

Incorrect term—#10-0

The wound was closed with a single tendo nylon suture. Celestone and Garamycin were injected subconjunctivally, TobraDex instilled in the eye and the eye patched and shielded.

PROOFREADING EXERCISE #3 KEY

Incorrect term—pterygium

PREOPERATIVE DIAGNOSIS
Peridium, right eye.

POSTOPERATIVE DIAGNOSIS
Peridium, right eye.

OPERATION
Excision of pterygium, right eye with mitomycin instillation and sliding conjunctival flap closure.

SURGEON
John Smith, MD.

Incorrect term—Peribulbar

ANESTHESIA
Local with standby.

Incorrect term—lid

PROCEDURE
Perivulvar anesthesia of the right eyelids and globe was obtained by injection of 2% Xylocaine. The right eye was sterilely prepped and draped. A lead speculum was inserted and additional anesthesia was obtained by subconjunctival Xylocaine. The pterygium was grasped with a forceps and an incision was made in clear cornea and carried out in the anterior stoma to the limbus. The pterygium was then cut free with Westcott scissors. Bleeding areas were meticulously cauterized.

Incorrect term—stroma

Incorrect term—limbus

Mitomycin 0.5 mg/mL was applied to the vascular area for 2 minutes and then copiously irrigated off. The conjunctiva was closed by incising along the lumbus, sliding the fat into the defect and closing with multiple, interrupted 8-0 Vicryl sutures.

Incorrect drug—TobraDex

Zoladex instilled in the eye and the eye patched and shielded. The patient tolerated the procedure well.

CHAPTER 18

Orthopedics/Chiropractic/Pain Management/Podiatry

OBJECTIVES CHECKLIST

A prepared exam candidate will know:

- ❑ Combining forms, prefixes, and suffixes related to the body system.
- ❑ Anatomy of the muscles and bones of the musculoskeletal system, including all 206 bones and the most common muscles and muscle groups of the human body.
- ❑ Types of bone found in the human body.
- ❑ Types of muscle found in the human body and the differences between each.
- ❑ Process of bone formation and the role of cartilage in the development of the bones of the skeleton.
- ❑ Anatomy and physiology of the supportive structures of the musculoskeletal system (tendons, ligaments, cartilage, etc.).
- ❑ Anatomy and physiology of the joints as well as the different types of joints.
- ❑ Physiology of the musculoskeletal system as it coordinates with the nervous system in mobility and ambulation.
- ❑ Terms used to describe position and direction.
- ❑ Imaging studies used in the identification and diagnosis of skeletal abnormalities, injuries, diseases, and malformations (congenital and traumatic).
- ❑ Laboratory studies used in the diagnosis and treatment of musculoskeletal disorders and diseases.
- ❑ Medications commonly prescribed for musculoskeletal symptoms, disorders, and diseases.
- ❑ Transcription standards pertaining to the specialty of orthopedics.

RESOURCES FOR STUDY

1. *The Language of Medicine*
   Chapter 15, Musculoskeletal System, pp. 559–628.
2. *H&P: A Nonphysician's Guide to the Medical History and Physical Examination*
   Chapter 12: Review of Systems: Neuromuscular, pp. 107–116.
   Chapter 26: Examination of the Back and Extremities, pp. 249–260.
3. *Human Diseases*
   Chapter 17: Musculoskeletal Disorders, pp. 259–274.
4. *Laboratory Tests & Diagnostic Procedures in Medicine*
   Section IV: Medical Imaging (Chapter 10: Plain Radiography, Chapter 11: Contrast Radiography, Chapter 12: Computed Tomography, Chapter 14: Magnetic Resonance Imaging, and Chapter 15: Nuclear Imaging), pp. 127–209.
5. *Understanding Pharmacology for Health Professionals*
   Chapter 14: Musculoskeletal Drugs, pp. 137–149.
   Chapter 26: Analgesic Drugs, pp. 296–310.
6. *AAMT Book of Style for Medical Transcription*
   Orthopedics, pp. 294–299.

SAMPLE REPORTS

The following five reports are examples of reports you might encounter while transcribing orthopedics, chiropractic, pain management, and podiatry.

HISTORY & PHYSICAL

HISTORY OF PRESENT ILLNESS
The patient is a 64-year-old female who was admitted to the hospital through the emergency room complaining of a nonhealing right foot ulcer. The patient denies any fever, chills, nausea, or vomiting at this time. The patient's vital signs are stable; the patient is afebrile.

CURRENT MEDICATIONS
See chart.

ALLERGIES
Denies having any drug allergies.

MEDICAL HISTORY
Diabetes, peripheral vascular disease.

SOCIAL HISTORY
The patient denies using tobacco, drugs or alcohol.

LABORATORY DATA ON ADMISSION
Chemistry profile was essentially within normal limits. Urinalysis is cloudy, slightly yellow, negative for ketones, glucose, blood, protein, nitrites, leukocytes. Normal urobilinogen. No RBCs or WBCs. CBC shows WBC 14,000, hemoglobin 11.4, hematocrit 34.6, and platelet count 394,000.

PHYSICAL EXAMINATION
VASCULAR EVALUATION OF THE RIGHT LOWER EXTREMITY: The patient has nonpalpable dorsalis pedis and posterior tibial pulses in the right lower extremity. A slight popliteal pulse is palpable in the right popliteal fossa. The temperature of the right lower extremity is cool to touch. The capillary refill time is negligible.
NEUROLOGICAL EVALUATION OF THE RIGHT LOWER EXTREMITY: The patient does have +5/5 muscle grading strength of the dorsiflexors and plantar flexors of the right lower extremity. However, the patient is unable to invert or supinate the right foot. There is a musculoskeletal deficit at the distal aspect of the right hallux, which will be evaluated by a radiograph. The patient uses assistance for ambulation and has a prosthesis of the left lower extremity. The patient has a markedly diminished Semmes-Weinstein 5.07 monofilament wire examination distal to the Lisfranc joint of the right lower extremity. Additionally, a 128-Hz tuning fork examination reveals that the patient's proprioceptive capacity at the first metatarsophalangeal joint, as well as at the right metatarsophalangeal joints, is markedly diminished. This examination is also diminished to the level of the medial and the lateral malleolus of the right lower extremity. The patient is unable to distinguish between sharp and dull at the distal aspects of digits 1–5 of the right foot.

(continued)

DERMATOLOGICAL EVALUATION OF THE RIGHT LOWER EXTREMITY: The epidermal segment is markedly hypertrophic, with severe scaling at the pretibial region of the right lower extremity. The epidermal/dermal segment of the right forefoot dorsally is also seen to have severe drying and scaling with fissuring and cracking present. These findings are most consistent with xerosis associated with autonomic neuropathy and the patient's long-standing history of diabetes. Additionally, the right hallux presents with a distal plantar wound, approximately 1.5 cm in diameter, with active drainage which is the consistency of a serous, yellow fluid. This is most consistent with a staphylococcal infection. However, a culture and sensitivity will immediately be taken of this region and sent to pathology for identification.

The right hallux nail plate has the eponychium intact with only the proximal one-third of the nail plate intact. This is consistent with a surgical procedure, which obviously was performed on the distal aspect of the right hallux and included some level of amputation, including the nail plate. The right hallux is edematous and erythematous, with a local cellulitis evident on the plantar aspect up to the level of the first metatarsophalangeal joint. The hallux wound depicts erythema around the margin as well as palpable and reproducible dolor on palpation to the region. The fluid is manually expressible. The web spaces are clear of any maceration or infection at this time. There is no lymphangitis, nor is there any lymphedema present.

IMPRESSION
1. Insulin-dependent diabetes mellitus with peripheral and autonomic neuropathic changes.
2. Ulcer, right hallux.
3. Peripheral vascular disease.
4. Diabetic dermopathy.
5. Diabetic neuropathy.

RECOMMENDATIONS
See chart for orders.

OPERATIVE REPORT

PREOPERATIVE DIAGNOSIS
Hypertrophic bone of 3rd and 4th digits.

POSTOPERATIVE DIAGNOSIS
Hypertrophic bone of 3rd and 4th digits.

PROCEDURE
Ostectomy of proximal phalanx, 3rd and 4th digits.

ANESTHESIA
Monitored anesthesia care.

DESCRIPTION OF PROCEDURE
The patient was transferred to the operating room in apparent good preoperative condition, and no contraindications to the proposed procedure were noted.

Attention was turned to the level of the patient's 3rd digit where an ostectomy was performed at the head of the proximal phalanx and the lateral aspect of the middle phalanx. Also, an incision was made at the dorsal level of the 4th digit where the ostectomies were made at the medial head of the proximal phalanx and the medial aspect of the middle phalanx on the 4th digit. All of these surgical areas where ostectomies were performed were rasped to smoothness and flushed with copious amounts of sterile saline. The soft tissue areas were then apposed and closed with 3-0 Vicryl material, as were the skin edges.

The patient appeared to have tolerated the procedure well and was removed from the operating room in apparent good postoperative condition.

OPERATIVE REPORT

PREOPERATIVE DIAGNOSIS
Right knee degenerative joint disease with degenerative meniscal tear.

POSTOPERATIVE DIAGNOSIS
Degenerative meniscal tear bilaterally, anterior cruciate ligament tear, and severe degenerative joint disease.

SURGEON
John Smith, MD.

ASSISTANT
Jane Smith, ARNP.

PROCEDURE
Diagnostic arthroscopy, bilateral partial meniscectomies, and chondroplasty of the medial femoral condyle, medial tibial plateau, lateral tibial plateau, and undersurface of the kneecap. Notchplasty was performed and craterization and saucerization of the bone to expose the anterior cruciate ligament, which was partially torn and gently débrided and tightened.

ANESTHESIA
General.

ESTIMATED BLOOD LOSS
Minimal.

COMPLICATIONS
None.

SPECIMENS
None.

DRAINS
None.

CULTURES
None.

IV FLUID
IV Ancef preoperatively.

DISPOSITION
To recovery room in stable condition.

HISTORY
The patient is a very pleasant 49-year-old white male well known to me, who in 1992 underwent a horrific car accident with open tib-fib fracture on the left side. He has had multiple surgeries and most recently, about 2 months ago, had a knee scope on the left side. MRIs showed that he had changes on the right side as well, and he has requested arthroscopy. All the complications and indications for the procedure were explained to the patient, and he voiced understanding. Informed consent was obtained.

(continued)

DETAILS OF PROCEDURE

The patient was brought to the operating room and placed on the table in supine fashion. After general anesthesia was induced, he was prepped and draped sterilely. Examination revealed a grossly stable knee. There was no pivot-shift, but he did have 1+ to 2+ positive Lachman. The knee was minimally swollen with palpable crepitus. At this point, standard 3-portal arthroscopy was performed, which revealed a rather large tear of the posterior horn of the medial meniscus and grade 3 changes on the medial femoral condyle, medial tibial plateau, and the undersurface of the patella. There were some grade 2 changes on the lateral tibial plateau and a small tear of the posterior horn of the lateral meniscus. At this point, bilateral partial meniscectomies were undertaken using the shaver, the upbiting rongeur, and the Oratec device. Notchplasty was performed using the shaver and a burr and the Oratec device to widen the arthritic notch to prevent impingement on the ACL. The ACL was gently débrided and tightened. Notchplasty consisted of craterization and saucerization of the bone of the lateral femoral condyle. This also helped to expose the tear of the posterior horn of the lateral meniscus. Chondroplasties were performed as stated previously. The gutters were clear. The knee was copiously irrigated. The portals were closed with interrupted nylon sutures. Then, 0.5% Marcaine with epinephrine and 10 mg of morphine were injected into the knee for postoperative pain control. He was placed in a bulky sterile dressing. He tolerated the procedure well and was sent to the recovery room in stable condition where he will be discharged to home when he is cleared by anesthesia. Followup will be in my office in 2 weeks. We have given him prescriptions for Darvocet, Keflex, and Ativan.

FOLLOWUP NOTE

HISTORY

Postoperative left wrist. The patient returns to the office today with limited complaints on the dorsoradial aspect of her hand. Her swelling is minimal. She was experiencing drainage from her second of two proximal pin sites but this has dried up. She is off the antibiotics, and she only takes an occasional Lortab for pain. She is out of her splint and sling but she needs to wear the Ace Wrap. Her ulnar-sided wrist pain is almost gone, only noting occasional shooting pain.

PHYSICAL EXAM

The patient is neurovascularly intact distally in her left upper extremity. Her pin sites are clean without drainage or erythema. She has full range of motion of her elbow. She pronates to 70 degrees and supinates to 45–50 degrees passively. She can flex her digits and has no soft-tissue swelling or destructive changes. She can nearly make a full fist and has good grip strength. She is nontender. Her ulnar styloid has no soft-tissue swelling.

IMAGING

Three views of the left wrist were obtained. Her hardware is in place without evidence of failure. There is minimal progression of callus formation. There is no loss of alignment. She has evidence of healing of her minimally displaced ulnar styloid fracture with calluses. Her fracture line is less apparent.

DIAGNOSES

1. Approximately 5-1/2 weeks status post ORIF of the left distal radius with additional fixator application of the left wrist.
2. Minimally displaced left ulnar styloid fracture.

TREATMENT RECOMMENDATIONS

1. I explained to the patient my impression and her treatment options. The plan is to remove her external fixator in 2 days. Based on the lack of her ulnar-sided symptoms at this point, and the fact that she is nontender over her styloid, I will hold off on delayed percutaneous pinning of her styloid fracture.
2. Will schedule her for Friday. She will be in a splint briefly postoperatively followed by fabrication of an Orthoplast orthosis.

OPERATIVE NOTE

PREOPERATIVE DIAGNOSIS
Chronic low back pain status post prior laminectomy, with postlaminectomy pain syndrome.

POSTOPERATIVE DIAGNOSIS
Chronic low back pain status post prior laminectomy with postlaminectomy pain syndrome.

PROCEDURES
1. Lumbar Racz catheter attempted neuroplasty at L4-5 and L5-S1.
2. Biplanar fluoroscopy.
3. Epidurograms.
4. Lysis of adhesions using Racz catheter and injection of Wydase to soften the scar tissue and to increase the lysis of adhesions.
5. Injection of local anesthetic, narcotic, steroid mixture.

SURGEON
John Smith, MD.

ASSISTANT
Mary Jones, ARNP.

JUSTIFICATION FOR PROCEDURE
This is a 60-year-old African-American male with chronic back pain and lumbar radiculopathy down the backs of his legs with a history of laminectomies. MRI findings showed status post L3-4 laminectomy for disk herniation with cephalad migration of disk material. There is also some evidence of canal stenosis, mainly congenital in etiology, at the same levels noted.

As a result of all this, we have decided to do a series of 3 lumbar Racz catheter neuroplasties with lysis of adhesions with the injection of Wydase to widen the spread of the narcotic/steroid mixture as well as to soften any scar tissue. It is hoped that we will be able to relieve any adhesions that might be compressing the respective nerve roots leading to his radiculopathy.

ANESTHESIA
Intravenous sedation due to the patient's apprehension.

PROCEDURE IN DETAIL
The patient was met in the preoperative area where extensive informed consent was obtained in writing. An IV was started in the dorsum of the hand, and the patient was taken to the procedure area where he was placed prone on the radiographic table with pillows below the abdomen. Other pressure points were padded, and monitors were placed to include EKG, Dinamap, and pulse oximetry. Nasal oxygen was given and intravenous sedation with propofol and Versed was started.

Once the desired level of sedation was achieved, the sacral and lower lumbar areas were prepped with Betadine solution and draped in a sterile fashion. Using biplanar fluoroscopy, the sacral cornu was identified and infiltrated with 2% Xylocaine plain.

(continued)

Next, a 16-gauge RK needle was inserted through the anesthetized area, and using biplanar fluoroscopic guidance, the needle was guided into the sacral foramen. Aspiration was carried out and was negative for any blood or cerebrospinal fluid. Next, a Brevi-XL 19-gauge 25-cm catheter was passed through the needle and up into the lower lumbosacral segment. The needle was advanced and at the L5-S1 interspace level was met with some obstruction. By gradual probing with the needle, we were able to advance it to the midbody of L5. At this point, an epidurogram was carried out by injecting Isovue-300 contrast material. The dye was noted to be pooled at the L5-S1 level, and it was then noted to spread in a caudal direction toward the coccyx area. There was no spread in a cephalad direction.

Again, gentle probing with the catheter tip was carried out and 300 units of Wydase was injected. After 2 to 3 minutes, again probing with the tip of the Racz catheter, we were able to advance the catheter up to the L4-5 interspace. Again, an epidurogram was carried out. This again showed dye pooling centrally in a loculated fashion, again suggestive of some adhesions, probably postsurgical, preventing the spread and possibly obliterating the epidural space. Film labeled #8 shows the initial epidurogram and film labeled #9 shows the second injection.

At this point, the Wydase was injected and, again, the spring-loaded tip of the Racz catheter was used to break up the adhesive processes. With this, the dye was noted to spread in a more cephalad direction, crossing the L4-5 level, getting up to the midbody of L4 and now spreading towards the lateral recesses. Again, the tip of the catheter was met with obstruction. Not wanting to puncture the dura, gentle probing was again carried out.

Having made progress from L5-S1 up to the midbody of L4, the decision was made not to carry out any further probing at this time. Therefore, 100 mcg of Fentanyl was injected. This was then followed by 80 mg of triamcinolone and 2 mL of 0.25% Chirocaine plain. The total volume was 6 mL plus the 2 mL for the Wydase, for a total of 8 mL. Film labeled #10 shows the final spread of the epidurogram, showing the area of adhesions lysed. This is available in hard copy on the chart. The lateral view confirmed confinement of the dye to the epidural space.

The needles and catheters were then removed, and the back was then cleansed of excess Betadine solution, and antibiotic ointment and dressings were applied. There were no complications noted and the patient tolerated the procedure well. He will be discharged when discharge criteria have been met, and he will be seen in followup in 3 weeks (1) to assess his level of improvement and (2) to perform the second procedure in this series.

REVIEW QUESTIONS

The goal of these questions is to test your knowledge in the areas of orthopedics, chiropractic, pain management, and podiatry.

Directions: Select the correct answer for each of the multiple-choice questions provided below. *Answers are provided at the end of this chapter.*

1. An abnormal outward curvature of a portion of the spine is called:
   A. Kyphosis
   B. Scoliosis
   C. Lordosis
   D. Osteoporosis
2. An abnormal sideways curvature of a portion of the spine is called:
   A. Kyphosis
   B. Scoliosis
   C. Lordosis
   D. Osteoporosis
3. Which of the following arthritis drugs does *not* contain aspirin (acetylsalicylic acid)?
   A. Ecotrin
   B. Celestone
   C. Dolobid
   D. Bufferin
4. When osteomalacia occurs in children the disease is called:
   A. Osteoporosis
   B. Scurvy
   C. Rickets
   D. Beriberi
5. Prevention of osteomalacia includes intake of sufficient:
   A. Vitamin C
   B. Vitamin E
   C. Vitamin B-12
   D. Vitamin D
6. Surgical repair of a broken bone is termed:
   A. Closed reduction
   B. Open reduction
   C. Scintiscan
   D. Fluoroscopy
7. If a pin is placed during surgical repair of a broken bone, what is done?
   A. Internal rotation
   B. External fixation
   C. Internal fixation
   D. External rotation
8. Allopurinol is a drug prescribed to treat:
   A. Arthritis
   B. Headaches
   C. Muscle spasm
   D. Gout
9. The removal of dead or damaged tissue from a wound is called:
   A. Conization
   B. Electrocautery
   C. Debridement
   D. Evisceration
10. Placement of CD-rods is typically done in treatment of:
    A. Scoliosis
    B. Total knee replacement
    C. Comminuted olecranon fracture
    D. Fracture of C1-2
11. Osteoporosis/osteopenia is the leading cause of:
    A. Death in the U.S.
    B. Multiple sclerosis
    C. Hip fracture
    D. Lou Gehrig disease
12. A tibial fracture classification system is:
    A. Salter-Harris
    B. Wilson-Cook
    C. Weber
    D. Watson-Jones

13. Which of these is used in the treatment of open wounds of the legs?
   A. Unna boots
   B. SCDs [sequential compression devices]
   C. Jobst boot
   D. Robert Jones dressing

14. The patient is a 72-year-old man admitted with hip fracture with a history of arthritis. Which of these medications is he likely to be taking?
   A. Celexa
   B. Cerebyx
   C. Celebrex
   D. Cenestin

15. The extensor pollicis brevis muscle is found in the:
   A. Ankle
   B. Forearm
   C. Back
   D. Neck

16. A right subacromial decompression would involve:
   A. The knee
   B. The eye
   C. The abdomen
   D. The shoulder

17. Which of these will be positive if a patient has osteomyelitis?
   A. Ceretec scan
   B. Technetium-99 SPECT scan
   C. MUGA scan
   D. VQ scan

18. The cervical spine consists of:
   A. 5 vertebrae
   B. 8 vertebrae
   C. 7 vertebrae
   D. 9 vertebrae

19. The correct medical term for the tailbone is the:
   A. Coccyx
   B. Thorax
   C. Humerus
   D. Malleolus

20. Carpals, metacarpals, and phalanges are found in the:
   A. Rib cage
   B. Hands
   C. Feet
   D. Spine

21. Spondylo- is the combining form meaning:
   A. Ankle
   B. Vertebra
   C. Knee
   D. Neck

22. Which of the following is a muscle located in the arm?
   A. Extensor carpi ulnaris
   B. Latissimus dorsi
   C. Sternocleidomastoid
   D. Rhomboid

23. The gastrocnemius muscle is located in the:
   A. Abdomen
   B. Thoracic cavity
   C. Leg
   D. Neck

24. The only movable bone in the skull is the:
   A. Mandible
   B. Ethmoid
   C. Maxilla
   D. Mastoid process

25. Osseous tissue is commonly called:
   A. Ligament
   B. Integument
   C. Bone
   D. Adipose

26. An abnormal inward curvature of a portion of the spine is called:
   A. Kyphosis
   B. Scoliosis
   C. Lordosis
   D. Hunchback

27. Which of the following tests is not used to assess the knee?
    A. Anterior drawer test
    B. Apley
    C. Lachman
    D. Romberg

28. Which of the following pharmacologic suffixes identifies a generic corticosteroid?
    A. -proxen
    B. -profen
    C. -sone
    D. -cycline

29. The medical term for the muscles located in the buttocks is:
    A. Quadriceps
    B. Gluteal
    C. Gastrocnemius
    D. Biceps

30. Chiropractors often diagnose sciatica in patients who complain of intermittent, shooting pain in the:
    A. Gluteal muscles going down one leg
    B. Gastrocnemius muscles going up one leg
    C. Trapezius muscles going into the chest
    D. Sternocleidomastoid muscles going into the jaw

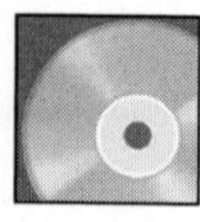

Please see the accompanying CD for additional review materials for this section.

PROOFREADING EXERCISES

These four proofreading exercises are provided to improve your skills in the areas of editing and effective identification and correction of errors in the medical record.

Directions: Identify and correct the transcription errors found in the exercises below. *Answers are provided at the end of this chapter.*

PROOFREADING EXERCISE #1

PREOPERATIVE DIAGNOSIS
Gangrene of 2nd and 3rd digits, left foot.

POSTOPERATIVE DIAGNOSIS
Gangrene of 2nd and 3rd digits, left foot.

PROCEDURE
Amputation of 2nd and 3rd digits, left foot.

ANESTHESIA
Monitored anesthesia care.

DESCRIPTION OF PROCEDURE
The patient was transferred to the operating room in apparent good preoperative condition and no contradictions to the proposed procedure were noted. However, the decision was made not to do a total foot amputation but only amputation of the 2nd and 3rd digits due to the advancing disease process in the patient's hand.

The initial incision was a transverse morsal incision going through the metatarsal phalangeal joints of the 2nd and 3rd digits. This incision was extended medially and laterally and then toward the planer surface to circumscribe the two digits. The extensor and flexor tendons were then excised, removing the 2nd and 3rd digits at the metatarsal phalangeal level. It was noted that the patient had vast necrotic tissue in the area of the amputation and, using Metzenbaum scissors, deep debridement was then performed. Also, cultures were taken aerobically and anaerobically to identify pathogens in the patient's foot.

(continued)

After debridement to a level of pliable tissue, the areas were then flushed with copious amounts of saline solution with Ancef, and with the use of 3-0 Vicryl suture material, the skin edges were then opposed and closed. The areas were dressed with antibiotic ointment and a dry, sterile dressing.

The patient appeared to have tolerated the surgical procedure well and was removed from the operating room apparently in good, postoperative condition.

PROOFREADING EXERCISE #2

PREOPERATIVE DIAGNOSIS
Right subcapital hip fracture.

POSTOPERATIVE DIAGNOSIS
Right subcapital hip fracture.

OPERATION
Right bipolar hip replacement.

SURGEON
John Smith, MD.

FIRST ASSISTANT
Mary Jones, MD.

ANESTHESIA
Spinal.

ESTIMATED BLOOD LOSS
100 mL.

COMPLICATIONS
None.

JUSTIFICATION FOR PROCEDURE
The patient is a 65-year-old male who fell, sustaining a right capitol hip fracture. The patient was medically cleared and then was taken to the operating room for definitive procedure.

PROCEDURE IN DETAIL
The patient was placed in the left lateral recumbent position and held in that position using an inflatable beanbag. The right hip and right lower extremity were then sterilely prepped and draped.

An incision was made over the lateral aspect of the right hip, curving slightly posterior. The incision was carried down through the subcutaneous tissue, and the tensor facial otto sharply divided.

(continued)

The muscles were bluntly dissected. A Charnley refractor was inserted to aid in retraction of the soft tissue. The short external rotators were identified and these were divided at the bone-tendon junction. A posterior capsulotomy was then performed. The patient was noted to have a subacute subcapital hip fracture. The hip was dislocated from the asa tabula. A femoral neck osteotomy was performed using an oscillating saw. The asa tabula had a trial with trial acetabular liners. Once the appropriate size was obtained, the femur was re-addressed. A box osteotome was used to osteotomize the proximal lateral aspect of the femur, followed by insertion of the canal finder, followed by reaming of the greater trochlear area, followed by insertion of successive broaches until the appropriate size was obtained. The patient was then fitted with trail head and neck prostheses. The hip was reduced on the operating table, and carried through a range of motion without any subluxation or dislocation. The hip was again dislocated with the aid of a bone hook, and the trial prostheses were removed.

The wound was copiously irrigated with pulse-irrigating antibiotic solution. The patient was then fitted with a size 10 humeral fracture stem from Biomet, with a standard 20-mm head and neck and a 42 outer-diameter bipolar cup. The hip was again reduced on the operating room table and taken through a range of motion without any sublimation or dislocation.

The wound was again copiously irrigated with pulse-irrigating antibiotic solution and the posterior capsule closed with #1 Vicryl suture. The short external rotators were re-attached to their insertion sight using #1 Vicryl suture. The tinsel fascia lata was closed with #1 Vicryl suture, the subcutaneous tissue was closed with 2-0 Vicryl suture, and the skin was closed with skin staples. The patient had a sterile dressing applied and was returned to the recovery room in stable condition.

PROOFREADING EXERCISE #3

CHIEF COMPLAINT
Low back pain and occasional left leg pain.

HISTORY OF PRESENT ILLNESS
I had the pleasure of seeing this patient for the first time at the pain center. He is a 45-year-old gentleman who gives a history of mainly back pain and left leg pain since being involved in a motor vehicle accident on 04/23/04. At that time, the patient was a restrained passenger. He began to have complaints of neck and back pain following the accident.

At this point in time, his chief complaint is that of back pain and some right leg pain. He continues to work and is employed as a painter. His pain is worse with standing or walking; bending or flexing the back also increases the pain. He does not report any weakness, but he does report some occasional tingling or numbness in the left lower extremity.

Treatments in the past have included various anti-inflammatories and narcotic analgesic medications with minimal relief, and he has also had chiropractic treatments and physical therapy. He has also been evaluated by the neurosurgeon. An MRI scan was performed showing a disk herniation at the L5-F1 level. There does not appear to be any neuroforaminal or final phimosis. He is here today for further evaluation and treatment.

PAST MEDICAL HISTORY
Sickle cell anemia.

PAST SURGICAL HISTORY
Noncontributory.

CURRENT MEDICATIONS
The patient does not have his medications with him at this time, but he will send us a list.

ALLERGIES
None.

(continued)

DIAGNOSTIC STUDIES
MRI results are as discussed above.

SOCIAL HISTORY
He sleeps for hours per night, has smoked 6 cigarettes per day for 8 years, drinks caffeine occasionally, drinks alcohol occasionally, and works as a painter.

PHYSICAL EXAMINATION
GENERAL: Well-developed, well-nourished gentleman in no acute distress.
HEENT: Pupils are equally round and reactive to light and accommodation, extraocular muscles are intact.
NECK: Supple, with full range of motion and negative jugular venous distension.
LUNGS: Clear.
CARDIOVASCULAR: Regular rate and rhythm.
MUSCULOSKELETAL: Full range of motion of all extremities. Good flexion and extension throughout the lumbar spine. Some reproduction of pain with extension. Minimal lumbar perisinus muscle tenderness, negative sacroiliac joint tenderness.
NEUROLOGICAL EXAMINATION: Deep tendon reflexes were 2+ throughout. Motor was 5/5 and sensory was intact.

IMPRESSION
Low back pain secondary to herniated nuclear prepulses at L5-S1.

PLAN
As discussed with the patient, we will be scheduling him for a fluoroscopically guided transforaminal injection bilaterally at the L5-F1 level. This appears to be the only pathology on the MRI scan. Following the first injection, if he obtains relief, we will consider a second injection in the series and, depending on how he is progressing, he will see the neurosurgeon to discuss other potential treatment options. Today, I will be giving him a prescription for a Mebaral Dosepak while we await scheduling for the lumbar epidermal.

PROOFREADING EXERCISE #4

HISTORY
Post-op right wrist. The patient returns to the office today indicating her wrist is feeling much better. She is not wearing her splint any longer. She is eager to return to work now. She has minimal soft-tissue swelling. She still notes some muscle soreness in the ulnar side of her wrist radiating both proximally and distillate. She is very pleased with her progress and her quick improvement.

PHYSICAL EXAM
The patient is neurovascularly intact distally in the right upper extremity. Her molar and dorsal incisions have healed. She has full range of motion of her elbow. She pronates passively 75° to 80° and supinates to 50° to 55°. Her wrist volar flexion is limited to 25° with discomfort in dorsal flexion to 60° with discomfort when she pushes up off the table. She is nontender over the ulnar styloid, and there is no point tenderness over her dorsal ulnar musculature and dorsal ulnar aspect of her hand.

IMAGING
Tree views of the right wrist out of the splint demonstrates her hardware is in place without evidence of failure of the screws. Her fracture line is less apparent and there is evidence of callous formation and healing, albeit slow. She has maintenance of her bowler tilt and radial length/height.

DIAGNOSIS
Approximately 2 months status post open reduction external fixation right distal radius fracture.

TREATMENT RECOMMENDATIONS
1. Continue to work on her home exercise program. If she does not find the occupational therapy beneficial after the first week, she should elevate and ice her wrist. If she is interested in resuming light weight training in her upper extremities, she needs to wear her clock up splint.
2. I will recheck her in 4-6 weeks to see how she is doing. I reassured her that the x-rays look good, but she is not entirely healed. She will likely feel soreness in the next month or two as she increases her functional abilities of the wrist.

ANSWER KEYS

REVIEW QUESTIONS ANSWER KEY

1. A
2. B
3. B
4. C
5. D
6. B
7. C
8. D
9. C
10. A
11. C
12. D
13. A
14. C
15. B
16. D
17. A
18. C
19. A
20. B
21. B
22. A
23. C
24. A
25. C
26. C
27. D
28. C
29. B
30. A

PROOFREADING EXERCISE #1 KEY

Incorrect term—contraindications

PREOPERATIVE DIAGNOSIS
Gangrene of 2nd and 3rd digits, left foot.

POSTOPERATIVE DIAGNOSIS
Gangrene of 2nd and 3rd digits, left foot.

PROCEDURE
Amputation of 2nd and 3rd digits, left foot.

ANESTHESIA
Monitored anesthesia care.

DESCRIPTION OF PROCEDURE
The patient was transferred to the operating room in apparent good preoperative condition and no contradictions to the proposed procedure were noted. However, the decision was made not to do a total foot amputation but only amputation of the 2nd and 3rd digits due to the advancing disease process in the patient's hand.

Incorrect word—foot

Incorrect term—dorsal

The initial incision was a transverse morsal incision going through the metatarsal phalangeal joints of the 2nd and 3rd digits. This incision was extended medially and laterally and then toward the planer surface to circumscribe the two digits. The extensor and flexor tendons were then excised, removing the 2nd and 3rd digits at the metatarsal phalangeal level. It was noted that the patient had vast necrotic tissue in the area of the amputation and, using Metzenbaum scissors, deep debridement was then performed. Also, cultures were taken aerobically and anaerobically to identify pathogens in the patient's foot.

Incorrect term—plantar

Use combined form—metatarsophalangeal

After debridement to a level of pliable ~~tissue~~, the areas were then flushed with copious amounts of saline solution with Ancef, and with the use of 3-0 Vicryl suture material, the skin edges were then opposed and closed. The areas were dressed with antibiotic ointment and a dry, sterile dressing.

The patient appeared to have tolerated the surgical procedure well and was removed from the operating room apparently in good, postoperative condition.

Incorrect term—viable

Incorrect word—apposed

PROOFREADING EXERCISE #2 KEY

PREOPERATIVE DIAGNOSIS
Right subcapital hip fracture.

POSTOPERATIVE DIAGNOSIS
Right subcapital hip fracture.

OPERATION
Right bipolar hip replacement.

SURGEON
John Smith, MD.

FIRST ASSISTANT
Mary Jones, MD.

ANESTHESIA
Spinal.

ESTIMATED BLOOD LOSS
100 mL.

COMPLICATIONS
None.

JUSTIFICATION FOR PROCEDURE
The patient is a 65-year-old male who fell, sustaining a right capitol hip fracture. The patient was medically cleared and then was taken to the operating room for definitive procedure.

Incorrect term—subcapital

PROCEDURE IN DETAIL
The patient was placed in the left lateral recumbent position and held in that position using an inflatable beanbag. The right hip and right lower extremity were then sterilely prepped and draped.

An incision was made over the lateral aspect of the right hip, curving slightly posterior. The incision was carried down through the subcutaneous tissue, and the tensor facial otto sharply divided. The muscles were bluntly dissected. A Charnley refractor

Incorrect term—fascia lata

Incorrect term—retractor

was inserted to aid in retraction of the soft tissue. The short external rotators were identified and these were divided at the bone-tendon junction. A posterior capsulotomy was then performed. The patient was noted to have a subacute subcapital hip fracture. The hip was dislocated from the asa tabula. A femoral neck osteotomy was performed using an oscillating saw. The asa tabula had a trial with trial acetabular liners. Once the appropriate size was obtained, the femur was re-addressed. A box osteotome was used to osteotomize the proximal lateral aspect of the femur, followed by insertion of the canal finder, followed by reaming of the greater trochlear area, followed by insertion of successive broaches until the appropriate size was obtained. The patient was then fitted with trail head and neck prostheses. The hip was reduced on the operating table, and carried through a range of motion without any subluxation or dislocation. The hip was again dislocated with the aid of a bone hook, and the trial prostheses were removed.

The wound was copiously irrigated with pulse-irrigating antibiotic solution. The patient was then fitted with a size 10 humeral fracture stem from Biomet, with a standard 20-mm head and neck and a 42 outer-diameter bipolar cup. The hip was again reduced on the operating room table and taken through a range of motion without any sublimation or dislocation.

The wound was again copiously irrigated with pulse-irrigating antibiotic solution and the posterior capsule closed with #1 Vicryl suture. The short external rotators were re-attached to their insertion sight using #1 Vicryl suture. The tinsel fascia lata was closed with #1 Vicryl suture, the subcutaneous tissue was closed with 2-0 Vicryl suture, and the skin was closed with skin staples. The patient had a sterile dressing applied and was returned to the recovery room in stable condition.

Incorrect term—acetabulum

Incorrect term—trochanter

Incorrect word—trial

Incorrect term—femoral

Incorrect term—subluxation

Incorrect word—site

Incorrect term—tensor

PROOFREADING EXERCISE #3 KEY

Incorrect side—left

CHIEF COMPLAINT
Low back pain and occasional left leg pain.

HISTORY OF PRESENT ILLNESS
I had the pleasure of seeing this patient for the first time at the pain center. He is a 45-year-old gentleman who gives a history of mainly back pain and left leg pain since being involved in a motor vehicle accident on 04/23/04. At that time, the patient was a restrained passenger. He began to have complaints of neck and back pain following the accident.

At this point in time, his chief complaint is that of back pain and some right leg pain. He continues to work and is employed as a painter. His pain is worse with standing or walking; bending or flexing the back also increases the pain. He does not report any weakness, but he does report some occasional tingling or numbness in the left lower extremity.

Treatments in the past have included various anti-inflammatories and narcotic analgesic medications with minimal relief, and he has also had chiropractic treatments and physical therapy. He has also been evaluated by the neurosurgeon. An MRI scan was performed showing a disk herniation at the L5-F1 level. There does not appear to be any neuroforaminal or final phimosis. He is here today for further evaluation and treatment.

Incorrect term—L5-S1

Should be 2 words—neural foraminal

Incorrect phrase—spinal stenosis

PAST MEDICAL HISTORY
Sickle cell anemia.

PAST SURGICAL HISTORY
Noncontributory.

CURRENT MEDICATIONS
The patient does not have his medications with him at this time, but he will send us a list.

ALLERGIES
None.

DIAGNOSTIC STUDIES
MRI results are as discussed above.

SOCIAL HISTORY
He sleeps for hours per night, has smoked 6 cigarettes per day for 8 years, drinks caffeine occasionally, drinks alcohol occasionally, and works as a painter.

Should be the number 4

PHYSICAL EXAMINATION
GENERAL: Well-developed, well-nourished gentleman in no acute distress.
HEENT: Pupils are equally round and reactive to light and accommodation, extraocular muscles are intact.
NECK: Supple, with full range of motion and negative jugular venous distension.
LUNGS: Clear.
CARDIOVASCULAR: Regular rate and rhythm.
MUSCULOSKELETAL: Full range of motion of all extremities. Good flexion and extension throughout the lumbar spine. Some reproduction of pain with extension. Minimal lumbar perisinus muscle tenderness, negative sacroiliac joint tenderness.
NEUROLOGICAL EXAMINATION: Deep tendon reflexes were 2+ throughout. Motor was 5/5 and sensory was intact.

Incorrect term—paraspinous

IMPRESSION
Low back pain secondary to herniated nuclear prepulses at L5-S1.

Incorrect phrase—nucleus pulposus

PLAN

As discussed with the patient, we will be scheduling him for a fluoroscopically guided transforaminal injection bilaterally at the L5-F1 level. This appears to be the only pathology on the MRI scan. Following the first injection, if he obtains relief, we will consider a second injection in the series and, depending on how he is progressing, he will see the neurosurgeon to discuss other potential treatment options. Today, I will be giving him a prescription for a Mebaral Dosepak while we await scheduling for the lumbar epidermal.

Incorrect drug—Medrol

Incorrect term—epidural

PROOFREADING EXERCISE #4 KEY

HISTORY
Post-op right wrist. The patient returns to the office today indicating her wrist is feeling much better. She is not wearing her splint any longer. She is eager to return to work now. She has minimal soft-tissue swelling. She still notes some muscle soreness in the ulnar side of her wrist radiating both proximally and distillate. She is very pleased with her progress and her quick improvement.

PHYSICAL EXAM
The patient is neurovascularly intact distally in the right upper extremity. Her molar and dorsal incisions have healed. She has full range of motion of her elbow. She pronates passively 75°–80° and supinates to 50°–55°. Her wrist volar flexion is limited to 25° with discomfort in dorsal flexion ~~to~~ 60° with discomfort when she pushes up off the table. She is nontender over the ulnar styloid, and there is no point tenderness over her dorsal ulnar musculature and dorsal ulnar aspect of her hand.

IMAGING
Tree views of the right wrist out of the splint demonstrates her hardware is in place without evidence of failure of the screws. Her fracture line is less apparent and there is evidence of callous formation and healing, albeit slow. She has maintenance of her bowler ~~tilt~~ and radial length/height.

DIAGNOSIS
Approximately 2 months status post open reduction external fixation right distal radius fracture.

Incorrect term—distally

Incorrect term—volar

Use combined form—dorsiflexion

Incorrect term—callus

Incorrect term—volar

Incorrect word—three

Incorrect word—internal

Incorrect term—cockup

TREATMENT RECOMMENDATIONS

1. Continue to work on her home exercise program. If she does not find the occupational therapy beneficial after the first week, she should elevate and ice her wrist. If she is interested in resuming light weight training in her upper extremities, she needs to wear her clock up splint.
2. I will recheck her in 4-6 weeks to see how she is doing. I reassured her that the x-rays look good, but she is not entirely healed. She will likely feel soreness in the next month or two as she increases her functional abilities of the wrist.

CHAPTER 19

Physical Medicine/ Rehabilitation

OBJECTIVES CHECKLIST

A prepared exam candidate will know the:

- ❑ Roles of each specialist in the field of physical medicine and rehabilitation, including physiatrists, physical therapists, occupational therapists, speech therapists, prosthetists, and orthotists.
- ❑ Diseases and conditions which can be treated by a physiatrist and therapists.
- ❑ Evaluations, tests, and devices used in physical therapy.
- ❑ Therapeutic modalities used in physical therapy.
- ❑ Evaluations, tests, and devices used in occupational therapy.
- ❑ Therapeutic modalities used in occupational therapy.
- ❑ Types of assistive devices used in occupational therapy.
- ❑ Terms used to describe anatomic planes, joint motions, and body movements.
- ❑ Common abbreviations used in physical and occupational therapy.

RESOURCE FOR STUDY

- *A Manual of Orthopaedic Terminology*
  Chapter 12: Physical Medicine and Rehabilitation: Physical Therapy and Occupational Therapy, pp. 347–356.
  Chapter 4: Tests, Signs and Maneuvers, pp. 119–140.
  Chapter 7: Prosthetics and Orthotics, pp. 169–188.
  Appendix A: Orthopaedic Abbreviations, pp. 371–370.
  Appendix B: Anatomic Positions and Directions, pp. 381–389.

SAMPLE REPORTS

The following five reports are examples of reports you might encounter while transcribing physical medicine and rehabilitation.

HISTORY AND PHYSICAL

CHIEF COMPLAINT

1. Status post hemilaminectomy L4-5 on the right and right L5-S1 diskectomy for lateral disk herniation L5-S1.
2. Weak right lower extremity.

HISTORY OF PRESENT ILLNESS

The patient fell in October of 2003 and developed severe pain and weakness into the right lower extremity as well as low back pain. He then had MRIs and the above-noted diagnoses and surgery. Since surgery he has been pain-free but is still very weak in the right lower extremity. He had this weakness prior to surgery. He denies any numbness or tingling. No bladder or bowel dysfunction. Cough, sneeze, or strain does not cause any pain. He is back to work.

He is not taking any medication for this condition at the present time. He is doing some walking exercises to strengthen his anterior tibialis.

PAST MEDICAL/SURGICAL HISTORY

Hypertension, glaucoma, BPH, no prior fractures, and he has never been diagnosed with cancer. He had a tonsillectomy as a child and a right inguinal hernia repair in the past.

FAMILY HISTORY

Negative for significant back problems.

SOCIAL HISTORY

He has been a widower for 10 years. He lives alone and has 7 children. He has never smoked, and he drinks 1 ounce of scotch per day.

ALLERGIES

None.

FITNESS PROGRAM

No set fitness program.

ACTIVITIES OF DAILY LIVING

Independent.

PHYSICAL EXAMINATION

This is an 80-year-old white male in no acute distress. He has a healing operative scar in the midline of the lumbar spine. There is no tenderness to palpation. He has 25% of lumbar spine flexion, no extension. He walks with a high-stepping gait on the right because of weakness. On muscle testing, the abdominals were 5/5, hip flexors were 5/5, hip adductors 3/5, gluteus maximus 5/5, quadriceps 4/5, anterior tibials 3/5, peroneals 3/5, toe extensors 3/5, gastrocnemius and soleus

(continued)

5/5. Knee jerk was 0/0, ankle jerk −2/0, and Babinski was downgoing bilaterally. He had a full range of motion of the hips and the knees but the hamstrings are tight.

EMG and nerve conduction studies done prior to surgery showed a severe, acute L5 radiculopathy on the right.

An MRI of lumbar spine showed degenerative disk disease at all levels, facet arthrosis, foraminal narrowing at all levels, and a lateral disk herniation at L5-S1.

CLINICAL IMPRESSION AND PLAN

1. Status post hemilaminectomy at L4-5 on the right and right L5-S1 diskectomy for lateral disk herniation right L5-S1.
2. Osteoarthritis of lumbar spine.
3. Persistent right lower extremity weakness.

The patient is already scheduled for physical therapy tomorrow, and I would appreciate the therapist instructing him regarding posture principles and body mechanics for the back, mainly focusing on strengthening exercises for the weakened hip abductor, quadriceps, and ankle group muscles. I also discussed with him an ankle-foot orthosis. His foot drop is also aggravated by the weak hip abductor. I would appreciate it if the therapist would try the ankle-foot orthosis with him and see how he likes it. Hopefully, he will be able to strengthen enough so he will not need the ankle-foot orthosis. I also recommend that he be instructed in the use of an exercise bike for fitness.

SPINE EVALUATION

DIAGNOSIS
Status post lumbar fusion.

PRECAUTIONS/CONTRAINDICATIONS
No bending or lifting.

MEDICATIONS
Coumadin and Zocor.

SUBJECTIVE
The patient reports that she had a fusion of L4-L5 using bone transplant and "nuts and bolts." This is the patient's third surgery on her back. She is now in a Velcro back support as needed. She also has an external bone stimulator. At the present time, patient complains of pain in the low lumbar area. If she applies pressure, it decreases discomfort. Also, she has pain in the left lumbosacral area and posterior left knee. Patient reports surgeries were due to degenerative bone disease in her lumbar spine.

PRIOR LEVEL OF FUNCTION
Prior to last surgery, the patient was in severe pain in the low back and left lower extremity and walked in extreme trunk flexion posture.

PAST MEDICAL HISTORY
Other than arthritis and back problems, past medical history is unremarkable. The patient did have first back surgery in 1992, a second back surgery in March of 1998.

SOCIAL HISTORY
The patient lives with her 13-year-old daughter. She is presently not working but is supposed to return to work at the end of August. She works as a telephone technician, and when she returns to work, she will work sitting at a computer.

RANGE OF MOTION/MUSCLE STRENGTH

Lumbar Flexion	Fingertips to superior knee joint line with discomfort in low back area.
Extension	To neutral.
Side bend right	Fingertips to mid thigh.
Left	Fingertips to mid thigh
Rotation right	Approximately 50% of normal with discomfort in the lower lumbar area.
Rotation left	Approximately 50% of normal with discomfort in the lower lumbar area.

The patient is able to walk on heels and toes without difficulty. She is able to do a full squat and return to standing without any difficulty. The right lower extremity demonstrates 4+/5 strength throughout except hip abduction and adduction, which are 4/5. Left hip flexion and extension 3/5. Left hip abduction and adduction 3/5. Knee flexion and extension 3/5. Abdominals 3−/5. Back extensors were not tested secondary to discomfort.

(continued)

NEUROLOGIC FINDINGS/COORDINATION/BALANCE

The patient reports that in the area of her left knee, in the dermatome of L4, there is decreased sensation. She reports initially after surgery it was totally numb in this area. Patient is unable to do single stance on left lower extremity longer than 1–2 seconds. She is, however, able to do single stance on right lower extremity approximately 5 seconds.

FUNCTIONAL MOBILITY

The patient reports that she is continuing to improve as the days go by. She is not allowed to do any bending or lifting at the present time. She is able to sleep at night. She is doing limited ADLs with discomfort felt constantly in the lower lumbar area.

POSTURE

The patient has scoliosis with right hip high, increased skin fold on the right, slight forward flexion at the waist as she stands and walks, tendency to keep weight shifted to right lower extremity due to pain in the left knee.

PALPATION

The patient is tender to palpation in the lower part of her lumbar incision. Incision has a deep appearance to it with only moderate tissue mobility.

SPECIAL TESTS

No special tests done on this date. It is noted that patient has tight hamstrings. She was able to do straight-leg raise only to 60 degrees, both left and right.

GAIT

On this date, patient has equal stride length and equal cadence both right and left lower extremity.

ASSESSMENT

The patient comes to the department status post lumbar fusion. She is showing a decrease in strength in left lower extremity and in trunk musculature. The patient will benefit from physical therapy in order to continue her rehabilitation following fusion of lumbar spine.

PLAN

1. Initially patient will be receiving aquatic exercises in order to increase strength and increase mobility.
2. Progressive home exercise program using dynamic lumbar stabilization program.
3. Patient will progress to land exercises again to increase strength, trunk stability, general mobility, and balance.
4. Hot packs or cold packs may be added as needed.

FREQUENCY

3 times per week.

PROJECTED LENGTH OF STAY

8 weeks.

REHAB POTENTIAL

Good for stated goals.

(continued)

PATIENT/FAMILY GOALS

Able to return to work without increased discomfort. Treatment plan was discussed with the patient who was in agreement with this plan.

4-WEEK TREATMENT GOALS

1. Patient to be independent in aquatic exercise program.
2. Have patient reporting a decrease in discomfort by 25–50%.
3. Increase AROM of trunk by 25% if possible.

8-WEEK TREATMENT GOALS

1. Have patient independent in dynamic lumbar stabilization program.
2. Have patient showing proper body mechanics for ADLs.
3. Decrease discomfort by 50%.
4. Have patient able to go through her day with only intermittent discomfort.
5. Have patient able to do activities for 30–45 minutes without having increased low back pain.

OCCUPATIONAL THERAPY REPORT

DIAGNOSIS
Left carpal tunnel syndrome; questionable left cubital tunnel.

PRECAUTIONS/CONTRAINDICATIONS
Shortness of breath with exertion, mitral valve prolapse, low blood pressure.

MEDICATIONS
Zoloft, Vioxx.

OCCUPATIONAL THERAPIST
Linda Jones, MS, OTR.

HISTORY
Patient states symptoms have progressively worsened over the past few years, with progressive worsening in December. She is experiencing severe paresthesias in left hand. She sought treatment with Dr. Smith, who issued a wrist support brace that she continues to wear during daytime hours. EMG testing 5/24 positive for carpal tunnel syndrome. MRI of cervical spine revealed bulging disk C4-6. She reports symptoms of "tingling" particularly when performing overhead tasks.

PRIOR LEVEL OF FUNCTION
Prior to December of 2000, she was able to perform all ADLs with no limitations.

PAST MEDICAL HISTORY
Sinus headaches, low blood pressure, fibromyalgia, severe back muscle spasms, spinal compression due to injury 1988, shortness of breath with exertion, mitral valve prolapse 20 years ago.

SOCIAL HISTORY
Patient is married. She enjoys golfing. She smokes 1 pack per day.

Occupation: Branch manager of a bank. Job duties entail several hours of computer work and writing, with which she reports she is experiencing significant difficulty. When symptoms are severe, she stops tasks, attempting to relieve symptoms. She continues to work full time.

CHIEF COMPLAINT
Numbness, "tingling" of left hand, difficulty with fine motor tasks, and hand weakness.

(continued)

UPPER EXTREMITY STATUS

ACTION	NORMAL	RIGHT AROM	STRENGTH	LEFT AROM	STRENGTH
Shoulder flexion	0–180°	WNL	5/5	WNL	
Shoulder abduction	0–180°				
Internal rotation	0–70°				
External rotation	0–90°				3+–4/5
Elbow flexion	0–150°				3+/5*
Elbow extension	0°				
Supination	0–80°			66°*	4/5
Pronation	0–80°			WFL	
Wrist extension	0–60°	0–60°		0–38°*	5/5
Wrist flexion	0–70°	0–70°		0–60°*	
Ulnar deviation	0–30°			WNL	
Radial deviation	0–20°			0–10°	

CLINICAL ASSESSMENT/HAND STATUS

Mild edema noted at the thenar eminence muscles. Hand intrinsics 4/5 bilaterally. Extensor pollicis brevis left 3+/5 with pain at MP joint, thumb abduction left 40°, right 50°.

SPECIAL TESTS

Finkelstein left positive, Phalen left positive, Tinel left positive. Palpation increases pain with light pressure to thenar eminence muscles and saddle joint. Demonstrates irritated radial nerve, cramping at wrist with fine motor tasks, pain with functional tasks 7/10.

GIRTH MEASUREMENTS

	RIGHT	LEFT
Wrist	N/A	17 cm
Distal palmar crease	N/A	21 cm
MCP heads	N/A	18.8 cm
Circumference of PIP joints	N/A	17 cm
IP joint	N/A	6.9 cm

(continued)

Fingertips to DPC: WNL.

Opposition: WNL.

Hand Strength: Dominant hand: Left.

Involved hand: Left.

	RIGHT	LEFT
Gross grasp	50,50,55	55,58,56
Lateral pinch	18	19
3 Pt. pinch	14	11
2 Pt. pinch	10	13

Coordination: Right and left intact with opposition testing.

Sensation: Right and left intact with light touch test. Two-point discrimination = deficits at forearm, proximally greater than distally 4.5–5 cm.

ADL Status: Independent. She is unable to manipulate clasp on jewelry secondary to prehension grasp or perform any bilateral power task such as opening jars. She struggles with manipulating buttons and zippers. Unable to pull up zipper on dress behind. Difficulty pulling on hosiery and don and doff bra.

ASSESSMENT
Patient presents as a 47-year-old female who is strongly left-hand-dominant. She has compromised left wrist and forearm range of motion, decreased strength, irritated radial nerve, positive Phalen and Finkelstein testing. EPB 3+/5, limited thumb mobility. Difficulty with ADL tasks which require grip or fine motor dexterity.

TREATMENT PLAN
Active and passive range of motion exercises, progressive wrist and hand strengthening, nerve/tendon glides, scar management and soft tissue mobilization, home exercise program. Modalities: Whirlpool, moist heat, paraffin dip, and cryotherapy p.r.n.

Frequency: 3 times per week.

Projected Length of Stay: 4 weeks.

Rehab Potential: Good for stated goals.

Patient/Family Goals: To increase hand function.

TREATMENT GOALS 4 WEEKS
1. Independent with upgraded home exercise program to increase range of motion and strength.
2. Demonstrate left wrist extension to 50° and radial deviation of 20°.
3. Demonstrate improvement in left thumb mobility to 50°.

SPINAL ASSESSMENT

DIAGNOSIS
Lumbar radiculopathy; left knee derangement.

PRECAUTIONS/CONTRAINDICATIONS
Cardiac precautions, hypertension, history of stroke.

MEDICATIONS
Celebrex and Neurontin.

SUBJECTIVE
Patient notes having intermittent back pain since 1996. Patient had a total knee replacement at that time and developed low back pain. X-rays subsequently showed a "broken back" that had not healed properly. Patient has followed up with a neurosurgeon and states that she was told her spinal cord was fraying out between her vertebrae, but her fractures have healed. Patient also has arthritis in her spine. Patient notes constant low back pain ranging 3 to 7 out of 10 to 10 out of 10, increasing with walking activities. Patient has pain which was initially in her right lower extremity but now has shifted to her left side. Patient states recent MRI showed pinched nerves in her low back. Patient has received physical therapy on and off since 1997, most recently 2 months ago. Patient also has complaints of left knee pain which is constant and increases with walking. Pain is at lateral aspect of knee and generally ranges 3 to 7 out of 10. Patient denies any locking, buckling, or clicking. Patient does not recall if she had an MRI of her left knee.

PRIOR LEVEL OF FUNCTION
Patient reports using a single-point cane since 1996 and then switched to a quad cane after mini strokes 2 years ago. Patient reports having occasional speech difficulties from her stroke, but no muscular weakness. Patient has had progressive increase in her back pain and lower extremity pain since 1996. During her course of physical therapy several months ago, patient was able to walk up to 8 minutes at 0.5 to 0.6 mph.

PAST MEDICAL HISTORY
1. Right total knee replacement in 1996
2. Open heart surgery September 2000.
3. Uterine cancer in 1986.
4. Mini strokes 2 years ago with residual speech difficulties.
5. Arthritis/joint pain.
6. Low back problems since 1996 as noted above.

SOCIAL HISTORY
Patient is married and lives in a mobile home with 5 steps to enter. Patient is employed at the university as an operator. She reports being in a disabled job description secondary to back and knee injuries. Recreational activities include gardening, flower arrangement, and crafts.

(continued)

RANGE OF MOTION/MUSCLE STRENGTH

Lumbar flexion	Fingertips to toes with complaints of hamstring pulling.
Lumbar extension	5° with complaints of pain into left lower extremity.
Side bend right	Fingertips to proximal patella with complaints of stiffness.
Side bend left	Fingertips to joint line with complaints of stiffness.
Rotation right	75% without pain.
Rotation left	75% with no complaints of pain.
Abdominal strength	4+/5
Back extensors	3+/5, assessed in standing position as patient is unable to tolerate prone.

AREA	RIGHT	LEFT
Knee strength		
Extension At 0°	4/5	4/5
at 45°	4/5	4/5
Flexion at 45°	4/5	4/5
at 90°	4/5	4/5

Area	Right LE AROM	PROM	Left LE AROM	PROM
Knee	1–110°	115°	3–115°	120°*

*End-range pain

AREA		RIGHT STRENGTH	LEFT STRENGTH
Hip	Flexion	4/5	4+/5
	Extension	4−/5	4/5
	Abduction		
	Adduction	3−/5*	3−/5*
	Dorsiflexion	WNL	WNL
	Plantar flexion	WNL	WNL

*with complaints of low back pain

NEUROLOGICAL FINDINGS/COORDINATION/BALANCE

Sensation grossly intact to light touch throughout bilateral lower extremities. Patient does report radiating pain in left hip, lateral thigh, lateral knee, and ankle, as well as into her groin. She denies any symptoms into her feet on the left. Patient reports numbness and tingling in her toes on the right and anterior thigh and shin.

Patellar and Achilles DTRs: Unable to elicit bilaterally.

(continued)

Functional Mobility: Patient reports inability to sleep on her back, to walk for prolonged periods or lifting activities due to low back pain. Patient has knee pain limiting walking and causing her pain, even ambulating using quad cane.

Posture: Patient is 5 feet 6 inches and 270 pounds. In standing, patient has hallux valgus bilateral feet, genu valgus bilaterally, forward head and rounding of shoulders.

Palpation: There is no joint line tenderness with palpation of left knee.

There is tenderness with palpation of left greater trochanteric region over L4, L5, and S1 spinous segments and in paraspinals.

SPECIAL TESTS

LUMBAR SPINE
Quadrant test: Negative for production of radicular symptoms. Provokes low back pain bilaterally.

Straight-leg raise: Negative for radicular symptoms of hamstring tightness.

FABER test: Positive.

KNEE
Varus test: Negative for joint line pain or gapping.

Valgus stress test: Positive for lateral joint line pain.

McMurray test: Provokes lateral joint line pain.

Gait: Patient ambulates with quad cane on right. There is increased lateral trunk sway over left lower extremity during stance phase and decreased stance time on right.

ASSESSMENT
Patient presents to physical therapy with complaints of lateral greater than medial left knee pain and with restrictions in extension, range of motion, and pain with maximal flexion. Patient does have tenderness in greater trochanteric region and along IT band which may be a contributing factor. Additionally, there is lateral joint line pain with McMurray testing for possible meniscal tear. Patient has additional complaints of low back pain and left greater than right radiculopathy. There is significant decrease in extension range of motion, decreased strength for pelvic stabilizing musculature, and decreased lower extremity strength evident. There is a decrease in intervertebral mobility and radicular symptoms consistent with degenerative changes of lumbar spine.

PLAN
1. Land-based and aquatic physical therapy for pelvic stabilizing exercises and lower extremity strengthening and flexibility exercises.
2. Jet massage in pool.
3. Pain modalities including moist heat pack, TENS, and possibly massage.
4. Home exercise program to enhance treatment.

Frequency: 3 times per week.

Projected Length of Stay: 4–6 weeks.

(continued)

Rehab Potential: Fair, noting chronic nature of patient's low back pain and diagnosis of internal derangement left knee which may not respond to conservative treatment.

Patient/Family Goals: Patient would like to diminish low back pain levels and left knee pain levels so that she is able to tolerate walking activities.

Treatment Goals: To be achieved in 4–6 weeks.

1. Patient to be independent with progression of land-based and aquatic physical therapy in order to continue independently at community pool as desired.
2. Improve pain-free lumbar extension at least 5°.
3. Improve strength for abdominals and back extensors at least one-half muscle grade to improve pelvic stabilization.
4. Improve strength for bilateral hip abduction, right hip extension, and bilateral knee flexion and extension at least one-half muscle grade.

OCCUPATIONAL THERAPY

DIAGNOSIS
Infantile hemiplegia.

ASSISTIVE DEVICES AND/OR BRACES
None.

PRECAUTIONS/ALLERGIES
None.

MEDICATIONS
None.

OCCUPATIONAL THERAPIST
Linda Jones, MS, OTR.

PHYSICAL HISTORY
The patient was born by emergency C-section 2 weeks premature. Apgar scale good. Mother states she began noticing delay with right lower extremity when the patient started to walk. She also began noticing that the patient was not using her right upper extremity for playing.

PAST MEDICAL HISTORY
Unremarkable. The patient is seen weekly by a chiropractor for adjustment since 14 months of age.

SOCIAL HISTORY
The patient is an only child to be entering kindergarten at Smithville Elementary.

CHIEF COMPLAINT
Not using right upper extremity.

EVALUATION
Upper Extremity Status: Left upper extremity within normal limits and strength is good throughout. Right: Difficulty with active movement above shoulder level. Strength: 2+ to 3/5.

COGNITIVE/PERCEPTUAL STATUS
Attention Span: Attention span good. Able to complete tasks as instructed without redirection.

Sequencing: Good.

Problem Solving: Excellent.

SELF HELP SKILLS
Feeding: Uses left to manipulate fork and spoon. She has difficulty with coordinating utensils and cutting her food.

(continued)

Dressing: Minimal to moderate assist with upper and lower extremity dressing.

Fastening: Unable to tie shoelaces, zip, or manipulate buttons. She is able to pull up zipper when initiated.

Bathing: Minimal to moderate assist with hair and body washing.

FINE MOTOR SKILLS AND BEHAVIORS
Intrinsics: Right equal to left, 2+/5. Grasp on writing tool weak using a cylindrical grasp. Using left for all fine motor activities today.

Functional Gross Motor Skills: Demonstrates difficulty stepping on/off step stool. Jumps, landing on left followed by right.

ASSESSMENT
The patient is a 5-year-old bright and happy child who has had delays in using right upper extremity functionally since birth. The patient demonstrates difficulty using appropriate grasp and prehension patterns during writing activities. Grasp is weak. She demonstrates difficulty coordinating right and left for scissor activities. Unable to use right functionally and prefers not to use right unless encouraged.

TREATMENT PLAN
Graded fine motor tasks including use of scissors, copying, tracing, gluing. Self-care tasks including fasteners and eye-hand coordination activities. Functional activities to improve overall upper extremity strengthening and grasp.

Frequency: 3 times per week.

Projected Length of Stay: 1 year.

Rehab Potential: Good.

Patient/Family Goals: To have better grip for writing.

Treatment Goals: For 6 months:
1. Caregiver/patient independent with home exercise program to provide continuity of care within home environment.
2. Able to cut a 12-inch straight line with 90% accuracy.
3. Able to button/unbutton 3 large buttons on button strip with no assistance.

REVIEW QUESTIONS

The goal of these questions is to test your knowledge in the areas of physical medicine and rehabilitation

Directions: Select the correct answer for each of the multiple-choice questions provided below. *Answers are provided at the end of this chapter.*

1. A physician who specializes in physical medicine and rehabilitation is called a/an:
   - A. Physical therapist
   - B. Occupational therapist
   - C. Physiatrist
   - D. Rehabilitation specialist
2. Hydrotherapy includes which of these modalities?
   - A. Paraffin
   - B. TENS
   - C. Diathermy
   - D. Iontophoresis
3. Which of the following is a form of electrical stimulation?
   - A. Iontophoresis
   - B. MENS
   - C. Diathermy
   - D. A & B
4. Which condition below would likely be treated by a physical medicine specialist?
   - A. A person with cholecystitis
   - B. An elderly person with a hip fracture
   - C. A person with an inoperable brain tumor
   - D. A diabetic with nephropathy
5. Which of the following might be utilized by a physical medicine practitioner?
   - A. An electrocardiogram
   - B. A cystoscope
   - C. An electroencephalogram
   - D. An electromyogram
6. Three-point gait refers to:
   - A. Ambulation with crutches
   - B. Ambulation with a walker
   - C. A shuffling gait
   - D. Ambulation with a lower extremity prosthesis
7. The medical professional who helps people improve their ability to perform activities of daily living and work tasks is called a/an:
   - A. Physical therapist
   - B. Fitness instructor
   - C. Workers' Compensation specialist
   - D. Occupational therapist
8. Physical therapists help to relieve pain using which modality?
   - A. Whirlpool therapy
   - B. Exploratory surgery
   - C. Use of a transcutaneous electrical nerve stimulation unit
   - D. Correction of electrolyte abnormalities
9. A diagnostic test used to assess the integrity of peripheral nerves by measuring the time required for an impulse to travel over a nerve segment is called:
   - A. NCV
   - B. EMG
   - C. Two-point discrimination
   - D. Proprioceptive testing
10. One example of low-impact therapy for individuals of all abilities would be:
    - A. Cross training
    - B. Jogging slowly
    - C. Anaerobic exercise
    - D. Aquatic therapy

11. Which of the following is not a parameter for assessing the function of a limb?
   A. ROM
   B. Sensation
   C. Strength
   D. Coordination

12. A combination of physical, occupational, and speech therapy; psychologic counseling; and social work directed toward helping patients maintain or recover physical capacities is the official definition of:
   A. Social work
   B. Physical therapy
   C. Occupational therapy
   D. Rehabilitation

13. Devices which provide support for damaged joints, ligaments, tendons, muscles, and bones are called:
   A. Orthotics
   B. Crutches
   C. Wheelchairs
   D. Braces

14. Devices which replace lost limbs or other body parts are called:
   A. Prosthetists
   B. Prostatics
   C. Prosthetics
   D. Prosthions

15. Passive, active-assistive, active describe:
   A. ROM exercises
   B. ADLs
   C. Speech exercises
   D. Massage techniques

16. A psychomotor defect in which the proper use of an object cannot be carried out is called:
   A. Aprosopia
   B. Aproctia
   C. Aphasia
   D. Apraxia

17. Impaired or absent comprehension or production of, or communication by, speech, writing, or signs, due to an acquired lesion of the dominant cerebral hemisphere is termed:
   A. Aphasia
   B. Aphanisis
   C. Aphalangia
   D. Apraxia

18. The goal of cardiac rehabilitation is to:
   A. Promote the formation of collateral circulation
   B. Prevent future heart attacks
   C. Help the patient recover quickly and improve physical functioning
   D. None of the above

19. Which of the following is not considered a physical therapy procedure?
   A. Codman exercise
   B. Accupressure
   C. Isokinetic exercise
   D. RICE

20. A dynamometer is used to:
   A. Measure muscle strength
   B. Measure ROM
   C. Measure sensation
   D. Measure ambulatory speed

21. Before treatment, an occupational therapist uses a variety of tests to assess the patient's abilities and deficits. These tests include:
   A. Crawford small parts dexterity
   B. Jebsen-Taylor hand function
   C. Minnesota rate of manipulation
   D. All of these

22. A painless awareness of an amputated limb possibly accompanied by mild tingling is termed:
   A. Prosthetic pain
   B. Mystery pain
   C. Phantom pain
   D. True pain

23. The therapeutic application of high-frequency currents using radiofrequency electromagnetic fields for therapeutic heating of tissues is called:
    A. Paraffin therapy
    B. Hydrotherapy
    C. Microwave therapy
    D. Short wave diathermy

24. The abbreviation FROM in the context of physical medicine and rehabilitation means:
    A. Fixed range of motion
    B. Full range of motion
    C. Fixed ratio of movement
    D. Frequent rapid ocular movements

25. Mechanical resistance devices may include:
    A. Weights, spring tension, and other techniques
    B. Treadmill and StairMaster
    C. TENS unit
    D. Cervical traction

26. A sense or perception, usually at a subconscious level, of the movements and position of the body and especially its limbs, independent of vision is called:
    A. Coordination
    B. Perception
    C. Cognition
    D. Proprioception

27. Transfer training is often used in the rehabilitation of hip fracture patients. This entails teaching the patient how to:
    A. Re-establish full ambulation
    B. Improve motor neuron skills
    C. Move safely from bed to chair, etc.
    D. Properly use orthotics

28. Training with parallel bars is often used in the rehabilitation of patients with:
    A. Proprioceptive disorders
    B. Impaired balance
    C. Motor neuron diseases
    D. Wheelchair status

29. This device is used by occupational therapists to measure gross movements of arm, hand, fingers, and fingertip dexterity:
    A. Purdue pegboard
    B. Jamar dynamometer
    C. Swiss ball
    D. Pulley

30. Assistive equipment might include:
    A. Sockdonners
    B. Reachers
    C. Splints
    D. A & B

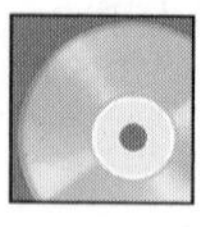

Please see the accompanying CD for additional review materials for this section.

PROOFREADING EXERCISES

These three proofreading exercises are provided to improve your skills in the areas of editing and effective identification and correction of errors in the medical record.

Directions: Identify and correct the transcription errors found in the exercises below. *Answers are provided at the end of this chapter.*

PROOFREADING EXERCISE #1

DIAGNOSIS
Rotator cuff dysfunction.

SUBJECTIVE
The patient returns to physical therapy today for follow up of progression. The patient reports that he has continued to have shoulder pain. He has been consistent with his exercise program 3–4 times a week. He has been able to progress to 35 pounds via bench press, but he is holding at 5 pounds for side lying external rotation as he feels he is having some difficulty with his papular muscles. The patient followed up with Dr. Smith of the department of physical medicine and rehabilitation, who has recommended progression to ultrasound and ion phoresis, but Dr. Smith's note was not available in the chart today.

OBJECTIVE
We will continue with physical therapy treatment including progression of therapeutic exercises and the addition of iontophoresis and ultrasound today. We discussed using ultrasound with the patient and iontophoresis including the contradictions. The patient is not allergic to Dexamethasone.

The patient received the following today:

Ultrasound x 8 minutes at 1.35 what/cm^2 continuous to anterior right shoulder near supraspinatus insertion.

The patient received iontophoresis using 2.5 mL of dexamethasone and a sound head at 3.0 microamps at a 40-microamps per minute rate, negative polarity with medicated pad at the area of most tenderness on the

(continued)

anterior shoulder and the disperser pad along the mid-humorous posteriorly. We will have the patient continue with his exercise program. I do not want him to advance at this point as his repetitions and resistance seem to be appropriate.

ASSESSMENT

The patient tolerated physical therapy well. He had very slight reddening underneath the medicated pad after the iontophoresis treatment but there was no subcutaneous water accumulation. We will continue with physical therapy with the following long term goals:

Patient will demonstrate improvement of horizontal adduction to 15 degrees on the right.

Patient will increase shoulder length by one-half grade.

Patient will return to fitness activities without pain greater then 2/10.

Patient will have punch, weightlifting, and fitness activities including the use of a training log 3–4 times a week without pain greater than 2/10.

PROOFREADING EXERCISE #2

DIAGNOSIS
Low back pain.

PRECAUTIONS/CONTRAINDICATIONS
Asthma.

MEDICATIONS
Celebrex.

SUBJECTIVE
The patient is a 17-year-old female who notes insipidus onset of low back discomfort approximately 3-1/2 months ago. The patient progressively worsened to the point where patient could barely bend forward and had pain rolling over in bed. The patient was initially treated by her family physician with Celexa after x-rays showed no abnormalities; however, her symptoms did not resolve. MRI ordered by her orthopedist, per patient, showed a herniated disk in her lumbar spine. The patient states her pain levels are improving, but she notes a constant ache and intermittent pain ranging up to 7/10 following activities. The patient currently has a mild extravasation which she attributes to having played whiffle ball last week. The patient does note several episodes of pain radiating into right buttock but no reticular symptoms at present.

PRIOR LEVEL OF FUNCTION
The patient notes no history of back pain and was unrestricted in activities such as basketball, volleyball, and occasional running.

PAST MEDICAL HISTORY
1. Asthma.
2. Right knee parcel patellar tendon tear 2000.

SOCIAL HISTORY
The patient is a senior in high school and lives with her family. She does not plan on participating in any other sports activities. Patient works approximately 20 hours a week in the house wares department at Sears. She is continuing to work full duty and states her job does not require any heavy lifting.

(continued)

RANGE OF MOTION/MUSCLE STRENGTH

AREA	MEASUREMENT
Lumbar flexion	Fingertips to proximal patella limited by right-greater-than-left lumbosacral region.
Extension	15° with pain throughout movement but not at in range.
Side bend right	Fingertips to distal patella with stretch noted on contralateral side but no pain.
Left	Fingertips to distill patella with stretch noted on contralateral side but no pain.
Rotation right	Within normal limits pain free.
Rotation left	Within normal limits pain free.

Lower extremity AROM within normal limits for hip, knee, and ankle.

Strength 5/5 throughout including EHL. The patient is able to heel walk and tow walk. Abdominals: Good minus with low back pain discomfort. Back extensors: Good minus without pain.

NEUROLOGIC FINDINGS/COORDINATION/BALANCE
Patellar and Achilles deep tendon reflexes equal and reactive bilaterally. Sensation intact to lite touch throughout all dermal tones bilateral lower extremities. The patient does note occasional episodes of pain radiating into right buttock.

FUNCTIONAL MOBILITY
Secondary to low back pain, the patient notes difficulty tolerating supine or prone lying with rolling over in bed. She is not able to participate in sports activities at prior functional level secondary to exacerbation of pain. The patient reports difficulty bending forward to put on pants and stockings.

POSTURE
In standing, patient exhibits increased lumbar lordosis and anterior pelvic tilt. There is founding of shoulders and the head is tipped forward. Levels of ileac crests are symmetrical. Level of right acronym (dominant upper extremity) is depressed with respect to left.

SPECIAL TESTS
Repeated flexion in standing: Increases low back pain but does not produce radicular symptoms.

(continued)

Repeated extension in standing: Diminishes low back pain slightly.

String testing: Negative for production of cervical radicular symptoms, inner vertebral mobility within normal limits throughout.

Straight-leg raze testing: Negative. Note: Hamstring tightness bilaterally at 65°.

GAIT
No significant alleviation noted.

ASSESSMENT
The patient is a 17-year-old female who presents to physical therapy with complaints of low back pain and, per patient, a positive MRI for lumbar disk herniation. On this date, the patient has significant limitation in flexion range of motion, hamstring tightness, and weakness of pelvic stabilizing musculature. Sensory motor exam is unremarkable.

PLAN
1. Extension-based pelvic sterilization exercises.
2. Hamstring stretching.
3. Accompanying HEB including postural education.
4. Pain modalities including ultrasound, possibly cold packs and moist heat packs.

FREQUENCY
2 times per week.

PROJECTED LENGTH OF STAY
3 to 4 weeks.

REHABILITATION POTENTIAL
Good.

(continued)

PATIENT/FAMILY GOALS

The patient would like to return to normal daily activities and recreational sports such as whiffle ball without exacerbation of pain.

4-WEEK TREATMENT GOALS

1. Patient to be independent with progression of home exercise program.
2. Improve pain-free trunk flexion at least finger tips to distal chin in order to increase ease with activities such as on/off socks/pants/stockings.
3. Diminish pain levels to 3/10 or less with performance of recreational sports activities.
4. Improve bilateral hamstring flexibility at least 5–10 degrees.

PROOFREADING EXERCISE #3

DIAGNOSIS
Knee tendonitis.

PRECAUTIONS/CONTRAINDICATIONS
Patient is on Coumadin. In 1995, patient had surgery for multiple aneurysms in the brain.

MEDICATIONS
Coded aspirin, Pravachol, Vioxx, Coumadin.

SUBJECTIVE
Patient reports that she had an operation on her left foot on 4/16/2001 to correct positioning of toes and to trim bunion on the left foot. Since that time, the patient has had persistent pain in the posterior speck of her left knee, posterior thigh, and up into both buttocks, left grader than right. She rates the pain as a 3/10 to a 6/10, describes it as an aching pain. She reports that she knows she has a faulty gait pattern but has been walking with a faulty gait pattern for approximately 5 years secondary to problems with her feet.

PRIOR LEVEL OF FUNCTION
Prior to 4/16/2001, pain in the knee was only intermittent, was not as constant or as sever as at present time.

PAST MEDICAL HISTORY
1. In 1995, patient underwent surgery for several aneurysms of the brain. Patient is on Coumadin at the present time.
2. Patient has a hammer toe and bunion on the right foot.

SOCIAL HISTORY
The patient is married. She is retired. Her hobbies are baby-sitting and gardening.

RANGE OF MOTION/MUSCLE STRENGTH
Active range of motion of both knees is within normal limits.

(continued)

She demonstrates 4 plus over 5 strength throughout knee flexion and extension. There is no pain with resistance to ether flexion or extension of the knee.

Patient is able to walk on heels and toes with only minor discomfort in for foot. Patient is able to do only a 50% squat and return to standing. Patient does show a decrease in strength in her hip vasculature.

Hip extension on the left is a 3+/5.

Hip abduction: 4/5.

Hip adduction: 3+/5.

Hip internal and external rotation: 3+/5.

NEUROLOGICAL FINDINGS/COORDINATION/BALANCE
DTRs were not tested on this date. Patient is able to do single dance on the right foot for approximately 3 seconds and able to do single dance on the left foot for 1–2 seconds.

Functional Motility: Patient reports that she is having difficulty baby-sitting secondary to pain in her knee; difficulty with sleeping; able to walk only 30 minutes and then must rest the knee secondary to pain; general decrease in activities.

Posture: Patient is 5 feet 2 inches tall, 135 pounds. She does have scoliosis of the spine. Kyphosis of the thoracic spine with forward head. Left shoulder is low, left hip is high as compared to the right. She has bilateral genus veris left greater than right, tibial torsion in the left lower leg, does have an onion both left and right.

Palpation: Patient is very tender to palpitation in the popliteal fossa of the left knee. There is no pain with palpation of the patellar tendon or any palpation of the hamstring insertions.

(continued)

SPECIAL TESTS
Faber test: Negative.

Straight-leg raise test: Negative but note the patient has decreased hamstring length. Is able to do straight-leg raise only to 65° both left and right and then feels hamstring tightness.

McMurray test: Negative.

Anterior-posterior drawer sign: Negative.

GAIT
Patient has an antalgic gait on the left. Tends to keep left foot flat as she goes through her ambulation but is able to do heel strike and toe off when given verbal queuing.

ASSESSMENT
Patient comes to the department with diagnosis of left knee tendonitis. She is complaining of pain in the poster aspect of her knee to the point that she has had decrease in functional activities and inability to sleep. Patient does show a faulty gait pattern in the left lower extremity. Patient is very tender to palpation in the posterior aspect of the left knee.

PLAN
1. Ultrasound to the posterior aspect of the left knee.
2. Progressive therapeutic exercise to work on strength and balance.
3. Gait trailing as appropriate.
4. Coal pack as needed.
5. Home exercise program.

Frequency: 3 times week.

Protected Length of Stay: 4 weeks.

Rehab Potential: Difficult to state at the present time.

(continued)

Patient/Family Goals: To be able to sleep at night and have decreased pain as she goes throughout her AVLs. Treatment plan was discussed with the patient who was in agreement with this plan.

Treatment Goals:
To be achieved in 4 weeks.
1. Have patient independent with HEP.
2. Increase single stance on left and right lower extremities for 5–10 seconds safely.
3. Increase ham string length in order to ease discomfort in knee.
4. Have patient able to walk 30–40 minutes without having increase in discomfort in the knee.

ANSWER KEYS

REVIEW QUESTIONS ANSWER KEY

1. C
2. A
3. D
4. B
5. D
6. A
7. D
8. C
9. A
10. D
11. D
12. D
13. A
14. C
15. A
16. D
17. A
18. C
19. D
20. A
21. D
22. C
23. D
24. B
25. A
26. D
27. C
28. B
29. A
30. D

PROOFREADING EXERCISE #1 KEY

DIAGNOSIS
Rotator cuff dysfunction.

SUBJECTIVE
The patient returns to physical therapy today for follow up of progression. The patient reports that he has continued to have shoulder pain. He has been consistent with his exercise program 3–4 times a week. He has been able to progress to 35 pounds via bench press, but he is holding at 5 pounds for side lying external rotation as he feels he is having some difficulty with his papular muscles. The patient followed up with Dr. Smith of the department of physical medicine and rehabilitation, who has recommended progression to ultrasound and ion phoresis, but Dr. Smith's note was not available in the chart today.

OBJECTIVE
We will continue with physical therapy treatment including progression of therapeutic exercises and the addition of iontophoresis and ultrasound today. We discussed using ultrasound with the patient and iontophoresis including the contradictions. The patient is not allergic to Dexamethasone.

The patient received the following today:

Ultrasound x 8 minutes at 1.35 what/cm² continuous to anterior right shoulder near supraspinatus insertion.

Use noun form—followup

Incorrect term—scapular

Incorrect term—iontophoresis

Incorrect term—contraindications

Generic name—use lowercase

Incorrect term—watts

The patient received iontophoresis using 2.5 mL of dexamethasone and a sound head at 3.0 microamps at a 40-microamps per minute rate, negative polarity, with medicated pad at the area of most tenderness on the anterior shoulder and the disperser pad along the mid-humorous posteriorly. We will have the patient continue with his exercise program. I do not want him to advance at this point as his repetitions and resistance seem to be appropriate.

Incorrect spelling—humerus

ASSESSMENT

The patient tolerated physical therapy well. He had very slight reddening underneath the medicated pad after the iontophoresis treatment, but there was no subcutaneous water accumulation. We will continue with physical therapy with the following long term goals:

Use hyphenated form—long-term

Patient will demonstrate improvement of horizontal adduction to 15 degrees on the right.

Patient will increase shoulder length by one-half grade.

Incorrect word—strength

Patient will return to fitness activities without pain greater then 2/10.

Incorrect word—than

Patient will have punch, weightlifting, and fitness activities, including the use of a training log, 3–4 times a week without pain greater than 2/10.

PROOFREADING EXERCISE #2 KEY

Incorrect term—insidious

DIAGNOSIS
Low back pain.

PRECAUTIONS/CONTRAINDICATIONS
Asthma.

MEDICATIONS
Celebrex.

SUBJECTIVE
The patient is a 17-year-old female who notes insipidus onset of low back discomfort approximately 3-1/2 months ago. The patient progressively worsened to the point where patient could barely bend forward and had pain rolling over in bed. The patient was initially treated by her family physician with Celexa after x-rays showed no abnormalities; however, her symptoms did not resolve. MRI ordered by her orthopedist, per patient, showed a herniated disk in her lumbar spine. The patient states her pain levels are improving, but she notes a constant ache and intermittent pain ranging up to 7/10 following activities. The patient currently has a mild extravasation which she attributes to having played whiffle ball last week. The patient does note several episodes of pain radiating into right buttock but no reticular symptoms at present.

Incorrect drug—Celebrex

Incorrect term—exacerbation

Incorrect term—radicular

PRIOR LEVEL OF FUNCTION
The patient notes no history of back pain and was unrestricted in activities such as basketball, volleyball, and occasional running.

Incorrect word—partial

PAST MEDICAL HISTORY
1. Asthma.
2. Right knee parcel patellar tendon tear 2000.

SOCIAL HISTORY

The patient is a senior in high school and lives with her family. She does not plan on participating in any other sports activities. Patient works approximately 20 hours a week in the housewares department at Sears. She is continuing to work full duty and states her job does not require any heavy lifting.

RANGE OF MOTION/MUSCLE STRENGTH

Area	Measurement
Lumbar flexion	Fingertips to proximal patella limited by right-greater-than-left lumbosacral region.
Extension	15° with pain throughout movement but not at in range.
Side bend right	Fingertips to distal patella with stretch noted on contralateral side but no pain.
Left	Fingertips to distill patella with stretch noted on contralateral side but no pain.
Rotation right	Within normal limits pain free.
Rotation left	Within normal limits pain free.

Lower extremity AROM within normal limits for hip, knee, and ankle.

Strength 5/5 throughout including EHL. The patient is able to heel walk and tow walk. Abdominals: Good minus with low back pain discomfort. Back extensors: Good minus without pain.

Incorrect word—end

Incorrect spelling—distal

Incorrect spelling—toe

NEUROLOGIC FINDINGS/COORDINATION/BALANCE
Patellar and Achilles deep tendon reflexes equal and reactive bilaterally. Sensation intact to lite touch throughout all dermal tones bilateral lower extremities. The patient does note occasional episodes of pain radiating into right buttock.

FUNCTIONAL MOBILITY
Secondary to low back pain, the patient notes difficulty tolerating supine or prone lying with rolling over in bed. She is not able to participate in sports activities at prior functional level secondary to exacerbation of pain. The patient reports difficulty bending forward to put on pants and stockings.

POSTURE
In standing, patient exhibits increased lumbar lordosis and anterior pelvic tilt. There is founding of shoulders and the head is tipped forward. Levels of ileac crests are symmetrical. Level of right acronym (dominant upper extremity) is depressed with respect to left.

SPECIAL TESTS
Repeated flexion in standing: Increases low back pain but does not produce radicular symptoms.

Repeated extension in standing: Diminishes low back pain slightly.

String testing: Negative for production of cervical radicular symptoms, inner vertebral mobility within normal limits throughout.

Straight-leg raze testing: Negative. Note: Hamstring tightness bilaterally at 65°.

GAIT
No significant alleviation noted.

Incorrect term—dermatomes

Incorrect spelling—iliac

Incorrect word—rounding

Incorrect term—acromion

Incorrect term—Spring

Incorrect word—intervertebral

Incorrect spelling—raise

Incorrect term—deviation

Use combined form—sensorimotor

ASSESSMENT
The patient is a 17-year-old female who presents to physical therapy with complaints of low back pain and, per patient, a positive MRI for lumbar disk herniation. On this date, the patient has significant limitation in flexion range of motion, hamstring tightness, and weakness of pelvic stabilizing musculature. Sensory motor exam is unremarkable.

Incorrect term—stabilization

PLAN
1. Extension-based pelvic sterilization exercises.
2. Hamstring stretching.
3. Accompanying HEB including postural education.
4. Pain modalities including ultrasound, possibly cold packs and moist heat packs.

Incorrect abbreviation—HEP (home exercise program)

FREQUENCY
2 times per week.

PROJECTED LENGTH OF STAY
3 to 4 weeks.

REHABILITATION POTENTIAL
Good.

PATIENT/FAMILY GOALS
The patient would like to return to normal daily activities and recreational sports such as whiffle ball without exacerbation of pain.

Incorrect term—shin

4-WEEK TREATMENT GOALS
1. Patient to be independent with progression of home exercise program.
2. Improve pain-free trunk flexion at least finger tips to distal chin in order to increase ease with activities such as on/off socks/pants/stockings.
3. Diminish pain levels to 3/10 or less with performance of recreational sports activities.
4. Improve bilateral hamstring flexibility at least 5–10 degrees.

Use combined form—fingertips

Incorrect terms—don/doff

PROOFREADING EXERCISE #3 KEY

Incorrect word—coated

DIAGNOSIS
Knee tendonitis.

PRECAUTIONS/CONTRAINDICATIONS
Patient is on Coumadin. In 1995, patient had surgery for multiple aneurysms in the brain.

MEDICATIONS
Coded aspirin, Pravachol, Vioxx, Coumadin.

Incorrect term—aspect

Incorrect word—greater

SUBJECTIVE
Patient reports that she had an operation on her left foot on 4/16/2001 to correct positioning of toes and to trim bunion on the left foot. Since that time, the patient has had persistent pain in the posterior speck of her left knee, posterior thigh, and up into both buttocks, left grader than right. She rates the pain as a 3/10 to a 6/10, describes it as an aching pain. She reports that she knows she has a faulty gait pattern but has been walking with a faulty gait pattern for approximately 5 years secondary to problems with her feet.

Incorrect spelling—severe

PRIOR LEVEL OF FUNCTION
Prior to 4/16/2001, pain in the knee was only intermittent, was not as constant or as sever as at present time.

Use combined form—hammertoe

PAST MEDICAL HISTORY
1. In 1995, patient underwent surgery for several aneurysms of the brain. Patient is on Coumadin at the present time.
2. Patient has a hammer toe and bunion on the right foot.

SOCIAL HISTORY
The patient is married. She is retired. Her hobbies are baby-sitting and gardening.

Incorrect format—4+/5

Incorrect spelling—either

RANGE OF MOTION/MUSCLE STRENGTH
Active range of motion of both knees is within normal limits.

She demonstrates 4 plus over 5 strength throughout knee flexion and extension. There is no pain with resistance to ether flexion or extension of the knee.

Incorrect spelling—forefoot

Incorrect term—musculature

Patient is able to walk on heels and toes with only minor discomfort in for foot. Patient is able to do only a 50% squat and return to standing. Patient does show a decrease in strength in her hip vasculature.

Hip extension on the left is a 3+/5.

Hip abduction: 4/5.

Hip adduction: 3+/5.

Hip internal and external rotation: 3+/5.

Incorrect word—stance

NEUROLOGICAL FINDINGS/ COORDINATION/BALANCE
DTRs were not tested on this date. Patient is able to do single dance on the right foot for approximately 3 seconds and able to do single dance on the left foot for 1–2 seconds.

Functional Motility: Patient reports that she is having difficulty baby-sitting secondary to pain in her knee; difficulty with sleeping; able to walk only 30 minutes and then must rest the knee secondary to pain; general decrease in activities.

Incorrect term—mobility

Incorrect term—genu varus

Posture: Patient is 5 feet 2 inches tall, 135 pounds. She does have scoliosis of the spine. Kyphosis of the thoracic spine with forward head. Left shoulder is low, left hip is high as compared to the right. She has bilateral genus veris left greater than right, tibial torsion in the left lower leg, does have an onion both left and right.

Incorrect term—bunion

Palpation: Patient is very tender to palpitation in the popliteal fossa of the left knee. There is no pain with palpation of the patellar tendon or any palpation of the hamstring insertions.

Incorrect term—palpation

SPECIAL TESTS
Faber test: Negative.

Straight-leg raise test: Negative but note the patient has decreased hamstring length. Is able to do straight-leg raise only to 65° both left and right and then feels hamstring tightness.

McMurray test: Negative.

Anterior-posterior drawer sign: Negative.

GAIT
Patient has an antalgic gait on the left. Tends to keep left foot flat as she goes through her ambulation but is able to do heel strike and toe off when given verbal queuing.

Incorrect spelling—cueing

ASSESSMENT
Patient comes to the department with diagnosis of left knee tendonitis. She is complaining of pain in the poster aspect of her knee to the point that she has had decrease in functional activities and inability to sleep. Patient does show a faulty gait pattern in the left lower extremity. Patient is very tender to palpation in the posterior aspect of the left knee.

Incorrect word—posterior

PLAN
1. Ultrasound to the posterior aspect of the left knee.
2. Progressive therapeutic exercise to work on strength and balance.

Incorrect word—cold

Incorrect term—training

3. Gait trailing as appropriate.
4. Coal pack as needed.
5. Home exercise program.

Frequency: 3 times week.

Protected Length of Stay: 4 weeks.

Rehab Potential: Difficult to state at the present time.

Incorrect abbreviation—ADLs

Patient/Family Goals: To be able to sleep at night and have decreased pain as she goes throughout her AVLs. Treatment plan was discussed with the patient who was in agreement with this plan.

Treatment Goals:
To be achieved in 4 weeks.

1. Have patient independent with HEP.
2. Increase single stance on left and right lower extremities for 5–10 seconds safely.
3. Increase ham string length in order to ease discomfort in knee.
4. Have patient able to walk 30–40 minutes without having increase in discomfort in the knee.

Use combined form—hamstring

CHAPTER 20

Endocrinology

OBJECTIVES CHECKLIST

A prepared exam candidate will know:

- ❑ All combining forms, prefixes, and suffixes related to endocrinology.
- ❑ Glands of the human body along with their location and primary function(s) in maintaining homeostasis.
- ❑ Hormones secreted by each gland as well as the hormones secreted by the pituitary gland that stimulate glandular function within the endocrine system.
- ❑ Primary diseases and conditions related to excessive and deficient secretions of the endocrine glands, along with the most common treatment modalities.
- ❑ Common laboratory tests ordered for endocrinologic conditions.
- ❑ Medications commonly prescribed for endocrinologic disorders, symptoms, and diseases.

RESOURCES FOR STUDY

1. *The Language of Medicine*
   Chapter 18: Endocrine System, pp. 719–768.
2. *Human Diseases*
   Chapter 15: Disorders of Metabolism, Nutrition, and Endocrine Function, pp. 223–240.
   Chapter 17: Musculoskeletal Disorders (Disorders of Joints), pp. 265–267.
3. *Laboratory Tests & Diagnostic Procedures in Medicine*
   Chapter 20: Chemical Examination of the Blood (Hormones and Blood Sugar), pp. 365–373, 377–378.
   Chapter 24: Laboratory Examination of Urine, Stool, and Other Fluids and Materials, pp. 441–442.
4. *The AAMT Book of Style for Medical Transcription*
   Diabetes Mellitus, pp. 129–132.
5. *Understanding Pharmacology for Health Professionals*
   Chapter 21: Endocrine Drugs, pp. 228–235.
   Chapter 22: Antidiabetic Drugs, pp. 236–242.

SAMPLE REPORTS

The following three reports are examples of reports you might encounter while transcribing endocrinology.

THYROID SONOGRAM

PROCEDURE/STUDY
Thyroid sonogram.

CLINICAL INDICATIONS
Enlarged thyroid gland.

TECHNIQUE
Ultrasound examination of the thyroid gland in the longitudinal and transverse planes using a high-resolution linear-array transducer was performed.

REFERENCED EXAM
None.

FINDINGS
There is irregularity of the contour and heterogeneous signal characteristic in both lobes of the thyroid gland consistent with a multinodular goiter. No prominent cystic components are identified. However, there are several small (4-mm and 6-mm) cystic components in the left lobe of the thyroid gland. Therefore, the appearance of the abnormality is most consistent with a multinodular goiter. The thyroid isthmus is prominent in size but within normal limits. No other acute abnormalities are identified.

IMPRESSION
Multiple bilateral nodules in the thyroid gland. The thyroid gland itself is minimally enlarged. There are several small areas of diminished signal intensity consistent with a cystic component. This most likely represents a multinodular goiter. Nonetheless, if there is no history of thyroid disease, then a radionuclide scan may be useful to confirm the presence of a multinodular goiter.

OFFICE VISIT

REASON FOR VISIT
Followup for thyroid cancer.

The patient is a pleasant 69-year-old woman who returns for followup. She had a thyroid biopsy done locally. This was suspicious for papillary or thyroid cancer. She underwent thyroidectomy on 12/17/2003. Multiple small nodules were noted in the thyroid; one was listed as 0.7 cm with a papillary appearance, located within the isthmus, closest to the right lobe. She had multiple colloid nodules and chronic thyroiditis, but it is unclear from her report whether there was more than one nodule that had papillary thyroid cancer. She reports she underwent a nuclear scan and then received 80 mCi of iodine ^{131}I on 1/14/2004. She then started Synthroid 137 mcg daily on 1/20/2004. She notes she did have typical hypothyroid symptoms and decreased energy, which are only now starting to improve. She was also taking calcium.

MEDICATIONS CURRENTLY
1. Synthroid 137 mcg daily.
2. Nexium.
3. Toprol.
4. Evoxac.
5. Folic acid.
6. Prednisone 30 mg a day.
7. Ambien.
8. Methotrexate.
9. Calcium.

PHYSICAL EXAM
An alert woman in no acute distress. Her blood pressure was 100/70. Her weight was 155. Thyroid exam showed no thyroid tissue palpable. No cervical lymphadenopathy. There was a well-healed neck scar. Cardiac exam showed a regular rhythm. Extremities showed no edema. Neurologic exam showed reflexes were normal. She had cushingoid changes.

IMPRESSION
Papillary thyroid cancer.

PLAN
I reviewed with the patient and her husband that she had appropriate treatment for her papillary thyroid cancer, including thyroidectomy and then subsequently 80 mCi of iodine ^{131}I therapy on 1/14/2004. I told her it was unclear to me by reading her report whether she only had a 0.7-cm nodule that was papillary thyroid cancer or whether there was more than one. I recommended she forward her pathology slides for pathology review. If she really only has one nodule that is under 1 cm, then I think thyroid hormone replacement with target TSH in the lower half of normal would be reasonable. On the other hand, if she had large nodules or multiple nodules, then lowering her TSH below normal would be considered. She has only been on Synthroid about 1 month.

(continued)

I suggested in 6 to 8 weeks after she initiated the Synthroid that she have her TSH, free T_4, and thyroglobulin measured. If she plans on having surgery for her kidneys, she should have her TSH and free T_4 measured before her surgery and ideally have normal thyroid tests before considering another surgery. She will try to get her outside pathology slides and nuclear medicine report forwarded to me. I told her I would be happy to review those, and I could give her a call once we have that information.

OFFICE VISIT

REASON FOR CONSULTATION
Hypercalcemia.

HISTORY
This is a 68-year-old female with a long-standing history of debilitating rheumatoid arthritis. She has had rheumatoid arthritis since age 22 and has been on chronic steroid treatment for the last 40+ years. She has had a history of kidney stones, which has required stent placement over the past several years. She was recently admitted with kidney stones and had urosepsis in the end of January 2005. At that time, apparently her calcium was in the normal range. On 01/31/2005, she was re-admitted with a history of confusion, decreased fluid intake, nausea, and vomiting. At the time of her admission, she was noted to have a creatinine greater than 4 and a calcium of 16. The patient has been on Fosamax and calcium in the past. She has had no previous history of hyperparathyroidism or malignancy. She has had a colostomy for several years. She was given IV fluids, Lasix, and was treated with pamidronate at the time of her admission on 01/31/2005. She had prompt resolution of her hypercalcemia, which went from a high of 16.1 down to the 9 range. Her calcium has since fallen into the range of 5 to 7 with a low albumin. She had one PTH level which was measured on 02/03/2005 at 94. At that time, her calcium was measured at 8.9. A 24-hour urine was obtained. Her serum protein electrophoresis was measured and was essentially unremarkable. The patient is now in the ICU receiving IV fluids and tube feedings. She has recently undergone a swallowing study which was negative.

PAST MEDICAL HISTORY
Her past medical history is significant for her rheumatoid arthritis, causing her to be wheelchair bound. She has significant ankle deformities and hand deformities as a result. She has had multiple kidney stones and hepatitis C. She has had a colostomy, hysterectomy, and appendectomy.

MEDICATIONS
Fosamax, prednisone, Premarin, Advair, Singulair.

SOCIAL HISTORY
She does not smoke. She occasionally drinks alcohol. She is married.

FAMILY HISTORY
Her mother and father are both deceased.

REVIEW OF SYSTEMS
As per medical review.

PHYSICAL EXAMINATION
Today, her blood pressure is 110/73. HEENT: Pupils are equal, round, reactive to light and accommodation. Extraocular movements are intact. The neck shows no thyromegaly. Chest is clear to auscultation. Cardiovascular: S1 and S2. Neurologic exam is grossly intact. Her extremities show multiple rheumatoid nodules on both hands. She has rheumatoid abnormalities of both her hands and her feet.

(continued)

LABORATORY DATA
Creatinine today is 1.3. Calcium is 7.3. Albumin 1.9. Phosphorus is 1.2. Magnesium is 1.8. Her Dilantin level is 15.

IMPRESSION
Hypercalcemia in a patient admitted with renal failure. The etiology of her renal failure is not clear, although it most likely is volume depletion in a patient on calcium and other medications. The patient currently has a low calcium and has received her pamidronate and intravenous fluids initially and now seems to be stabilized as far as this is concerned. It is possible that the kidney stones were a result of her hyperparathyroidism, although I am not convinced that it is the underlying cause of either her kidney stones or her hypercalcemia. Patients who have colostomy, particularly, can have problems with kidney stones also.

PLAN
1. I will discuss these issues with the patient's internist and nephrologist.
2. Consider repeating a complete workup once the patient is out of the ICU and an outpatient, as this would give us a better understanding of her overall calcium balance to see if her levels of PTH are elevated at a time when her calcium is also elevated.
3. Finally, because of all these other complicating variables, I think it is important to have her stable medically before we embark upon any sort of workup or consideration of treatment options. At the present time I do not think that there is any need for any other agents to lower her calcium, as her calcium is in the normal range now. In addition, her kidney function is now normal, and we would expect that to maintain her calcium within the normal range. The plan will be to obtain the workup as an outpatient.

REVIEW QUESTIONS

The goal of these questions is to test your knowledge in the area of endocrinology.

Directions: Select the correct answer for each of the multiple-choice questions provided below. *Answers are provided at the end of this chapter.*

1. Diabetes insipidus is caused by insufficient levels of:
   A. Insulin
   B. Sugar
   C. Sodium
   D. ADH (antidiuretic hormone)

2. The endocrine cells which produce insulin are located in the:
   A. Pineal gland
   B. Circle of Willis
   C. Islets of Langerhans
   D. Adrenal glands

3. Which test can be used to monitor blood sugar control over a 2-month period?
   A. 24-hour urine collection
   B. Hemoglobin A_{1c}
   C. CA-125
   D. Serum calcitonin

4. A patient who has a blood sugar of 450 is:
   A. Hypokalemic
   B. Hypernatremic
   C. Hyperglycemic
   D. Hypoglycemic

5. A patient with restlessness, nervousness, palpitations, and weight loss would be evaluated for:
   A. Cushing syndrome
   B. Addison disease
   C. Hyperthyroidism
   D. Diabetes mellitus

6. Bulging of the eyes, as seen is hyperthyroidism, is called:
   A. Exophthalmos
   B. Megalophthalmos
   C. Anophthalmos
   D. Microphthalmos

7. What are the two primary forms of diabetes mellitus?
   A. Type A and type B
   B. Type 1 and type 2
   C. Insulitis and insipidus
   D. Mellitus and insulitis

8. Which of the following is not a cause of hypothyroidism?
   A. Hashimoto thyroiditis
   B. Iodine deficiency
   C. Deficiency of TSH
   D. Deficiency of ACTH

9. Together with the central nervous system, the endocrine system regulates the body's metabolism to maintain:
   A. Homeostasis
   B. Autonomic responses
   C. Neural pathways
   D. Hormonal pathways

10. The laboratory tests done to determine if ovarian function has slowed down or ceased are:
    A. ACTH and TSH
    B. TSH and FSH
    C. FSH and LH
    D. T_3 and T_4

11. The master endocrine gland which controls the other endocrine glands is the:
    A. Pituitary gland
    B. Hypothalamus
    C. Adrenal gland
    D. Pancreas

12. The adrenal glands are located:
    A. Behind the liver
    B. In the brain
    C. In the throat
    D. On top of the kidneys

13. Which gland is responsible for the "fight or flight" response?
    A. The pancreas
    B. The thyroid
    C. The pituitary
    D. The adrenals

14. Which gland is responsible for releasing oxytocin to stimulate labor?
    A. The pancreas
    B. The thyroid
    C. The pituitary
    D. The adrenals

15. Another term for hyperthyroidism is:
    A. Hashimoto thyroiditis
    B. Thyrotoxicosis
    C. de Quervain disease
    D. Addison disease

16. There are four parathyroid glands and their primary function is to:
    A. Regulate calcium levels in the serum
    B. Regulate chloride and prevent syncope
    C. Control metabolic activity and protein synthesis
    D. Produce insulin and control blood sugar

17. Addison disease is an example of hypofunction of the:
    A. Pituitary
    B. Adrenals
    C. Parathyroids
    D. Thyroid

18. This hormone will cause calcium to move from the serum into the bones, helping to regulate serum calcium levels and strengthen bones:
    A. Calcitonin
    B. Calciferol
    C. Calcine
    D. Calan

19. The adrenal gland secretes:
    A. Corticosteroids
    B. PTH
    C. Insulin
    D. Glucagon

20. An endemic goiter is caused by the lack of _______ in the diet.
    A. Calcium
    B. Chloride
    C. Iodine
    D. Magnesium

21. The adrenal medulla secretes:
    A. Calcitonin
    B. Glucagon
    C. Adrenaline and noradrenaline
    D. TSH

22. The pituitary gland is located within the:
    A. Sella turcica
    B. Kidneys
    C. Throat
    D. Chest

23. Oral hypoglycemics are used in the treatment of:
    A. Type 1 diabetes mellitus
    B. Type 2 diabetes mellitus
    C. Diabetes insipidus
    D. Ketoacidosis

24. One outward manifestation of hypothyroidism is:
    A. An enlarged thyroid gland
    B. Unexplained weight gain
    C. Weight loss despite increased appetite
    D. Heat intolerance

25. A primary complication of diabetes characterized by improper burning of fats instead of sugar is called:
    A. Ketoacidosis
    B. Diabetes insipidus
    C. SIADH
    D. Insulin shock

26. A life-threatening form of metabolic acidosis in diabetics is termed:

A. TSH
B. PKU
C. DKA
D. ADHD

27. Which of these is a long-acting insulin?

A. Amaryl
B. Lamictal
C. Metformin
D. Insulin glargine

28. Growth hormone is the common name for which adrenal hormone?

A. Somatostatin
B. Follicle-stimulating hormone
C. Prolactin
D. Adrenocorticotropic hormone

29. Which of the following is not secreted by the thyroid gland?

A. Thyroxine
B. Triiodothyronine
C. Calcitonin
D. Thyroid-stimulating hormone

30. After the closure of the growth plates, excessive somatotropin secretion causes:

A. Dwarfism
B. Acromegaly
C. Cushing disease
D. Addison disease

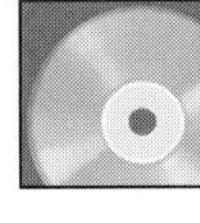

Please see the accompanying CD for additional review materials for this section.

PROOFREADING EXERCISES

These three proofreading exercises are provided to improve your skills in the areas of editing and effective identification and correction of errors in the medical record.

Directions: Identify and correct the transcription errors found in the exercises below. *Answers are provided at the end of this chapter.*

PROOFREADING EXERCISE # 1

PROBLEM #1: Idiopathic hypocalciuria with secondary hyperparathyroidism.

The patient's urea calcium had decreased down to 375 mg in a 24-hour specimen. Her parathyroid hormone also normalized with the hydrochlorothiazide use. Her parathyroid scan showed faint radiotracer in the region of the lower pole of the right lobe, and a parathyroid adenoma could not be excluded. Her bone sensory was normal.

I reviewed with the patient that I believe she has a secondary hypoparathyroidism due to her renal leek of calcium and that hydrochlorothiazide treatment would be the best option to decrease her urinary calcium excretion and normalize her thyroid status. She reports she has started taking it about once every third day, because she notes skipped heartbeats when she takes it regularly. Her passive medium was in the lower end of normal at 3.7. Therefore, I recommended that she take potassium chloride 10 million equivalents daily along with the hydrochlorothiazide to see if she will be able to tolerate taking the hydrochlorothiazide every day. I suggested she have a followup urinary calcium again after she has been taking the hydrochlorothiazide regularly and, if her urinary calcium has not normalized, then the hydrochlorothiazide dose could be adjusted upward further if needed and tolerated.

PROBLEM #2: Impaired glucose tolerance/hypotriglyceridemia.

Glucose was 117, fasting A1c was normal. Triglycerides to 33, cholesterol 170. I recommended to the patient that she restrict sugars and saturated fat in the diet and try to lose some weight. In addition, physical activity will help improve her glucose and tolerance and hypertriglyceridemia.

(continued)

PROBLEM #3: Thyroid hormone replacement.

PSH was normal on her current dose of Synthroid which I encouraged her to continue.

PROBLEM #4: Kidney stones/proteinuria.

The patient's serum ureic acid is mildly elevated along with urinary uric acid and calcium. Her urinary protein was 215. She has not been to see the neurologist, but I did strongly encourage her to see the neurologist regarding her kidney stones and proteinuria to see if there are additional measures that would be helpful to prevent recurrent kidney stones.

PROOFREADING EXERCISE # 2

REASON FOR REFERRAL: Hypocalcemia.

HISTORY OF PRESENT ILLNESS
The patient is a pleasant, 26-year-old, family medicine resident physician who reports that his calcium was first reported to be mildly elevated back in 1996. He has not had any further workup other than au pair thyroid hormone measured last fall. He denies taking any calcium supplements. He does take may lox a couple of times a week. He has not taken any vitamin A or vitamin D supplements. He denies using lithium or thiazide diuretics. There is no family history of hypercalcemia or parathyroid disorders. He reports he has never had a kidney stone, and he had an ultrasound that showed no kidney stones. He fractured his clavicle playing football but has had no other fractures. He denies any bone pain other than occasional joint pain in his hands. He does have some intermittent abdominal discomfort for which he notes Maalox helps. He has never had any radiation treatment. He does have a history of sauriasis but has not used any Accutane or vitamin A derivatives.

PAST MEDICAL HISTORY
Psoriasis, gastroesophageal reflux, Gilbert disease.

MEDICATIONS
Maalox as needed, multivitamins, and vitamin C.

FAMILY HISTORY
Type II diabetes in his father.

SOCIAL HISTORY
No tobacco or alcohol.

PHYSICAL EXAMINATION
Alert gentleman in no acute distress. Blood pressure: 110/60. Weight: 742 kg. Thyroid normal. No cervical lymphadenopathy. Lungs clear. Spine exam showed no cytosis. Cardiac examination regular rhythm. Abdomen showed no hepatosplenomegaly. Skin exam did show some sporadic plaques.

(continued)

LABORATORY DATA

Calcium 10, 10.5, and 10.6, parathyroid hormone 10 when his calcium was 10.4, phosphorus 4.1, creatinine 1.0, alkaline phosphatase normal.

IMPRESSION AND PLAN

Intermittent hypercalcemia, known since about 1996.

I recommended to the patient that we pursue additional tests to rule out other potential causes of his hypercalcemia. I have suggested a TSH, protein electrophoresis, iron, eyed calcium, repeat parathyroid hormone, vitamin D levels, ace level, and a chest x-ray to screen for sarcoidosis. He certainly does not have evidence of familiar hypocalciuric hypercalcemia given his generous urinary calcium. If these are all normal, he may have a very mild hyperparathyroidism, since his PPH is inappropriately normal given a mild elevation in calcium. If these additional screening studies are normal, we did discuss the option of a parathyroid scan also versus a coarse of observation. The patient will think about this but would like to proceed with the laboratory testing and chest x-ray.

PROOFREADING EXERCISE # 3

REASON FOR CONSULTATION
Hyponatremia.

HISTORY AND FINDINGS
This is a 74-year-old female who presented with hyponatremia. She had previously had a sodium which was in the normal range. She presented with significant weight loss, bronchiectasis, and progressive mental confusion and delirium. She has reported to have poor aural intake for several weeks prior to her admission. She was noted on admission to have a sodium of 12.5. She subsequently has been on fluid restriction for the past 3–4 days, and her sodium has remained in the same range. She probably has not had a very rigorous fluid restriction based upon the I/O data. She has normal thyroid function studies including TFH. We do not have the results of a cordis at all.

PAST MEDICAL HISTORY
Significant for hypertension, diverticulitis, chronic cough with bronchiectasis, community-aspired pneumonia, osteoporosis. Her present medications include inhalers.

FAMILY HISTORY
Unremarkable.

SOCIAL HISTORY
She does not smoke. She does not drink alcohol.

REVIEW OF SYSTEMS
Otherwise as per medical review.

PHYSICAL EXAMINATION
GENERAL: She is a very pour historian. VITAL SIGNS: Blood pressure 136/70, pulse 70. CHEST: Clear to auscultation and percussion. CARDIOVASCULAR: Normal S1, S2. NECK: Shows no thyromegaly.

LABORATORY DATA
Sodium 125, potassium 41, chloride 86, bicarbonate 36, calcium 8.7.

(continued)

IMPRESSION
Hyponatremia in a patient currently hospitalized for confusion. The patient's sodium is unchanged. Her confusion is somewhat better. It is not clear as to the cause of her initial hypernatremia, although it appears to be syndrome of an appropriate antidiuretic hormone secretion based upon the high urine molality. She also received intravenous fluids of normal saline which did not improve her sodium. I believe that the best option at the present time would be to treat her with strict fluid restriction. In addition, we will rule out adrenal and sufficiency with foramen cortisol. We will then also recheck her serum and urine os malady.

PLAN
Restrict her fluid intake to 750 mL per day and obtain calorie counts. Recheck serum urine osmolality and cortisol.

ANSWER KEYS

REVIEW QUESTIONS ANSWER KEY

1. D
2. C
3. B
4. C
5. C
6. A
7. B
8. D
9. A
10. C
11. A
12. D
13. D
14. C
15. B
16. A
17. B
18. A
19. A
20. C
21. C
22. A
23. B
24. A
25. A
26. C
27. D
28. A
29. D
30. D

PROOFREADING EXERCISE #1 KEY

PROBLEM #1: Idiopathic hypocalciuria with secondary hyperparathyroidism.

The patient's urea calcium had decreased down to 375 mg in a 24-hour specimen. Her parathyroid hormone also normalized with the hydrochlorothiazide use. Her parathyroid scan showed faint radiotracer in the region of the lower pole of the right lobe, and a parathyroid adenoma could not be excluded. Her bone sensory was normal.

I reviewed with the patient that I believe she has secondary hypoparathyroidism due to her renal leek of calcium and that hydrochlorothiazide treatment would be the best option to decrease her urinary calcium excretion and normalize her thyroid status. She reports she has started taking it about once every third day, because she notes skipped heartbeats when she takes it regularly. Her passive medium was in the lower end of normal at 3.7. Therefore, I recommended that she take potassium chloride 10 million equivalents daily along with the hydrochlorothiazide to see if she will be able to tolerate taking the hydrochlorothiazide every day. I suggested she have a followup urinary calcium again after she has been taking the hydrochlorothiazide regularly and, if her urinary calcium has not normalized, then the hydrochlorothiazide dose could be adjusted upward further if needed and tolerated.

Incorrect term—urinary

Incorrect term—density

Incorrect term—hyperparathyroidism

Incorrect spelling—leak

Incorrect term—parathyroid

Incorrect term—potassium

Incorrect term—milliequivalents, abbreviated mEq

PROBLEM #2: Impaired glucose tolerance/hypotriglyceridemia.

Glucose was 117, fasting A1c was normal. Triglycerides to 33, cholesterol 170. I recommended to the patient that she restrict sugars and saturated fat in the diet and try to lose some weight. In addition, physical activity will help improve her glucose and tolerance and hypertriglyceridemia.

PROBLEM #3: Thyroid hormone replacement.

PSH was normal on her current dose of Synthroid which I encouraged her to continue.

PROBLEM #4: Kidney stones/proteinuria.

The patient's serum ureic acid is mildly elevated along with urinary uric acid and calcium. Her urinary protein was 215. She has not been to see the neurologist, but I did strongly encourage her to see the neurologist regarding her kidney stones and proteinuria to see if there are additional measures that would be helpful to prevent recurrent kidney stones.

Incorrect punctuation—117 fasting,

Incorrect value—233

Incorrect abbreviation—TSH

Incorrect term—nephrologist

Incorrect prefix—hypertri-glyceridemia

Incorrect term—intolerance

Incorrect term—uric acid

PROOFREADING EXERCISE #2 KEY

REASON FOR REFERRAL: Hypocalcemia.

Incorrect prefix—hypercalcemia

HISTORY OF PRESENT ILLNESS

The patient is a pleasant, 26-year-old, family medicine resident physician who reports that his calcium was first reported to be mildly elevated back in 1996. He has not had any further workup other than au pair thyroid hormone measured last fall. He denies taking any calcium supplements. He does take may lox a couple of times a week. He has not taken any vitamin A or vitamin D supplements. He denies using lithium or thiazide diuretics. There is no family history of hypercalcemia or parathyroid disorders. He reports he has never had a kidney stone, and he had an ultrasound that showed no kidney stones. He fractured his clavicle playing football but has had no other fractures. He denies any bone pain other than occasional joint pain in his hands. He does have some intermittent abdominal discomfort for which he notes Maalox helps. He has never had any radiation treatment. He does have a history of sauriasis but has not used any Accutane or vitamin A derivatives.

Incorrect term—a parathyroid

Incorrect term—Maalox

Incorrect term—psoriasis

PAST MEDICAL HISTORY

Psoriasis, gastroesophageal reflux, Gilbert disease.

MEDICATIONS

Maalox as needed, multivitamins, and vitamin C.

FAMILY HISTORY

Type II diabetes in his father.

Incorrect format—Type 2

SOCIAL HISTORY

No tobacco or alcohol.

Incorrect term—kyphosis

Incorrect term—psoriatic

Should be flagged as value is too high

PHYSICAL EXAMINATION

Alert gentleman in no acute distress. Blood pressure: 110/60. Weight: 742 kg. Thyroid normal. No cervical lymphadenopathy. Lungs clear. Spine exam showed no cytosis. Cardiac examination regular rhythm. Abdomen showed no hepatosplenomegaly. Skin exam did show some sporadic plaques.

LABORATORY DATA

Calcium 10, 10.5, and 10.6, parathyroid hormone 10 when his calcium was 10.4, phosphorus 4.1, creatinine 1.0, alkaline phosphatase normal.

IMPRESSION AND PLAN

Intermittent hypercalcemia, known since about 1996.

I recommended to the patient that we pursue additional tests to rule out other potential causes of his hypercalcemia. I have suggested a TSH, protein electrophoresis, iron, eyed calcium, repeat parathyroid hormone, vitamin D levels, ace level, and a chest x-ray to screen for sarcoidosis. He certainly does not have evidence of familiar hypocalciuric hypercalcemia given his generous urinary calcium. If these are all normal, he may have a very mild hyperparathyroidism, since his PPH is inappropriately normal given a mild elevation in calcium. If these additional screening studies are normal, we did discuss the option of a parathyroid scan also versus a coarse of observation. The patient will think about this but would like to proceed with the laboratory testing and chest x-ray.

Incorrect words—ionized

Incorrect spelling—course

Incorrect format—ACE

Incorrect word—familial

Incorrect abbreviation—PTH

PROOFREADING EXERCISE #3 KEY

Incorrect word—oral

Flag—value too far out of range

Incorrect abbreviation —TSH

Incorrect term—cortisol

Incorrect word—acquired

REASON FOR CONSULTATION
Hyponatremia.

HISTORY AND FINDINGS
This is a 74-year-old female who presented with hyponatremia. She had previously had a sodium which was in the normal range. She presented with significant weight loss, bronchiectasis, and progressive mental confusion and delirium. She has reported to have poor aural intake for several weeks prior to her admission. She was noted on admission to have a sodium of 12.5. She subsequently has been on fluid restriction for the past 3–4 days, and her sodium has remained in the same range. She probably has not had a very rigorous fluid restriction based upon the I/O data. She has normal thyroid function studies including TFH. We do not have the results of a cordis at all.

PAST MEDICAL HISTORY
Significant for hypertension, diverticulitis, chronic cough with bronchiectasis, community-aspired pneumonia, osteoporosis. Her present medications include inhalers.

FAMILY HISTORY
Unremarkable.

SOCIAL HISTORY
She does not smoke. She does not drink alcohol.

REVIEW OF SYSTEMS
Otherwise as per medical review.

Incorrect spelling—poor

PHYSICAL EXAMINATION
GENERAL: She ~~is a very~~ pour historian. VITAL SIGNS: Blood pressure 136/70, pulse 70. CHEST: Clear to auscultation and percussion. CARDIOVASCULAR: Normal S1, S2. NECK: Shows no thyromegaly.

Flag—value too far out of range

LABORATORY DATA
Sodium 125, potassium 41, chloride 86, bicarbonate 36, calcium 8.7.

IMPRESSION
Hyponatremia in a patient currently hospitalized for confusion. The patient's sodium is unchanged. Her confusion is somewhat better. It is not clear as to the cause of her initial hypernatremia, although it appears to be syndrome of an appropriate antidiuretic hormone secretion based upon the high urine molality. She also received intravenous fluids of normal saline which did not improve her sodium. I believe that the best option at the present time would be to treat her with strict fluid restriction. In addition, we will rule out adrenal and sufficiency ~~with~~ foramen cortisol. We will then also recheck her serum and urine os malady.

Incorrect prefix—hypo

Incorrect term—osmolality

One word—inappropriate (delete an)

One word—insufficiency (delete and)

Incorrect word—4 AM

Incorrect term—osmolality

PLAN
Restrict her fluid intake to 750 mL per day and obtain calorie counts. Recheck serum urine osmolality and cortisol.

Missing word—serum and urine

CHAPTER

21

Psychiatry/Psychology

OBJECTIVES CHECKLIST

A prepared exam candidate will know the:

- ❑ Combining forms, prefixes, and suffixes related to psychiatry and psychology.
- ❑ Role and function of the psychiatrist, psychologist, and other specialists within the discipline of mental health.
- ❑ Clinical signs, symptoms, and disorders related to psychiatry and mental illness.
- ❑ Substances associated with abuse and dependence.
- ❑ Clinical and diagnostic procedures and therapeutic techniques used in the identification and treatment of mental diseases and disorders.
- ❑ Medications and drug therapies commonly used to treat psychiatric disorders.
- ❑ Terminology and format related to recording a mental status examination, including testing and classification systems related to mental evaluation and diagnosis.
- ❑ Role of the *Diagnostic and Statistical Manual of Mental Disorders, Fourth Edition* (DSM-IV) in identifying and classifying psychiatric disorders.
- ❑ Multi-axial system used in diagnosing psychiatric patients.

RESOURCES FOR STUDY

1. *The Language of Medicine*
   Chapter 22: Psychiatry, pp. 887–924.
2. *H&P: A Nonphysician's Guide to the Medical History and Physical Examination*
   Chapter 13: Review of Systems: Psychiatric, pp. 117–124.
   Chapter 28: The Formal Mental Status Examination, pp. 273–280.
3. *Human Diseases*
   Chapter 20: Mental Disorders, pp. 315–332.
4. *Understanding Pharmacology for Health Professionals*
   Chapter 25: Psychiatric Drugs, pp. 279–295.
5. *The AAMT Book of Style for Medical Transcription*
   Global assessment of functioning (GAF) scale, p. 75.
   Global assessment of relational functioning (GARF) scale, p. 76.
   Social and occupational functioning assessment scale (SOFAS), p. 79.
   Psychiatric diagnoses, pp. 133–134.

SAMPLE REPORTS

The following five reports are examples of reports you might encounter while transcribing psychiatry and psychology.

CONSULTATION

IDENTIFICATION DATA
The patient is a 33-year-old African-American male with no prior psychiatric contacts. He was admitted to the inpatient mental health service by Dr. Jones secondary to an acute overdose. The patient apparently overdosed on Pamelor and Tylenol (approximately 15 tablets). The patient was intending to hurt himself secondary to his recent divorce.

CHIEF COMPLAINT
"Yeah, I've been depressed."

HISTORY OF PRESENT ILLNESS
The patient is a 33-year-old African-American male with no prior psychiatric contact who was admitted to the inpatient mental health service through the courtesy of Dr. Jones secondary to a possible overdose. The patient stated, "I took the pills but then I called my pastor."

The patient relates that he has been depressed over the past few years secondary to his mother dying. Shortly after his mother's death 2 years ago, he relates that he discovered he was adopted and he became even more despondent. Early last month, his wife of 3 years filed for divorce, and that has been worsening his mood. He apparently moved to Indiana after the divorce "to find a job" but moved back to Iowa over the past week and moved into his mother's old home. He states that he has been living in a home with no running water and no utilities and has been increasingly despondent secondary to this. He states that he took the pills "without thinking." The patient also reported drinking about a 24-ounce can of beer prior to taking the overdose, stating, "I just got more depressed after I drank." The patient also has a history of cannabis use but denies recent use.

The patient requests discharge and is enthusiastic about the job that he has waiting for him in Iowa. The patient relates that he went through orientation on the job last Thursday and felt that his life was taking a turn for the better, but he then became acutely depressed on the day prior to admission, drank some alcohol, and took the pills. The patient states, "I did it without thinking, and after I took the pills, I called my pastor right away. Then I called my cousin and they told me to come to the hospital."

PAST PSYCHIATRIC HISTORY
The patient has a history of depression, by his report, over the past 2 years. The patient reports decreased interest in daily activities but has no sleep disturbance, and his appetite has been "fine." He has some guilt about not being able to provide for his biological children in a consistent fashion and occasionally feels helplessness. There are no feelings of hopelessness or worthlessness. The patient is actually hopeful about the future, and there are no psychotic symptoms in evidence and no manic symptoms either. The patient downplays his cannabis use and denies alcohol use on a regular basis.

(continued)

PAST MEDICAL HISTORY
The patient denies any active medical problems, but he is status post overdose with 15 tablets of Pamelor and Tylenol, as above. The patient does have a history of a gunshot wound to the left shoulder, which the patient describes as an "accident" after he got into an argument with someone. He states he has no access to handguns or firearms and states that the mother of his biological children has all of his firearms. He is reluctant to allow disclosure of information regarding why he is in the hospital.

SOCIAL/FAMILY HISTORY
The patient was born in Ohio and raised in this area. He was raised by his adoptive mother. He had no contact with his biological parents. He has a twelfth-grade education. He also went to college and studied pre-law at the local community college. He has worked in the past doing various jobs and plans to start work tomorrow as previously mentioned. His 3 children with his previous girlfriend include a daughter, age 12, and two sons, ages 8 and 10.

INVENTORY OF ASSETS
The patient is physically healthy, has gainful employment, a supportive pastor, a supportive cousin, and supportive ex-girlfriend.

MENTAL STATUS EXAMINATION
In general, the patient appears cooperative, pleasant, and interactive. Psychomotor activity is within normal limits. Speech is normal in amount and tone. Mood is "better." Affect is bright. The patient denies suicidal or homicidal ideations, plans, or intents. He also denies auditory or visual hallucinations, and he has concrete plans for the future, including starting his job tomorrow morning in Iowa. He states that he has a "good job" with "good benefits" and states, "Someone like me will not have this opportunity again."

He was alert and oriented x3. The patient is very emotional about the overdose attempt and is also ashamed, stating, "I don't know what I was thinking." The patient was able to recall 3/3 items after 1 minute and 3/3 items after 5 minutes. Serial sevens were intact. Abstractions are concrete.

ADMITTING DIAGNOSES
Axis I Adjustment disorder with mixed disturbance of emotions and conduct; rule out major depression, not otherwise specified.
Axis II None.
Axis III Please refer to the internal medicine notes.
Axis IV Recent divorce. Recent occupational history, which has actually improved, and death of his mother 2 years ago.
Axis V Global assessment of functioning = 75–80. Highest in the past year not known.

PLAN
At the present time, the patient will be discharged to the outpatient setting. The patient denied suicidal or homicidal ideation and does not pose a threat to himself or others, and this seems to have been an impulsive gesture after drinking alcohol and possible use of cannabis. In addition, the patient states he has concrete plans for the future, including starting to work tomorrow morning at his new job.

(continued)

The patient will be started on Wellbutrin SR 150 mg p.o. q.a.m. for 3 days and increased to 150 mg b.i.d. thereafter. The patient will receive a 2-week supply of this medication through my office in the form of samples. The risks, benefits, and side effects of the medications were discussed with the patient, and he gave informed consent to treatment.

The patient will follow up with Comprehensive Mental Health or my office after discharge within 2 weeks.

The patient was advised to go to the nearest emergency room if he has any suicidal thoughts, and the patient was strongly recommended to abstain from alcohol and drug use.

CONSULTATION

IDENTIFICATION DATA
Please refer to her detailed mental status assessment and diagnosis.

CHIEF COMPLAINT
Please refer to her detailed mental status assessment and diagnosis.

HISTORY OF PRESENT ILLNESS
Please refer to her detailed mental status assessment and diagnosis.

DIAGNOSES UPON DISCHARGE
Axis I Major depression with psychotic features as well as cocaine abuse.
Axis II Personality disorder; not otherwise specified.
Axis III History of colostomy secondary to perforated diverticulum, as well as gastroesophageal reflux disease and hypertension.
Axis IV Chronic mental illness and multiple medical issues.
Axis V Global assessment of functioning = 20–25; highest in the past year 55–60.

HOSPITAL COURSE
This patient was admitted to the inpatient psychiatric service for evaluation and treatment of suicidal ideation as well as cocaine abuse. The patient was increasingly depressed secondary to news that her colostomy would be irreversible, and she verbalized suicidal thoughts. The patient was placed on routine precautions after being admitted on April 22 and started on Xanax 0.5 mg t.i.d., Remeron 15 mg nightly, and Prozac 20 mg q.a.m. She was also started on Zyprexa 5 mg at 8:00 p.m. on April 23. Surgical nursing was consulted for ostomy supplies. Zyprexa was increased to 7.5 mg at 8:00 p.m. on April 25, and she continued to be monitored for depressive symptoms. A GI consultation was ordered for Dr. Jones to see the patient for abdominal pain on April 26. Social work referred the patient to ARTS, as the patient was reluctant to go to our inpatient treatment program. She was also referred to the partial hospitalization program.

She was discharged to her home on April 30 with her husband and was scheduled to follow up with Dr. Jones within 2 weeks of discharge and to follow up at her regular hospital for colostomy care the day after discharge from this facility.

At the time of discharge, the patient denied suicidal or homicidal ideation, her psychotic symptoms have cleared, and she was more interactive, pleasant, and no longer tearful.

MEDICATIONS UPON DISCHARGE
Remeron 15 mg nightly, Prevacid 30 mg q.d., Norvasc 5 mg q.d., Colace 100 mg b.i.d., Metamucil b.i.d., Prozac 20 mg q.a.m., Zyprexa 7.5 mg nightly, Premarin 0.625 mg q.d., and Xanax 0.5 mg t.i.d.

PROGNOSIS AT TIME OF DISCHARGE
Guarded, secondary to the patient's substance abuse issues, minimizing of symptoms, and sporadic compliance. At the time of discharge, the patient was strongly advised to abstain from the use of cocaine secondary to its deleterious effects on her health, and the patient agreed to follow with the inpatient program for relapse prevention.

CONSULTATION

HISTORY OF PRESENT ILLNESS
The patient is a 59-year-old female admitted on an emergency basis because of a confusional state, irritability, walking out of her home, not sleeping, and feeling very anxious. The patient was taken to the emergency room 2 days ago, her blood sugar and other medical problems were checked, and she was sent back home. Then her sister, with whom she had been living, called on April 22, 2004, to report that at odd hours the patient walks out of the house, apparently in a confused state, and she is not eating or sleeping well. She is also not making much sense most of the time.

I recommended admission, but the patient declined to go to the hospital, so her sister brought her to the office this morning. She appeared to be drowsy, lethargic, mumbling to herself, and hearing voices. However, she is under the impression that she has some medical problems and that her diabetes is out of control. Therefore, she wants to go to the medical floor. Her blood sugar has been pretty stable, according to the sister. Finally, the patient agreed to be admitted to the psychiatric floor.

PAST PSYCHIATRIC HISTORY
The patient has a long history of having had psychiatric problems. She has had one admission here in 2002. Prior to that, she was living in Alabama and had multiple admissions there. She has had psychotic symptoms practically all of her adult life. During the past 6 months, she has grown quite resistant to taking her psychotropic medications. These consist of Risperdal 3 mg b.i.d. and Depakote-ER 500 mg, 3 nightly. Her Risperdal was reduced at her request because she claimed she was sleeping too much, but the reality was that she sleeps through the day and stays up at night. Her Depakote was decreased about 1 month ago, but this was again because of complaints that she was gaining weight, etc. She did not want to take Depakote any longer. I had warned both the patient and her sister that she might have increased symptoms, and not surprisingly, within 2 weeks, she began deteriorating, getting confused, and hearing voices.

FAMILY HISTORY
Unchanged from previous admissions.

REVIEW OF SYSTEMS
The patient offers no specific complaints, but she thinks her tiredness, confusion, drowsiness, etc., are because of her diabetes.

PHYSICAL EXAMINATION
HEAD: Normocephalic.
NECK: Supple.
CHEST: Symmetrical.
LUNGS: Clear to percussion and auscultation.
HEART: No murmur.
ABDOMEN: Soft and nontender; no organs or masses palpable.
NEUROLOGICAL EXAMINATION: Gait and coordination normal.

(continued)

MENTAL STATUS EXAMINATION

The patient looks older than her stated age. She is glum and wary. She mumbles often and has difficulty in expressing her thoughts in a relevant fashion. She is not able to answer questions appropriately. She is reasonably oriented to date, place, and person. Sensorium, in that sense, is fairly clear, but she lacks clarity of thinking. She looks very depressed, somewhat perplexed, and is mildly confused. She always has excessive worry about things. Insight and judgment are poor.

DIAGNOSES

Axis I Schizoaffective disorder, depressed-type, with acute relapse.

Axis II None.

Axis III Type 2 diabetes mellitus, hypertension, coronary artery disease, obesity, hypothyroidism, history of chronic obstructive pulmonary disease, and history of congestive cardiac failure.

Axis IV Psychosocial stressors: None.

Axis V Global assessment of functioning at the time of admission: 55.

CONSULTATION

SUMMARY OF INFORMATION
The patient is a 42-year-old male who was admitted to this facility with a variety of complaints, not the least of which was a low mood, agitation, and getting into violent fights. He said he had to come and get checked out to see for himself. He wanted to know if he handled things responsibly. These were his words, which are a bit unusual for this man. Of course, he has had several years of college training, and we have worked rather hard with him trying to get a stable place for him to live because none of his family seems to take any interest in him.

FAMILY HISTORY
His father has diabetes and his mother is hypertensive. He has a brother with HIV and a sister who is supposedly bipolar, just as he is.

He had been doing fairly well with his once-a-month office visits and his occasional need for long-acting medicines, but recently he has become quite irritable, easily agitated, takes umbrage at the slightest thing, mopes around a great deal, and is noncompliant in general.

He has had no injuries or operations since the last time we saw him. Medications have been given, and his caretaker has seen to it that he at least gets his medicine. Whether he actually swallows it or not is a different story, and she cannot be sure of this one way or the other.

PHYSICAL EXAMINATION
GENERAL: He is very well developed and well nourished, with good muscle structure, good station and gait.
VITAL SIGNS: He is 180 pounds now. He had been about 160 before we got him stabilized. He is 5 feet 10 inches. He has a blood pressure of 124/64. Temperature, pulse, and respiratory rate are normal.
HEENT: No masses of the head, neck, chest, or abdomen. Extraocular movements are normal. He is quite expressive when he wants to be. Sometimes be becomes a bit grandiloquent and is hard to follow. He has the notion that he and his family are better off than they really are, and yet he cannot explain the fact that no one comes to visit him and no one will take him in.
CHEST: Lungs are clear.
HEART: No murmurs are appreciated.
ABDOMEN: Normal and very muscular.
EXTREMITIES: His extremities are also muscular.

MENTAL STATUS EXAMINATION
Aside from having some hostile display, irritability, and attitudes of being withdrawn, he has not had gross hallucinations, though there seems to be a paranoid delusional system simmering in him at this point. He is rather flippant in his affect except when he is trying to explain himself. He thinks he has business to take care of and does not think that this hospital stay should be very long. Indeed, it probably will not be.

PLAN
The patient will be admitted, and we will make sure that he gets restarted on his medications. We will contact his boarding home caretaker to make sure there is medicine at the house upon discharge.

(continued)

READMISSION DIAGNOSIS

Axis I Schizoaffective disorder.
Axis II Paranoid personality.
Axis III No pathology.
Axis IV Questionable compliance with treatment protocols.
Axis V Current global assessment of functioning is 50.

CONSULTATION

CHIEF COMPLAINT/HISTORY OF PRESENT ILLNESS
The patient is a 20-year-old female with ingestion of an overdose of aspirin because she wanted to kill herself after an argument with her mother about 15 minutes prior to presentation in our emergency room.

CURRENT MEDICATIONS
Unknown at this time.

ALLERGIES
Unknown.

PHYSICAL EXAMINATION
VITAL SIGNS: Temperature 96.3, pulse 120, respirations 24, blood pressure 146/68. She is morbidly obese.
GENERAL: The patient appears to be in some distress.
HEENT: Normocephalic. Eyes normal. ENT normal.
NECK: Supple.
CHEST: Clear.
HEART: Tachycardia.
ABDOMEN: Soft and nontender.
GENITALS: Deferred.
RECTAL: Deferred.
EXTREMITIES: Limbs are normal.
NERVOUS SYSTEM: No sign of focal deficit. No sign of meningismus.

DIAGNOSTIC STUDIES
Her salicylate level was 6 mg/dL. Tylenol level was less than 10.

EMERGENCY DEPARTMENT COURSE
The patient was given 50 g of charcoal mixed with sorbitol, and a normal saline IV was started to run at 125 mL/hr. She also received Zantac 300 mg and Maalox 1 ounce. Dr. Jones was consulted, and the patient will be admitted for an aspirin overdose in a suicide attempt. The psychiatrist will evaluate her with regard to her suicide attempt.

FINAL DIAGNOSES
Aspirin overdose.
Suicide attempt.
Morbid obesity.

REVIEW QUESTIONS

The goal of these questions is to test your knowledge in the areas of psychiatry and psychology.

Directions: Select the correct answer for each of the multiple-choice questions provided below. *Answers are provided at the end of this chapter.*

1. A psychiatric assessment includes how many axes?
   A. Two
   B. Three
   C. Four
   D. Five

2. Which of the following is an adult intelligence assessment test?
   A. WISC
   B. WAIS
   C. MMPI
   D. BSI-18

3. *Catatonic, disorganized-type, undifferentiated-type,* and *paranoid-type* are descriptors for which of the following disorders:
   A. Schizoaffective disorder
   B. Schizophrenia
   C. Bipolar disorder
   D. Major depression

4. An anxiety disorder is characterized by:
   A. Mental symptoms (disturbance of memory and identity that hide the anxiety of unconscious conflicts)
   B. A persistent false belief that is not due to any other mental disorder
   C. Conditions marked by a prolonged emotion (such as depression) that dominates a person's life
   D. Troubled feelings, unpleasant tensions, distress, and avoidance behavior

5. If a patient has an obsessive-compulsive disorder, they have:
   A. One or more manic episodes alternating with depressive episodes
   B. Recurrent thoughts and repetitive acts that dominate their behavior
   C. Withdrawal symptoms when a drug is discontinued abruptly
   D. Psychosis marked by withdrawal from reality into an inner world of disorganized thinking and conflict

6. Under which general psychiatric disorder would a patient with multi-infarct dementia be classified?
   A. Anxiety disorder
   B. Organic mental disorder
   C. Personality disorder
   D. Mood disorder

7. Delirium tremens is a condition brought on by:
   A. Dementia
   B. Ingestion of alcohol and drugs
   C. Withdrawal after prolonged bouts of heavy alcohol ingestion
   D. The aging process

8. Which of these psychoactive substances is an opioid drug?
   A. Cannabis
   B. Haldol
   C. Heroin
   D. Thorazine

9. Schizophrenia is characterized by withdrawal from reality into an inner world of disorganized thinking and conflict. Which is a characteristic of schizophrenia?
   A. Calm behavior
   B. Manic mood
   C. Depressed mood
   D. Delusions

10. Which of the following is a form of treatment for severe depression using electrical currents?
    A. Group therapy
    B. Free association

C. Electroconvulsive therapy
D. CBT

11. Bulimia is an eating disorder characterized by:
A. Excessive dieting because of emotional factors
B. Binge eating followed by vomiting and laxative abuse
C. Troubled feelings, unpleasant tension, distress, and avoidance behavior
D. Exaggerated concern with one's physical health and exaggeration of normal sensations and minor complaints

12. Which of these classes of drugs is not used to treat depression?
A. SSRIs
B. MAO inhibitors
C. Tricyclics
D. Benzodiazepines

13. Affect is the emotional response associated with an experience. It can be described as:
A. Fair
B. Impaired
C. Constricted
D. Autistic

14. In describing a patient's appearance, such as their hair or clothing, the most likely term would be:
A. Unkempt
B. Unkept
C. Shabby
D. Poor

15. Involuntary movement, a potentially irreversible side effect of taking antipsychotic drugs such as Haldol and Thorazine, is called:
A. Kinesia
B. Habituation
C. Pica
D. Tardive dyskinesia

16. Hypnotics, a class of drugs, are used to:
A. Treat ADHD
B. Treat OCD
C. Induce sleep
D. Place the patient in a trance

17. Which of the following would describe the manic phase of bipolar disorder?
A. Sad, worried
B. Euphoric, expansive, or irritable
C. Down in the dumps, fatigued
D. Dissociated

18. Anxiety disorders involve unpleasant tension, distress, palpitations, and sweating disproportionate to the circumstances. Which of the following is an anxiety disorder?
A. Anorexia nervosa
B. Agraphesthesia
C. SAD
D. Agoraphobia

19. Common signs of anxiety include:
A. Trembling, restlessness, and muscle tension
B. Nonsensical speech
C. Agitated behavior
D. Hostile attitude

20. A person with obsessive compulsive syndrome suffers severe anxiety if they:
A. Are in an enclosed space
B. Fail to perform a repetitive behavior such as hand washing
C. Have to repeat an action more than once
D. Disappoint someone

21. One of the symptoms of ADHD (attention-deficit hyperactive disorder) is:
A. Grandiosity
B. Inhibition
C. Anxiety
D. Distractibility

22. Trichotillomania (compulsive hair pulling) may fall within the spectrum of:
A. Attention-deficit hyperactive disorder
B. Obsessive compulsive disorder
C. Panic disorder
D. Anxiety disorder

23. Which of the following is not associated with dementia?
    A. Multiple infarctions
    B. Parkinsonism
    C. Alzheimer disease
    D. Bulimia

24. The mental disorder most closely associated with persistent sadness is:
    A. Anxiety
    B. Depression
    C. Bipolar disorder
    D. Dependent personality trait

25. Psychedelic drugs such as LSD can produce:
    A. Bradykinesia
    B. Visual hallucinations
    C. Resting tremors
    D. Cogwheeling

26. Psychomotor agitation is an excessive motor activity associated with a feeling of inner tension. It can manifest in such behavior as:
    A. Pacing back and forth
    B. Shuffling gait
    C. Unsteady ambulation
    D. Smiling expression

27. Which of the following is an example of a selective serotonin reuptake inhibitor?
    A. Prozac
    B. Lithium
    C. Prolixin
    D. Cannabis

28. THC (delta-9-tetrahydrocannabinol) is the chemical name for the psychoactive ingredient in the street drug:
    A. Heroin
    B. Cocaine
    C. Marijuana
    D. Crack

29. A form of therapy used to change behavior patterns and responses by training and repetition is called:
    A. Psychoanalysis
    B. Play therapy
    C. Cognitive behavioral therapy
    D. Hypnosis

30. Having physical symptoms that cannot be explained by an actual physical disorder is called:
    A. Schizophrenia
    B. Somnambulism
    C. Sundowning
    D. Somatization

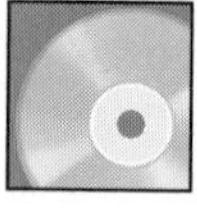

Please see the accompanying CD for additional review materials for this section.

PROOFREADING EXERCISES

These three proofreading exercises are provided to improve your skills in the areas of editing and effective identification and correction of errors in the medical record.

Directions: Identify and correct the transcription errors found in the exercises below. *Answers are provided at the end of this chapter.*

PROOFREADING EXERCISE #1

HISTORY OF PRESENT ILLNESS
The patient is here today for psychotherapy medication management. The chart was reviewed, medications were reviewed and the staff were consulted. The patient was seen on an individual basis. The patient was found in the activity room. He said that he continued to be very depressed with poor energy but wishes to be involved in activities on the unit. However, when he is in the activity room, he watches the television, is isolated and with drawn.

The patient continues to have pyrenoid ideations. He wants to know why other people want to hurt him. The patient reported odd story hallucinations. The patient is verbalizing feelings of helplessness, hopelessness, and worthlessness, mainly related to his obvious problems.

MENTAL STATUS EXAMINATION
The patient is sad and worried. He is alert and oriented to person, place, and time. The patient's mood is depressed, anxious, and the effective response is coherent with the mood. Auditory hallucinations are present. Attention and concentration is decreased. Memory seems to be preserved. There are ideas of paranoid-type present. The insight is poor and the judgement is impaired.

DIAGNOSTIC IMPRESSION
Schizoaffective disorder.

MEDICATIONS
Risperdal 1 mg p.o. b.i.d., Wellbutrin 100 mg p.o. b.i.d., and Ambien 100 mg p.o. nightly.

(continued)

PLAN
The patient continues to need in patient treatment. The patient will therefore stay in the hospital until there is further stabilization of her mental condition. The patient is unable at this time to be placed in a less restrictive environment.

PROOFREADING EXERCISE #2

EVALUATION PROCEDURES
Clinical Interview of Patient, Review of Records.

REASON FOR REFERRAL
Pain extending past the usual healing time, depression, increased stressors due to postoperative complications.

CHIEF COMPLAINT
The patient complains of chronic contractible back pain which led to surgery in December of 2004. She had a fusion at L5-S1 and slightly improved but continued to have low back pain. She was admitted to the hospital in January 2005 due to a postoperative wound infection. She was discharged from the hospital around the end of January and her pain level since the surgery ranges from 4–6 out of 10. She complains today of a depressed mood developing after the postoperative infection occurred.

HISTORY OF PRESENT INJURY
The patient suffered an on-the-job injury in July of 2001. She underwent spinal surgery in September of 2002 but the pain continued after that time. She underwent a series of lumbar epidural steroid infections with minimal improvement. I saw her for psychological evaluation in September 2003 and recommended her for participation in a chronic pain management program. She completed that program successfully in November 2003. Her pain coping skills improved, but her pain showed no appreciable decrease, and there was little improvement in her overall functioning. In August of 2004, she was referred back to her surgeon for additional evaluation. Dr. Jones felt she was a good candidate for surgery to remove her hardware, and she subsequently underwent surgery for that purpose in December 2004 with the outcome and sequel E as noted above.

CURRENT MEDICATION
Darvocet 500 mg 1–2 q.6 h. for pain, Effector 225 mg per day, Neupogen 600 mg 1 q.6 h. p.r.n. sharp, burning pain, fluconazole 150 mg 1 per day p.r.n., rifampin 300 mg 2 per day.

(continued)

CURRENT FUNCTIONING

The patient is not presently working. Her self-report of current functioning on the Vestry Disability Scale completed 2/04/2005 would place her in the "crippled" range of functioning. On a typical day, she spends her time at home in sedimentary activities. She states she is able to take care of all personal needs unassisted. She states she does "nothing" for fun and her social activities are limited to her family. She describes disturbed sleep, and even with medication, has less than 4 hours of continuous sleep each night. After waking, she notes it may take her 2–3 hours to return to sleep.

SUBJECTIVE MOOD EXPERIENCE

The patient describes her current mood as "depressed." She notes it is slightly improved with increased antidepressant medication. Her scores on the Brief Symptom Inventory-18 completed 02/04/2005 are elevated with somatotropin, depression, anxiety, and global severity entities to be elevated above the 95th centile as compared to the community population.

DIAGNOSIS

Axis I

1. Adjustment disorder with depressed mood, acute, secondary to postoperative complications.
2. Pain disorder associated with both psychological factors and a general medical condition, chronic.

Axis II No diagnosis.

Axis III Obtained from medical record:

1. Lumbar reticular syndrome with right sciatica, status post lumbar interbody fusion at L5-S1 in 2002 and 12/2004 with postoperative wound infection (primary).
2. Chronic intractable pain secondary to frail back surgery syndrome.
3. Depression secondary to chronic intractable pain.

Axis IV Sever: Pain, disability, functional limitations, significant complications from medical care.

Axis V Current GAF = 55. Highest GAF in the Past Year = 70.

(continued)

RECOMMENDATIONS
In addition to her current antidepressant medication, the patient would benefit from conservative behavioral therapy. The therapy would focus on helping her deal with her current emotional distress, develop a cents of a future for herself, and reinforce her previously learned coping skills. I recommend an initial trial of therapy once weekly for 8 weeks and evaluate her progress at the end of that time.

PROOFREADING EXERCISE #3

REASON FOR ADMISSION
Combination drug dependency ("crack" cocaine, marijuana, and alcohol).

HISTORY OF PRESENT ILLNESS
The patient is a 41-year-old white male who was admitted for the first time to St. Jude treatment program with the diagnosis of combination drug redundancy ("crack" cocaine, marijuana, and alcohol). The patient stated that he started using marijuana when he was 13-years-old and has been using "crack" for the past 10 years. He usually smokes the cocaine and denies intravenous drug use or sorting the drug. He stated he drinks alcohol only on weekends and usually this is limited to beer.

He stated he came by himself because he wanted to get help for his drug use. He stated he is having significant martial problems and has been placed on probation at his job. He has noticed his memory is ensnared and often he feels anxious or jittery.

PAST MEDICAL/SURGICAL HISTORY
He denied any history of diabetes, hypertension, asthma, or seizures.

ALLERGIES
No known allergies.

MEDICATIONS
None at this time.

SOCIAL HISTORY
He has a 20 pack/year history of cigarette smoking. His alcohol use usually includes a 12-pack on weekends. He works as a mechanic, is married, and has 2 children. He has 2 years of college.

FAMILY HISTORY
No family history of drug abuse.

REVIEW OF SYSTEMS
The patient denied any chest pain, shortness of breath, abdominal pain, or diarrhea.

(continued)

PHYSICAL EXAMINATION
GENERAL: This is a medium-built male who is awake, alert, and oriented x3. He is pleasant but unkept.
VITAL SIGNS: Temperature 98, pulse 68, respirations 20, and blood pressure is 126/72. He weighs 212 pounds and is 6′0″ tall.
SKIN: Normal, without cyanosis or ulcerations.
HEENT: The head is normocephalic without lesions. Pupils are equal and reactive. Extraocular muscles are intact. Oral mucosa is high.
LUNGS: The lungs are clear to auscultation and percussion.
CARDIOVASCULAR: Tachycardia without gallops or murmurs.
ABDOMEN: Soft; bowel sounds present.
EXTREMITIES: No edema. Pulses are equal and symmetrical.
NEUROLOGICAL: There are no vocal deficits. The patient is oriented to time, place, and self. His judgment is intact, and he is experiencing no hallucinations or paranoid illusions.

IMPRESSION
This is a 41-year-old white male admitted for the first time to a drug treatment program with a diagnosis of combination drug dependency. He has developed a trance to marijuana, as he has progressively increased the amount and frequency of his intake in order to feel high.

PLAN
We will admit the patient to the drug treatment program as per treatment protocols with further diagnosis and treatment as appropriate.

ANSWER KEYS

REVIEW QUESTIONS ANSWER KEY

1. D	6. B	11. B	16. C	21. D	26. A
2. B	7. C	12. D	17. B	22. B	27. A
3. B	8. C	13. C	18. D	23. D	28. C
4. D	9. D	14. A	19. A	24. B	29. C
5. B	10. C	15. D	20. B	25. B	30. D

PROOFREADING EXERCISE #1 KEY

HISTORY OF PRESENT ILLNESS
The patient is here today for psychotherapy medication management. The chart was reviewed, medications were reviewed and the staff were consulted. The patient was seen on an individual basis. The patient was found in the activity room. He said that he continued to be very depressed with poor energy but wishes to be involved in activities on the unit. However, when he is in the activity room, he watches the television, is isolated and with drawn.

The patient continues to have pyrenoid ideations. He wants to know why other people want to hurt him. The patient reported odd story hallucinations. The patient is verbalizing feelings of helplessness, hopelessness, and worthlessness, mainly related to his obvious problems.

MENTAL STATUS EXAMINATION
The patient is sad and worried. He is alert and oriented to person, place, and time. The patient's mood is depressed, anxious, and the effective response is coherent with the mood. Auditory hallucinations are present. Attention and concentration is decreased. Memory seems to be preserved. There are ideas of paranoid-type present. The insight is poor and the judgement is impaired.

DIAGNOSTIC IMPRESSION
Schizoaffective disorder.

MEDICATIONS
Risperdal 1 mg p.o. b.i.d., Wellbutrin 100 mg p.o. b.i.d., and Ambien 100 mg p.o. nightly.

Use combined form—withdrawn

Incorrect verb—was

Incorrect term—paranoid

Incorrect term—auditory

Incorrect spelling—affective

Incorrect spelling—judgment

Incorrect dose—most likely 10 mg

Use combined form—inpatient

PLAN

The patient continues ~~to need~~ in patient treatment. The patient will therefore stay in the hospital until there is further stabilization of her mental condition. The patient is unable at this time to be placed in a less restrictive environment.

Gender change—his

PROOFREADING EXERCISE #2 KEY

EVALUATION PROCEDURES
Clinical Interview of Patient, Review of Records.

REASON FOR REFERRAL
Pain extending past the usual healing time, depression, increased stressors due to postoperative complications.

CHIEF COMPLAINT
The patient complains of chronic contractible back pain which led to surgery in December of 2004. She had a fusion at L5–S1 and slightly improved but continued to have low back pain. She was admitted to the hospital in January 2005 due to a postoperative wound infection. She was discharged from the hospital around the end of January, and her pain level since the surgery ranges from 4–6 out of 10. She complains today of a depressed mood developing after the postoperative infection occurred.

HISTORY OF PRESENT INJURY
The patient suffered an on-the-job injury in July of 2001. She underwent spinal surgery in September of 2002 but the pain continued after that time. She underwent a series of lumbar epidural steroid infections with minimal improvement. I saw her for psychological evaluation in September 2003 and recommended her for participation in a chronic pain management program. She completed that program successfully in November 2003. Her pain coping skills improved, but her pain showed no appreciable decrease, and there was little improvement in her overall functioning. In August of 2004, she was referred back to her surgeon for additional evaluation. Dr. Jones felt she was a good candidate for surgery to remove her hardware, and she subsequently underwent

Incorrect term—intractable

Incorrect term—injections

Incorrect drug—Neurontin

Incorrect term—sequelae

surgery for that purpose in December 2004 with the outcome and sequel E as noted above.

CURRENT MEDICATION

Darvocet 500 mg 1–2 q.6 h. for pain, Effector 225 mg per day, Neupogen 600 mg 1 q.6 h. p.r.n. sharp, burning pain, fluconazole 150 mg 1 per day p.r.n., rifampin 300 mg 2 per day.

Not a valid drug name—Effexor

Incorrect term—Oswestry

CURRENT FUNCTIONING

The patient is not presently working. Her self-report of current functioning on the Vestry Disability Scale completed 2/04/2005 would place her in the "crippled" range of functioning. On a typical day, she spends her time at home in sedimentary activities. She states she is able to take care of all personal needs unassisted. She states she does "nothing" for fun and her social activities are limited to her family. She describes disturbed sleep, and even with medication, has less than 4 hours of continuous sleep each night. After waking, she notes it may take her 2–3 hours to return to sleep.

Incorrect term—sedentary

SUBJECTIVE MOOD EXPERIENCE

The patient describes her current mood as "depressed." She notes it is slightly improved with increased antidepressant medication. Her scores on the Brief Symptom Inventory-18 completed 02/04/2005 are elevated with somatotropin, depression, anxiety, and global severity entities to be elevated above the 95th centile as compared to the community population.

Missing prefix—percentile

Incorrect term—somatization

Incorrect term—indices

DIAGNOSIS

Axis I

1. Adjustment disorder with depressed mood, acute, secondary to postoperative complications.

2. Pain disorder associated with both psychological factors and a general medical condition, chronic.

Axis II No diagnosis.

Axis III Obtained from medical record:

1. Lumbar reticular syndrome with right sciatica, status post lumbar interbody fusion at L5–S1 in 2002 and 12/2004 with postoperative wound infection (primary).
2. Chronic intractable pain secondary to frail back surgery syndrome.
3. Depression secondary to chronic intractable pain.

Axis IV Sever: Pain, disability, functional limitations, significant complications from medical care.

Axis V Current GAF = 55. Highest GAF in the Past Year = 70.

RECOMMENDATIONS

In addition to her current antidepressant medication, the patient would benefit from conservative behavioral therapy. The therapy would focus on helping her deal with her current emotional distress, develop a cents of a future for herself, and reinforce her previously learned coping skills. I recommend an initial trial of therapy once weekly for 8 weeks and evaluate her progress at the end of that time.

Incorrect term—radicular

Incorrect word—failed

Incorrect word—severe

Incorrect term—cognitive

Incorrect word—sense

PROOFREADING EXERCISE #3 KEY

REASON FOR ADMISSION
Combination drug dependency ("crack" cocaine, marijuana, and alcohol).

HISTORY OF PRESENT ILLNESS
The patient is a 41-year-old white male who was admitted for the first time to St. Jude treatment program with the diagnosis of combination drug redundancy ("crack" cocaine, marijuana, and alcohol). The patient stated that he started using marijuana when he was 13-years-old ~~and~~ has been using "crack" for the past 10 years. He usually smokes the cocaine and denies intravenous drug use ~~or~~ sorting the drug. He stated he drinks alcohol only on weekends and usually this is limited to beer.

Incorrect term—dependency

No hyphens required

Incorrect word—snorting

He stated he came by himself because he wanted to get help for his drug use. He stated he is having ~~significant~~ martial problems and has been placed on probation at his job. He has noticed his memory ~~is~~ ensnared and often he feels anxious or jittery.

Incorrect word—marital

Incorrect term—impaired

PAST MEDICAL/SURGICAL HISTORY
He denied any history of diabetes, hypertension, asthma, or seizures.

ALLERGIES
No known allergies.

MEDICATIONS
None at this time.

SOCIAL HISTORY
He ~~has a~~ 20 pack/year history of cigarette smoking. His alcohol use usually includes a 12-pack on weekends. He works as a mechanic, is married, and has 2 children. He has 2 years of college.

Incorrect format—20-pack-year

FAMILY HISTORY
No family history of drug abuse.

REVIEW OF SYSTEMS
The patient denied any chest pain, shortness of breath, abdominal pain, or diarrhea.

PHYSICAL EXAMINATION
GENERAL: This is a medium-built male who is awake, alert, and oriented x3. He is pleasant but unkept.

Incorrect word—unkempt

VITAL SIGNS: Temperature 98, pulse 68, respirations 20, and blood pressure is 126/72. He weighs 212 pounds and is 6'0" tall.

Incorrect format—6 feet tall

SKIN: Normal, without cyanosis or ulcerations.
HEENT: The head is normocephalic without lesions. Pupils are equal and reactive. Extraocular muscles are intact. Oral mucosa is high.

Incorrect word—dry

LUNGS: The lungs are clear to auscultation and percussion.
CARDIOVASCULAR: Tachycardia without gallops or murmurs.
ABDOMEN: Soft; bowel sounds present.
EXTREMITIES: No edema. Pulses are equal and symmetrical.
NEUROLOGICAL: There are no vocal deficits. The patient is oriented to time, place, and self. His judgment is intact, and he is experiencing no hallucinations or paranoid illusions.

Incorrect term—focal

Incorrect term—delusions

IMPRESSION
This is a 41-year-old white male admitted for the first time to a drug treatment program with a diagnosis of combination drug dependency. He has developed a trance to marijuana, as he has progressively increased the amount and frequency of his intake in order to feel high.

Incorrect term—tolerance

PLAN
We will admit the patient to the drug treatment program as per treatment protocols with further diagnosis and treatment as appropriate.

CHAPTER

22

Pulmonology

OBJECTIVES CHECKLIST

A prepared exam candidate will know:

- ❑ Combining forms, prefixes, and suffixes related to the body system.
- ❑ Anatomical structures of the respiratory system.
- ❑ Physiologic process of respiration and the pathway of air from the nose to the lung capillaries.
- ❑ Difference between external (pulmonary) respiration and internal (cellular) respiration.
- ❑ Physiologic role of oxygen and carbon dioxide exchange and the correlation to acid-base balance in the body.
- ❑ Terminology and definitions related to auscultated breath sounds.
- ❑ Signs, symptoms, and diseases related to the respiratory system.
- ❑ Diagnostic studies used in the diagnosis and treatment of respiratory symptoms, disorders, and diseases.
- ❑ Respiratory therapies.
- ❑ Imaging studies used in the identification and diagnosis of respiratory diseases.
- ❑ Laboratory studies used in the diagnosis and treatment of respiratory symptoms, disorders, and diseases.
- ❑ Common medications prescribed for respiratory symptoms, disorders, and diseases.
- ❑ Transcription standards related to pulmonary and respiratory terms.

RESOURCES FOR STUDY

1. *The Language of Medicine*
   Chapter 12: Respiratory System, pp. 441–186.
2. *H&P: A Nonphysician's Guide to the Medical History and Physical Examination*
   Chapter 9: Review of Systems: Respiratory, pp. 83–88.
   Chapter 24: Examination of the Lungs, pp. 227–234.
3. *Human Diseases*
   Chapter 10: Diseases of the Respiratory System, pp. 141–152.
4. *Laboratory Tests & Diagnostic Procedures in Medicine*
   Chapter 4: Measurement of Temperature, Rates, Pressures and Volumes (Respiratory Measurements), pp. 48–50.
   Chapter 7: Visual Examinations of the Eyes, Ears, Nose and Respiratory Tract, pp. 95–106.
   Chapter 10: Plain Radiography (Chest X-ray), pp. 137–138.
   Chapter 20: Chemical Examination of the Blood (Acid-Base Balance, pp. 357–360, and Arterial Blood Gases, p. 362).
5. *Understanding Pharmacology for Health Professionals*
   Chapter 18: Pulmonary Drugs, pp. 192–204.
6. *The AAMT Book of Style for Medical Transcription*
   Pulmonary and Respiratory Terms, pp. 338–340.

SAMPLE REPORTS

The following four reports are examples of reports you might encounter while transcribing pulmonology.

FOLLOWUP REPORT

HISTORY OF PRESENT ILLNESS
The patient is a 56-year-old white female with rheumatoid arthritis and bronchiectasis. She had a right upper lobe cavity develop on CT scan. When I saw her in January, she had had an upper respiratory tract infection. She felt better with antibiotics, and then as she came off the antibiotics her symptoms worsened. By phone, I prescribed Avelox for 21 days. She is 1 week into her therapy and feels significantly better. On a scale of 1–10 (with 10 being normal), she is about a 7 or 8 now, in her opinion, and previously had been as low as a 4, by her description, when she first became ill. She has not had any hemoptysis. She had chills but they resolved. No sweats. No fevers. No chest pain. Appetite is acceptable but not quite at normal. She has also had Mycobacterium avium (MAI) in her sputum. She has never had cyclic antibiotics because she has had minimal symptoms and normal PFTs. Her most recent set of PFTs in January 2004, despite fairly extensive radiographic studies, was unremarkable.

PHYSICAL EXAMINATION
Physical exam today is unremarkable.

DIAGNOSTIC STUDIES
A CT scan of the thorax today, compared with January, shows that the cavitary lesion in the right upper lobe has not significantly changed other than more opacity within the cavity suggesting retained secretions. She has diffuse bronchiectatic changes throughout including all areas of confluence.

ASSESSMENT
I had a very long discussion with her today regarding bronchiectasis and its interaction with MAI and the difficulties in treating MAI, including 18 months of therapy with triple-drug combinations. Because she is clinically feeling well, her PFTs are normal, and her exercise tolerance has always been good, our current plan is to continue with the Avelox until it is completed at 21 days. We will check sputum for MAI between now and then, and I will see her back in 1 month with CT and PFTs at that time.

I have given her a web site to look for information regarding nontuberculous mycobacterium and have discussed the disease in great detail with her. I highlighted the controversies with regard to management and the appropriate timing of beginning antimycobacterial therapy. I also discussed our lack of good knowledge regarding temporal changes in PFTs over time.

I will see the patient in 1 month. I have invited her to call me if she develops any interim problems. She appears to be agreeable to this plan and is anxious to proceed as outlined.

CONSULTATION

HISTORY OF PRESENT ILLNESS

The patient is a 73-year-old white female originally from Europe. She is seeking evaluation here at the clinic for left upper abdominal pain. She is in seen in the pulmonary clinic today for evaluation of chronic lung disease. She is a previous smoker, having smoked until 2 years ago. She also has a history of childhood "bronchitis" and also previous pneumonia. She has cough and dyspnea but not much in the way of phlegm production. It sounds as if she may have also had a positive tuberculin skin test, but never had active TB as far as she is aware. The remainder of her history and physical examination is as documented by her primary care physician. I highlight that she is on nocturnal oxygen, but she is not wearing it during the day. She is only on inhalers with beta agonists and ipratropium. She is not on any inhaled steroid. She has had deleterious side effects with systemic steroids.

PHYSICAL EXAMINATION

Physical exam today is limited by her discomfort. Lung exam is most notable for very diminished breath sounds and a few wheezes with poor air exchange throughout.

DIAGNOSTIC STUDIES

Chest x-ray shows changes of hyperinflation with increased retrosternal air space and a flattened hemidiaphragm. PFTs show severe obstructive lung disease with relatively preserved diffusion capacity and some reversibility. The ratio is 37.7. FEV_1 is 0.87, which is 37% of predicted, and it increases to 1.08 or 24% after bronchodilators. Lung volumes show increased TLC and increased RV/TLC. Diffusion capacity is 61% and resting saturation is 88%.

ASSESSMENT AND PLAN

Chronic obstructive lung disease with some reversibility and mildly reduced diffusion capacity. I do not suspect her pain has anything to do with her lung disease. I am uncertain if her underlying lung disease is a fixed asthma, bronchiectasis, or changes of chronic bronchitis, although her clinical history does not suggest that. I would like to perform a CT scan to better characterize her lung disease. If it appears that this is predominantly bronchiectasis, there will not be strong indications for inhaled corticosteroids. However, if this is asthma that still maintains reversibility, then proceeding with inhaled steroids in addition to other therapies would be of benefit. Next, I am not certain that her Singulair is offering her much benefit, and discontinuation of this would be appropriate.

BRONCHOSCOPY

PROCEDURE PERFORMED
Bronchoscopy.

PREOPERATIVE DIAGNOSIS
Nodular density in the right lower lobe, etiology uncertain.

POSTOPERATIVE DIAGNOSIS
Nodular density in the right lower lobe, etiology uncertain.

FINDINGS
No endobronchial lesions seen.

INDICATIONS FOR PROCEDURE
This is a patient with what appears to be neurofibromatosis and was found to have a density in the right midlung field, felt by the radiologist to be in the lower lobe. Bronchoscopy is being done for further evaluation. He has a past smoking history. He came in with left-sided pleurisy.

PREOPERATIVE MEDICATIONS
Demerol 30 mg IM plus atropine 0.6 mg IM.

DESCRIPTION OF PROCEDURE
The patient was brought to Endoscopy, where topical anesthesia was administered. The bronchoscope was introduced through the right transnasal approach. The nasopharynx appeared normal. The vocal cords were normal. The trachea, main carina, right mainstem, right upper lobe, right middle lobe, and right lower lobe segments appeared normal. No lesions were seen. The left mainstem and left upper lobe segments appeared normal. There was some mild extrinsic compression of the left lower lobe orifice. There was no evidence of any endobronchial lesions seen. The bronchoscope was then reintroduced into the right upper lobe where the areas were reexamined, and no lesions were seen. The bronchoscope was then reintroduced into the right lower lobe where multiple washings were taken from the right basilar segments and the superior segment of the right lower lobe. Brushings were taken from the superior segment of the right lower lobe and sent for cytology also.

COMPLICATIONS
None so far. A postprocedure chest x-ray is pending.

SPECIMENS
1. Bronchial washings from the right lower lobe are being sent for routine culture and sensitivity, fungal culture, acid-fast bacillus smear, acid-fast bacillus culture, and routine viral cultures, since the patient did have some left chest pain on admission.
2. Bronchial brushings from the superior segment of the right lower lobe were sent for cytology.

CONDITION TO RECOVERY
Stable.

EXAMINATION PRE-PROCEDURE
Lungs were clear to auscultation and percussion. Heart had a regular rhythm with no murmurs, rubs, or gallops.

(continued)

EXAMINATION POST-PROCEDURE
Lungs were clear to auscultation and percussion. Heart had a regular rhythm with no murmurs, rubs or gallops.

TELEMETRY
Sinus rhythm throughout without any arrhythmias. Oxygen saturation was well above 90% throughout the procedure on 50% oxygen via mask. Postprocedure on room air, the oxygen saturation was 96%. The blood pressure did increase during the procedure, but the patient indicated that he felt fine.

DISPOSITION
The patient will have a postprocedure chest x-ray done and will be monitored over the next few hours.

PULMONARY FUNCTION STUDIES

PROCEDURE
Pulmonary function testing.

LUNG VOLUMES
There is a moderate decrease in FVC. There is a marked reduction in TLC, RV, and FRC.

LUNG FLOWS
Moderate decrease in FVC, marked reduction in FEV_1, mild reduction in FEV_1/FVC. Marked decrease in FEF $_{25-75\%}$.

RESPONSE TO BRONCHODILATORS
There is a significant improvement in the FEV_1 and FEF $_{25-75\%}$ post-bronchodilator administration.

MVV AND PEF
None.

FLOW VOLUME LOOP
No evidence of upper airway obstruction.

DIFFUSING CAPACITY
Marked reduction in lung diffusion. The corrected DLCO [DL/VA] is moderately reduced.

ARTERIAL BLOOD GASES
None.

IMPRESSION
1. This study is suggestive of severe restrictive lung disease.
2. No evidence of upper airway obstruction.
3. Significant response to bronchodilators was seen.
4. Moderate reduction in the corrected DLCO [DL/VA].
5. The patient's obesity is probably related to the decrease in lung diffusion, at least in part.
6. At least a mild degree of coexisting airway obstruction is suspected. Clinical correlation is indicated.
7. The marked reduction in FRC and other lung volumes may be erroneous. Clinical correlation is indicated.

REVIEW QUESTIONS

The goal of these questions is to test your knowledge in the area of pulmonology.

Directions: Select the correct answer for each of the multiple-choice questions provided below. *Answers are provided at the end of this chapter.*

1. Which of these is used for treatment of tuberculosis?
   A. Robaxin
   B. Robitussin
   C. Rocephin
   D. Rifampin

2. Which of these is part of an arterial blood gas?
   A. FEV
   B. FVC
   C. pCO_2
   D. PFT

3. To further evaluate bilateral pulmonary infiltrates, a CT of the chest could be done using:
   A. HIDA solution
   B. High resolution
   C. Respiratory quotient
   D. High-dose dilution

4. A heavy smoker with pulmonary bullae develops a pneumothorax on the left; a short while later he develops a pneumothorax on the right. He could be said to have:
   A. Bilateral pneumothoraxes
   B. Pneumothorax simplex
   C. Bilateral pneumothoraces
   D. Iatrogenic pneumothorax

5. Which of these can be done at the time of bronchoscopy?
   A. Bronchiectasis
   B. Bronchoalveolar lavage
   C. Ventilation-perfusion lung scan
   D. Paracentesis

6. Which of these is part of the lung?
   A. Hilum
   B. Stapes
   C. Ventricle
   D. Tarsus

7. Which of the following is a genetic disease which causes accumulation of thick mucus leading to recurrent respiratory infections?
   A. Multiple sclerosis
   B. Chronic obstructive pulmonary disease
   C. Cystic fibrosis
   D. Tuberculosis

8. The most common pulmonary opportunistic infection seen in AIDS patients is:
   A. Epstein-Barr
   B. Pneumocystis jiroveci (P. carinii)
   C. Candidiasis
   D. RSV

9. In the lungs, the chief respiratory unit for gas exchange is called the:
   A. Alveolus
   B. Bronchi
   C. Carina
   D. Hilum

10. The material that lubricates the pleural surfaces is called:
    A. Pleural fluid
    B. Alveolar fluid
    C. Visceral fluid
    D. Serous fluid

11. The area between the lungs is called the:
    A. Azygos space
    B. Anterior thoracic cage
    C. Mediastinum
    D. Pericardial sac

12. While the posterior thoracic cage consists of the vertebral column and 12 pairs of ribs, the anterior thoracic cage consists of the:
    A. Sternum and xiphoid process
    B. Ribs 1–10 and the xiphoid process
    C. Ribs 1–8 and the xiphoid process
    D. Manubrium, sternum, and xiphoid process

13. An individual presents to the ER with difficulty breathing. He is gasping for air and the skin between his ribs sucks in with every breath. This is called:
    A. Suprasternal pulsations
    B. Posterior retractions
    C. Subcostal retractions
    D. Forced expiration

14. Accessory muscles of respiration include:
    A. Pectorals, sternocleidomastoids, and scalenes
    B. Trapezius, pectorals, and buccinators
    C. Sternocleidomastoids, scalenes, and diaphragm
    D. Diaphragm, pterygoid, and pectorals

15. How many lobes does the right lung have?
    A. Two
    B. Three
    C. Six
    D. Four

16. The abbreviation FEV_1 stands for forced expiratory volume. What does the subscript 1 mean?
    A. In the first breath
    B. In one breath
    C. In one second
    D. The first stage of the test

17. When oxygen passes into the bloodstream, it binds with hemoglobin to form which of the following?
    A. Red blood cells
    B. Carbon dioxide
    C. Oxyhemoglobin
    D. White blood cells

18. Which classification of drugs is used to improve respiratory function?
    A. Mucolytics
    B. Hemostatics
    C. Immunostimulants
    D. Keratolytics

19. One medication used to prevent bronchial asthma attacks is:
    A. Benzodiazepine
    B. Guaifenesin
    C. Imipramine
    D. Cromolyn sodium

20. The arterial blood gas values pCO_2 and pO_2 are reported in which of the following units:
    A. mm
    B. cm
    C. mmHg
    D. mL

21. The creation of an opening into the trachea through the neck is called a:
    A. Tracheostomy
    B. Thoracotomy
    C. Thoracentesis
    D. Thoracostomy

22. Which condition below is characterized by diffuse interstitial pulmonary fibrosis?
    A. Adult respiratory distress syndrome
    B. Asbestosis
    C. Sudden infant death syndrome
    D. Status asthmaticus

23. One predisposing factor for developing COPD is:
    A. Recurrent respiratory infections
    B. Alcoholism
    C. Intravenous drug abuse
    D. X-ray exposure as a child

24. Another commonly used term for asthma is:
    A. Extrinsic allergic reaction
    B. Reactive airway disease
    C. Intrinsic irritant syndrome
    D. Pleuritic paroxysmal syndrome

25. An accumulation of air in the pleural cavity that leads to partial or complete lung collapse is termed:
    A. Dyspnea
    B. Pneumonia
    C. Pneumothorax
    D. Hemothorax

26. In the early stages of pulmonary edema, the patient may present with which constellation of symptoms?
    A. Tachypnea, PND, and dyspnea on exertion
    B. Decreased blood pressure, bradycardia, and thirst
    C. Paroxysmal nocturnal dyspnea, hematemesis, and rales
    D. Tension pneumothorax, hemoptysis, and hematemesis

27. Which of the following is not a bronchodilator?
    A. Ipratropium
    B. Terbutaline
    C. Albuterol
    D. Vanceril

28. Tuberculosis is transmitted through:
    A. The fecal-oral route
    B. Contact with blood
    C. Inhalation of infected droplets
    D. Dirty needles

29. A pulmonary thromboembolism can be caused by:
    A. A hypercoagulable state
    B. DVT
    C. Prolonged immobilization
    D. All of these

30. A pleural effusion is:
    A. The presence of fluid in the pleural space
    B. Pockets of mucus in the lungs of a cystic fibrosis patient
    C. Leakage of air into the pleural space
    D. Excessive sputum production

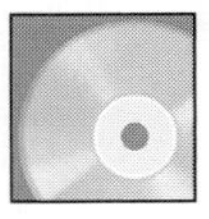

Please see the accompanying CD for additional review materials for this section.

PROOFREADING EXERCISES

These three proofreading exercises are provided to improve your skills in the areas of editing and effective identification and correction of errors in the medical record.

Directions: Identify and correct the transcription errors found in the exercises below. *Answers are provided at the end of this chapter.*

PROOFREADING EXERCISE #1

HISTORY

I had the pleasure of seeing this female patient on June 10, 2004, for an evaluation of dyspnea and exercise limitations. Her evaluation here was extensive and included an echocardiogram, a Cardiolyte study, a chest CT using pulmonary embolus protocols, an arterial blood gas, and cardiopulmonary exercise testing. Together, these studies show that she has essentially normal cardiopulmonary function. The only objective abnormality found on this testing was a mild reduction in diffusion capacity at 70% of predicted. Oxygenation, however, was maintained. An arterial blood gas showed excellent oxygenation with a $PA0_2$ on room air of 87. Chest CT did not demonstrate any significant parenchymal disease or any evidence of thromboembolic disease. There was minimal scaring in the left lung apex. Echocardiogram demonstrated good left and right ventricular function with normal size. There was mild diastolic dysfunction, grade 1, noted. There was no significant valvular disease. The left atrium was not enlarged. Estimated right ventricular systolic pressure was normal at 32 mmHg. Cardiopulmonary stress testing demonstrated no ventilatory limit to exercise. Heart rate response to exercise was inadequate.

She was evaluated by our group. We felt she had an allergy to dust mites. A note was made of an eosinophil count of 78. The absolute eosinophil count here was within the normal range at 0.09 x 1000 with 0.50 x 1000 as the upper limit of normal. Total white count was 7.9. Inspiratory flow up did not demonstrate any suggestion of proximal airway obstruction. A note was made of a decreased MEV relative to the FEV_1.

A methyl choline challenge study did not suggest any evidence of asthma. There was only a 5% decline in FEV_1 after methyl choline; however, a bronchial dilator was used earlier in the day.

(continued)

I do not find any overwhelming cardiopulmonary dysfunction as the ideology of her dyspnea. The inadequate heart rate response on beta-blocking medication may be contributing to her symptoms. In the absence of ongoing atrial fibrillation and lack of left atrial enlargement, discontinuation of a beta-blocking agent may be appropriate. Additionally, the evidence for asthma was unconvincing. Admittedly, the methacholine was done in the presence of bronchodilators given earlier in the day, but I do not suspect her symptoms are due to intermittent asthma with baseline good pulmonary function. Continuation of her medication therapy for house dust, mite allergy and associated allergic rhinoconjunctivitis with basal steroid and antihistamine is appropriate. I do not see a clear role for Xolair therapy in her management. She is implementing the appropriate dust mite measures at home.

She was evaluated by a cardiologist because of a nondiagnostic exercise stress test, and showed good LB function by imaging studies. He did not feel that further evaluation of cardiac disease was appropriate. It was noted that her lipid profile was unfavorable, and therapy with a lipid lowering agent would be appropriate.

She was evaluated because of difficulty palpating peripheral pulses. He felt that she did not have evidence of significant large-vessel or vascular disease. Ankle bronchial indices were acceptable. He recommended screening ultrasound because of a family history of an aortic aneurysm. This was performed and was unremarkable.

Together we explored whether or not her deep-vain stimulators could be affecting her sensation of dyspnea. I have discussed this with neurosurgery. He felt that the thalamic location of these stimulators would preclude that as a contributor to her symptoms.

PROOFREADING EXERCISE #2

CHIEF COMPLAINT
Respiratory insufficiency.

HISTORY OF PRESENT ILLNESS
In summary, this is a 74-year-old male who has ALS as well as a possible tumor of the spinal canal that has not been proven by tissue biopsy. He has had a previous history of destructive sleep apnea treated with CTAP prior to his diagnosis of ALS and subsequently has been managed on BiPAP 12 and 5 for respiratory insufficiency with ALS. Overall, he has tolerated that well. At rest during the day, he does not have any significant respiratory insufficiency signs. At night, he sleeps well; however, last night he had an episode where he woke up while wearing BiPAP and felt he was not getting adequate breathes. He took the mask off and still felt as if he were "breathing in a vacuum." Rescue was called and with the initiation of supple mental oxygen and evaluation in the ER, he ultimately felt okay again. Laboratory studies at that time were remarkable for an elevated CO_2 at 33 and an INR of 1.8. I should note that he is on Coumadin for a previous DVC but it is subtherapeutic.

PHYSICAL EXAMINATION
Examination is limited by the patient's lack of mobility. He is in a wheelchair. He is not in any respiratory dress. His lung exam is significant for basal air crackles and diminished breath sounds throughout.

DIAGNOSTIC STUDIES
I reviewed a new chest x-ray from later in the day which shows small lung volumes. No further laboratory testing. PSTs are not yet scanned into the computer but show no evidence of obstruction. They do, however, show restriction and diminished respiratory pressures and normal DL_{CO} when corrected for alveolar volume.

ASSESSMENT
1. Amyotrophic lateral sclerosis (ALS).
2. Respiratory insufficiency chronic secondary to #1.
3. Central abdominal obesity on exam.

(continued)

4. Episode of respiratory insufficiency, acute, for reasons that are not entirely clear.
5. Previous DVT on Coumadin with a subtherapeutic INR.

PLAN
1. Overnight oximetry to assess oxygenation on BiPAP at the current settings. If this shows periods of anemia, I would evaluate in the sleep lab overnight with a titration study on BiPAP and the addition of supplemental oxygen as needed.
2. I am unclear as to the ideology of his acute respiratory insufficiency. Thromboembolic disease is a possibility, although his rapid improvement makes me less suspicious of that; however, I would check viral CT scan of the chest and an arterial blood gas.
3. Followup in the pulmonary clinic as needed.

PROOFREADING EXERCISE #3

HISTORY OF PRESENT ILLNESS
The patient is a 64-year-old lady referred by her primary care physician for evaluation of shortness of breath which has been off and on for the past 2 years. The patient has been intubated in the past secondary to a spell of acute shortness of breath in 1994. She has not required any other mechanical ambulatory support since then. The patient has been feeling worse in the last 2 weeks, having acute shortness of breath for which the patient was started on Advil by her primary care physician at the dose of 200/50 along with antibiotics for 5 days. The patient had severe chest tightness but did not go to the hospital. The patient is not on lone oxygen, denies chronic cough, and denies any significant cough at the present time. Denies any chest pain or hemoptysis, and denies any other symptoms except those mentioned above.

PAST MEDICAL HISTORY
Positive for hypertension for the past 2 years, hyperlipidemia for at least 5 years, and peptic ulcer disease since 1985.

PAST SURGICAL HISTORY
Negative.

FAMILY HISTORY
Positive for asthma in her mother. There is no history of PE.

SOCIAL HISTORY
Married. Denies any chronic alcohol intake. Former smoker who quit 10 years ago but had been smoking at least one pack per day for 30 years.

ALLERGIES
Not allergic to any medication.

(continued)

REVIEW OF SYSTEMS
See attached evaluation form for review of systems. There is no history of nausea or vomiting. Stable appetite, no significant weight loss.

RESPIRATORY: The patient has been wheezing off and on for the last 2 weeks, but better over the last few days. Has been complaining of shortness of breath. Denies any history of pulmonary embolism, no history of tuberculosis.

PHYSICAL EXAMINATION:
VITAL SIGNS: On physical examination, the patient is afebrile. Blood pressure is 110/70. Heart rate is regular at 88. Respiratory rate is nonlabored at 20. Height is at 5′3″. Weight is at 133 pounds.
CEPHALIC: Eyes: Normal conjunctivae. Pupils equally reactive to light and accommodation. Ears, Nose, and Throat: Normal aural examination, normal tympanic membranes, no sinus tenderness.
NECK: No jugular venous distention of the neck, no thyromegaly, no cervical adenopathy.
RESPIRATORY/CHEST: There is no significant chest deformity, except for mild cytosis of the spine. There is decreased air entry in both bases with prolonged expiratory phase, mild end expiratory wheezes in both bases without any grackles. There is no substernal detraction, no interchondral retraction.
CARDIOVASCULAR: The patient has a regular rate and rhythm, no S_3 or S_4 gallop. There is no murmur that I could appreciate.
ABDOMEN: Soft and nontender. Bowel sounds are present. There is no hepatomegaly and no splenomegaly.
NEUROLOGICAL: The patient is alert and oriented.
MUSCULOSKELETAL: The patient has a normal ambulatory status in the office with stable O_2 maturation with minimal exertion at 92% with baseline at 94% on room air. There is no scoliosis but mild kyphosis.
SKIN AND LYMPHATIC: There is no cervical adenopathy, no rash over the face and hands, no clubbing of the fingers, no cyanosis of the lips or fingers.

(continued)

DATA

Stereometry has been done in the office which showed severely increased FEV_1 at 0.95 liters or 42% of the predicted value, with decreased FEV_1/FVC at 53% and decreased FVC at 1.79 liters or 62% of the predicted value with a low volume loop suggestive of severe airflow obstruction at the level of the small airway with normal aspiratory flow.

The patient had a chest x-ray done which showed no specific infiltrates, hyperinflation consistent with asthma/COPD, with increased bilateral hila suggestive of pulmonary hypotension per report. Films are not available for review.

IMPRESSION

1. Resolving chronic obstructive pulmonary disease (COCD) exacerbation.
2. Status post infectious bronchitis with appropriate antibiotic treatment.
3. Dyspnea secondary to #1 and #2.
4. Pulmonary hypertension per chest x-ray report.

PLAN

Will get full pulmonary function tests with diffusion capacity to assess the severity of the patient's potential emphysema in the context of a 30-pack-year smoking history. Will get an echocardiogram for further evaluation of the patient's acute and chronic shortness of breath and get a chest CT scan with audiogram as the patient is at risk for pulmonary embolism. The patient has been advised to increase her Advair to 500/50, one puff p.o. b.i.d. I will give her some Spiriva for probable empyema. The patient is on Lotronex nebulization treatments and has been advised to continue taking them 3–4 times a day as needed.

ANSWER KEYS

REVIEW QUESTIONS ANSWER KEY

1. D
2. C
3. B
4. C
5. B
6. A
7. C
8. B
9. A
10. D
11. C
12. D
13. C
14. A
15. B
16. C
17. C
18. A
19. D
20. C
21. A
22. B
23. A
24. B
25. C
26. A
27. D
28. C
29. D
30. A

PROOFREADING EXERCISE #1 KEY

Incorrect spelling—Cardiolite

Incorrect spelling—scarring

Incorrect abbreviation—MVV

Incorrect term—flow loop

HISTORY

I had the pleasure of seeing this female patient on June 10, 2004, for an evaluation of dyspnea and exercise limitations. Her evaluation here was extensive and included an echocardiogram, a Cardiolyte study, a chest CT using pulmonary embolus protocols, an arterial blood gas, and cardiopulmonary exercise testing. Together, these studies show that she has essentially normal cardiopulmonary function. The only objective abnormality found on this testing was a mild reduction in diffusion capacity at 70% of predicted. Oxygenation, however, was maintained. An arterial blood gas showed excellent oxygenation with a $PA0_2$ on room air of 87. Chest CT did not demonstrate any significant parenchymal disease or any evidence of thromboembolic disease. There was minimal scaring in the left lung apex. Echocardiogram demonstrated good left and right ventricular function with normal size. There was mild diastolic dysfunction, grade 1, noted. There was no significant valvular disease. The left atrium was not enlarged. Estimated right ventricular systolic pressure was normal at 32 mmHg. Cardiopulmonary stress testing demonstrated no ventilatory limit to exercise. Heart rate response to exercise was inadequate.

She was evaluated by our group. We felt she had an allergy to dust mites. A note was made of an eosinophil count of 78. The absolute eosinophil count here was within the normal range at 0.09 x 1000 with 0.50 x 1000 as the upper limit of normal. Total white count was 7.9. Inspiratory flow up did not demonstrate any suggestion of proximal airway obstruction. A note was made of a decreased MEV relative to the FEV_1.

Incorrect term—methacholine

A methyl choline challenge study did not suggest any evidence of asthma. There was only a 5% decline in FEV_1 after methyl choline; however, a bronchial dilator was used earlier in the day.

Incorrect word—etiology

Incorrect term—bronchodilator

I do not find any overwhelming cardiopulmonary dysfunction as the ideology of her dyspnea. The inadequate heart rate response on beta-blocking medication may be contributing to her symptoms. In the absence of ongoing atrial fibrillation and lack of left atrial enlargement, discontinuation of a beta-blocking agent may be appropriate. Additionally, the evidence for asthma was unconvincing. Admittedly, the methacholine was done in the presence of bronchodilators given earlier in the day, but I do not suspect her symptoms are due to intermittent asthma with baseline good pulmonary function. Continuation of her medication therapy for house dust, mite allergy and associated allergic rhinoconjunctivitis with basal steroid and antihistamine is appropriate. I do not see a clear role for Xolair therapy in her management. She is implementing the appropriate dust mite measures at home.

Incorrect punctuation—no comma

Incorrect term—nasal

She was evaluated by a cardiologist because of a nondiagnostic exercise stress test, and showed good LB function by imaging studies. He did not feel that further evaluation of cardiac disease was appropriate. It was noted that her lipid profile was unfavorable, and therapy with a lipid lowering agent would be appropriate.

Incorrect abbreviation—LV

She was evaluated because of difficulty palpating peripheral pulses. He felt that she did not have evidence of significant large-vessel or vascular disease. Ankle-bronchial indices were acceptable. He recommended screening ultrasound because of a family history of an aortic aneurysm. This was performed and was unremarkable.

Incorrect term—brachial

Incorrect term—brain

Together we explored whether or not her deep-vain stimulators could be affecting her sensation of dyspnea. I have discussed this with neurosurgery. He felt that the thalamic location of these stimulators would preclude that as a contributor to her symptoms.

PROOFREADING EXERCISE #2 KEY

CHIEF COMPLAINT
Respiratory insufficiency.

HISTORY OF PRESENT ILLNESS
In summary, this is a 74-year-old male who has ALS as well as a possible tumor of the spinal canal that has not been proven by tissue biopsy. He has had a previous history of destructive sleep apnea treated with CTAP prior to his diagnosis of ALS and subsequently has been managed on BiPAP 12 and 5 for respiratory insufficiency with ALS. Overall, he has tolerated that well. At rest during the day, he does not have any significant respiratory insufficiency signs. At night, he sleeps well; however, last night he had an episode where he woke up while wearing BiPAP and felt he was not getting adequate breathes. He took the mask off and still felt as if he were "breathing in a vacuum." Rescue was called and with the initiation of supple mental oxygen and evaluation in the ER, he ultimately felt okay again. Laboratory studies at that time were remarkable for an elevated CO_2 at 33 and an INR of 1.8. I should note that he is on Coumadin for a previous DVC but it is subtherapeutic.

PHYSICAL EXAMINATION
Examination is limited by the patient's lack of mobility. He is in a wheelchair. He is not in any respiratory dress. His lung exam is significant for basal air crackles and diminished breath sounds throughout.

DIAGNOSTIC STUDIES
I reviewed a new chest x-ray from later in the day which shows small lung volumes. No further laboratory testing. PSTs are not yet scanned into the computer but show no evidence of obstruction.They do, however, show restriction and diminished respiratory pressures and normal DL_{CO} when corrected for alveolar volume.

Incorrect term—obstructive

Incorrect abbreviation—CPAP

Single word—supplemental

Incorrect spelling—breaths

Incorrect abbreviation—DVT

Incorrect term—basilar

Incorrect word—distress

Incorrect abbreviation—PFTs

Incorrect punctuation—set off with commas

Spell out abbreviations in the Assessment—deep vein thrombosis

Incorrect term—hypoxemia

Incorrect term—etiology

Incorrect term—spiral

ASSESSMENT

1. Amyotrophic lateral sclerosis (ALS).
2. Respiratory insufficiency chronic secondary to #1.
3. Central abdominal obesity on exam.
4. Episode of respiratory insufficiency, acute, for reasons that are not entirely clear.
5. Previous DVT on Coumadin with a subtherapeutic INR.

PLAN

1. Overnight oximetry to assess oxygenation on BiPAP at the current settings. If this shows periods of anemia, I would evaluate in the sleep lab overnight with a titration study on BiPAP and the addition of supplemental oxygen as needed.
2. I am unclear as to the ideology of his acute respiratory insufficiency. Thromboembolic disease is a possibility, although his rapid improvement makes me less suspicious of that; however, I would check viral CT scan of the chest and an arterial blood gas.
3. Followup in the pulmonary clinic as needed.

PROOFREADING EXERCISE #3 KEY

Incorrect term—ventilatory

Incorrect drug—Advair

Incorrect word—home

HISTORY OF PRESENT ILLNESS
The patient is a 64-year-old lady referred by her primary care physician for evaluation of shortness of breath which has been off and on for the past 2 years. The patient has been intubated in the past secondary to a spell of acute shortness of breath in 1994. She has not required any other mechanical ambulatory support since then. The patient has been feeling worse in the last 2 weeks, having acute shortness of breath for which the patient was started on Advil by her primary care physician at the dose of 200/50 along with antibiotics for 5 days. The patient had severe chest tightness but did not go to the hospital. The patient is not on lone oxygen, denies chronic cough, and denies any significant cough at the present time. Denies any chest pain or hemoptysis, and denies any other symptoms except those mentioned above.

PAST MEDICAL HISTORY
Positive for hypertension for the past 2 years, hyperlipidemia for at least 5 years, and peptic ulcer disease since 1985.

PAST SURGICAL HISTORY
Negative.

FAMILY HISTORY
Positive for asthma in her mother. There is no history of PE.

SOCIAL HISTORY
Married. Denies any chronic alcohol intake. Former smoker who quit 10 years ago but had been smoking at least one pack per day for 30 years.

ALLERGIES
Not allergic to any medication.

REVIEW OF SYSTEMS
See attached evaluation form for review of systems. There is no history of nausea or vomiting. Stable appetite, no significant weight loss.

RESPIRATORY
The patient has been wheezing off and on for the last 2 weeks, but better over the last few days. Has been complaining of shortness of breath. Denies any history of pulmonary embolism, no history of tuberculosis.

PHYSICAL EXAMINATION:
VITAL SIGNS: On physical examination, the patient is afebrile. Blood pressure is 110/70. Heart rate is regular at 88. Respiratory rate is nonlabored at 20. Height is at 5′3″. Weight is at 133 pounds.
CEPHALIC: Eyes: Normal conjunctivae. Pupils equally reactive to light and accommodation. Ears, Nose, and Throat: Normal aural examination, normal tympanic membranes, no sinus tenderness.
NECK: No jugular venous distention of the neck, no thyromegaly, no cervical adenopathy.
RESPIRATORY/CHEST: There is no significant chest deformity, except for mild cytosis of the spine. There is decreased air entry in both bases with prolonged expiratory phase, mild end expiratory wheezes in both bases without any grackles. There is no substernal detraction, no interchondral retraction.
CARDIOVASCULAR: The patient has a regular rate and rhythm, no S_3 or S_4 gallop. There is no murmur that I could appreciate.
ABDOMEN: Soft and nontender. Bowel sounds are present. There is no hepatomegaly and no splenomegaly.
NEUROLOGICAL: The patient is alert and oriented.
MUSCULOSKELETAL: The patient has a normal ambulatory status in the office with stable O_2 maturation with minimal exertion at 92% with baseline at 94% on room air. There is no scoliosis but mild kyphosis.

Incorrect term—kyphosis

Incorrect term—retraction

Incorrect term—crackles

Incorrect term—intercostal

Incorrect term—saturation

Incorrect term—spirometry

Incorrect suffix—decreased

SKIN AND LYMPHATIC: There is no cervical adenopathy, no rash over the face and hands, no clubbing of the fingers, no cyanosis of the lips or fingers.
DATA: Stereometry has been done in the office which showed severely increased FEV_1 at 0.95 liters or 42% of the predicted value, with decreased FEV_1/FVC at 53% and decreased FVC at 1.79 liters or 62% of the predicted value with a low volume loop suggestive of severe airflow obstruction at the level of the small airway with normal aspiratory flow.

Incorrect term—inspiratory

Incorrect word—flow

The patient had a chest x-ray done which showed no specific infiltrates, hyperinflation consistent with asthma/COPD, with increased bilateral hila suggestive of pulmonary hypotension per report. Films are not available for review.

Incorrect suffix—hypertension

Incorrect abbreviation—COPD

IMPRESSION

1. Resolving chronic obstructive pulmonary disease (COCD) exacerbation.
2. Status post infectious bronchitis with appropriate antibiotic treatment.
3. Dyspnea secondary to #1 and #2.
4. Pulmonary hypertension per chest x-ray report.

PLAN

Will get full pulmonary function tests with diffusion capacity to assess the severity of the patient's potential emphysema in the context of a 30-pack-year smoking history. Will get an echocardiogram for further evaluation of the patient's acute and chronic shortness of breath and get a chest CT scan with audiogram as the patient is at risk for pulmonary embolism. The patient has been advised to increase her Advair to 500/50, one puff p.o. b.i.d. I will give her some Spiriva for probable empyema. The patient is on Lotronex nebulization treatments and has been advised to continue taking them 3–4 times a day as needed.

Incorrect term—angiogram

Incorrect term—emphysema

Incorrect drug—Xopenex

CHAPTER 23

Urology

OBJECTIVES CHECKLIST

A prepared exam candidate will know:

- ❑ Combining forms, prefixes, and suffixes related to the urological system.
- ❑ Anatomical structures of the urinary system.
- ❑ Anatomical structures of the male reproductive system.
- ❑ Physiology of waste removal and urine production.
- ❑ Physiology of sperm production and the sequence of structures through which sperm passes, from the seminiferous tubules to exiting the body.
- ❑ Sequence of structures through which urine is produced and eliminated from the body, from glomerular filtration to micturition.
- ❑ Role of the kidneys as endocrine organs and the purpose and function of the substances secreted.
- ❑ Signs, symptoms, and diseases related to the urinary system.
- ❑ Signs, symptoms, and diseases related to the male reproductive system, including sexually transmitted diseases.
- ❑ Imaging studies used in the identification and diagnosis of urinary and male reproductive diseases and disorders.
- ❑ Laboratory studies used in the diagnosis and treatment of urinary disorders and male reproductive symptoms, disorders, and diseases.
- ❑ Common medications prescribed for urinary and male reproductive symptoms, disorders, and diseases.
- ❑ Transcription standards related to urology.

RESOURCES FOR STUDY

1. *The Language of Medicine*
   Chapter 7: Urinary System, pp. 213–252.
   Chapter 9: Male Reproductive System, pp. 305–332.
2. *H&P: A Nonphysician's Guide to the Medical History and Physical Examination*
   Chapter 11: Review of Systems: Genitourinary, pp. 97–106.
   Chapter 25: Examination of the Abdomen, Groins, Rectum, Anus, and Genitalia, pp. 235–248.
3. *Human Diseases*
   Chapter 12: The Excretory System, the Male Reproductive System, and Sexually Transmitted Diseases, pp. 173–188.
4. *Laboratory Tests & Diagnostic Procedures in Medicine*
   Chapter 8: Endoscopy: Examination of the Digestive Tract and Genitourinary System, pp. 107–118.
   Chapter 20: Blood Chemistry (Osmolality, Electrolytes and Acid-Base Balance, Minerals, and Waste Products), pp. 371–400.
   Chapter 24: Examination of Urine, Stool, and Other Fluids and Materials, pp. 437–454.
5. *Understanding Pharmacology for Health Professionals*
   Chapter 12: Urinary Tract Drugs, pp. 102–714.
   (Review anti-infectives for the treatment of STDs).
6. *The AAMT Book of Style for Medical Transcription*
   Gleason tumor grade, p. 53.
   Jewett classification of bladder carcinoma, p. 54.
   Specific gravity, p. 233.
   Urinalysis, p. 407.

SAMPLE REPORTS

The following five reports are examples of reports you might encounter while transcribing urology.

OPERATIVE REPORT

PREOPERATIVE DIAGNOSES
1. Urethral stricture.
2. Hypospadias.
3. Urethrocutaneous fistula.

POSTOPERATIVE DIAGNOSES
1. Urethral stricture.
2. Hypospadias.
3. Urethrocutaneous fistula.

PROCEDURE
1. Retrograde urethrogram.
2. Cystoscopy.
3. Placement of suprapubic catheter.
4. Placement of scrotal drains.

ANESTHETIC
General.

HISTORY
The patient is a 59-year-old gentleman with a history of a previous urethroplasty of the pendulous urethra who was seen in the office with urinary retention, urinary tract infection, and dysuria with a slow urinary stream. Attempts at dilation in the office were frustrated by patient discomfort and a very tight, pendulous urethra. The patient is scheduled now for cystoscopy, urethral dilation, and urethrogram.

The patient was aware of the potential for bleeding, infection, pain, and numbness, as well as bladder, bowel, or other organ injury.

PROCEDURE IN DETAIL
General anesthesia was given by the anesthesia staff. The patient was placed in a left lateral oblique position by rotating the table. A 14-French Foley catheter was placed in the fossa navicularis, actually more proximally due to a coronal hypospadias. There was also evidence of a urethrocutaneous fistula at the penoscrotal junction. Contrast material was injected in a retrograde fashion under fluoroscopy. There appeared to be some extravasation of the contrast at the distal urethra; otherwise, this was a fairly normal-appearing urethra.

The catheter was removed and the patient was placed in the dorsal lithotomy position. A 17-French panendoscope was introduced into the urethra with difficulty due to poor visualization of the actual urethra. There was a false passage, which appeared at about the level of the penoscrotal junction, but I was able to feed a filiform stylet into the appropriate channel. This was followed alongside by the 17-French panendoscope.

(continued)

The prostatic urethra appeared to have a markedly elongated median lobe. The bladder neck was slightly elevated, and the interior of the bladder revealed median lobe intrusion into the lumen. The trigone was difficult to see due to floating debris and bladder wall trabeculation. There did not appear to be any neoplasia. There appeared to be some acellular debris floating in the bladder. The scope was removed along with the filiform stylet.

My feeling was that the 17-French scope did pass, and I felt it would be fairly reasonable to expect a 16-French coude tip Foley catheter to follow the same tract; however, this was not the case. The tissue in the penoscrotal junction was quite friable and allowed for passage of the coude tip Foley in different directions except for the proper channel. Attempts at trying to relocate the proper channel by the cystoscope and passage of the filiform stylet again were unsuccessful, with a progressively enlarging scrotum from accumulation of irrigant solution.

At this point, I elected to discontinue irrigating and looking for the urethra with the cystoscope, as tissue plane dissection was continuing. I did locate the bladder suprapubically with a spinal needle and instilled it through a 30-mL syringe until it presented a large enough target so that I could safely place a Rush-type suprapubic catheter blindly into this distended bladder. This was accomplished and the balloon was inflated to 10 mL. There was prompt return of the irrigant solution. The catheter was placed for gravity drainage.

Following this, I did make stab wounds in the scrotum to allow for placement of Penrose drains for dependent drainage of the accumulated irrigation solution. This has been dressed with 4 x 4s, ABDs and the mesh shorts.

At this point, the procedure was ended, anesthesia was ended, and the patient was returned to the recovery room in satisfactory condition.

It should be noted that previous urine cultures were growing gram-positive organisms. The patient received 2 g of Ancef IV piggyback during the course of the procedure.

OPERATIVE REPORT

PREOPERATIVE DIAGNOSIS
Right kidney stone.

POSTOPERATIVE DIAGNOSIS
Right kidney stone.

OPERATION
1. Right stent placement.
2. Right extracorporeal shock-wave lithotripsy.

ANESTHESIA
General.

COMPLICATIONS
None.

DRAINS
6-French, 26-cm stent.

INDICATIONS FOR THE PROCEDURE
The patient is a 35-year-old male who presented with a right kidney stone, and after discussing all options, risks, and complications, including hemorrhage, sepsis, perforation, need for nephrostomy tube, hypertension, etc., he decided to undergo ESWL with stent placement.

FINDINGS
On cystoscopy, the urethra appeared normal. The prostate appeared bilobar. The ureteral orifice was quickly localized and the stent glided all the way up the ureter without difficulty. Following this, the patient was taken to the ESWL suite.

PROCEDURE IN DETAIL
The patient was taken to the operating suite, and under satisfactory general anesthesia, he was prepped and draped in the usual sterile fashion using Betadine soap.

The 21-French cystoscope was introduced into the bladder. The right ureteral orifice was quickly localized, and a glide wire was threaded all the way up under fluoroscopic control. This was followed by insertion of a 6-French, 26-cm stent that curled up nicely in the renal pelvis and in the bladder after removing the glide wire.

The bladder was then emptied, and the patient was taken to the lithotripsy suite, where the treatment was carried out with 2400 shock waves to the right kidney. Fragmentation appeared to be excellent. The patient tolerated the procedure well and was transferred to the recovery room in good condition.

OPERATIVE REPORT

PREOPERATIVE DIAGNOSIS
Right renal mass.

POSTOPERATIVE DIAGNOSIS
Right renal mass.

PROCEDURE
Right radical nephrectomy.

ANESTHESIA
General endotracheal anesthesia.

DESCRIPTION OF THE PROCEDURE
After being properly identified and consented, the patient was taken to the operating room and placed under general endotracheal anesthesia. Under sterile conditions, a 16-French Foley catheter was placed.

The patient was positioned in the right flank position with the table flexed, and the right flank was prepped and draped. A skin incision overlying the 12th rib was made. The incision was taken down through the subcutaneous fat, and the muscles overlying the flank were incised. The incision was taken down onto the rib. The intercostal muscles were separated from the upper portion of the 12th rib using Bovie electrocautery, and the tip of the rib was dissected away from its attachments.

Once all the muscles of the flank were divided and the tip of the rib was mobilized, we entered the Gerota space right where it meets the tip of the 12th rib. We then used the periosteal elevator to remove the diaphragmatic pleural attachments to the posterior aspect of the 12th rib. Using Bovie electrocautery to remove the intercostal muscles from the superior portion of the 12th rib, and using the periosteal elevator as described, the rib was completely mobilized away from the muscles, pleura and diaphragm, all the way to the posterior aspect of this rib, and the intercostal ligament was identified and incised with Metzenbaum scissors.

At this point, the pleura was identified as well as the peritoneum. The peritoneum was swept away medially from the Gerota fascia, and the diaphragmatic and pleural attachments to the Gerota fascia were dissected away as well. The Burford retractor was placed in between the 11th and 12th ribs and the Gerota space exposed appropriately.

Once proper exposure of the right kidney and Gerota fascia was accomplished, we incised the Gerota fat and entered into the perinephric fat. The perinephric fat was then dissected away from the kidney using Bovie electrocautery, and the kidney was mobilized posteriorly, superiorly, and inferiorly, away from the fat, using right-angle dissection and Bovie electrocautery. We then mobilized the anterior aspect of the kidney.

The ureter was identified inferior to the kidney and it was isolated, with a vessel loop placed around it. Once the kidney was completely mobilized up to the hilum, we identified the right renal artery, and from a posterior dissection, we were able to completely dissect it out and place a vessel loop around it. From an anterior approach, we then dissected out the right renal vein, and we were able to put a vessel loop around that as well.

(continued)

At this point, 12.5 g of mannitol was given IV. The right renal artery and renal vein were clamped using Fogarty clamps, a bowel bag was placed around the kidney, and slush ice was placed around the kidney. The kidney was cooled for 10 minutes, and then we approached the renal mass.

Bovie electrocautery was used to circumscribe the renal mass, and then the Bovie cautery was used to continue the dissection around the renal mass deep into the renal substance. We cut into several segmental veins as well as the collecting system and realized that this tumor was just too deep to resect with a partial nephrectomy, and we decided that we would perform a radical nephrectomy as a curative cancer procedure.

The bowel bag was removed and the ice was removed. A right-angle clamp was placed on the right renal artery, and #0 silk ties were placed, two on the patient's side and one on the specimen side, and the artery was divided. We then placed #0 silk sutures around the right renal vein, two ties on the patient's side and one on the specimen side, and the renal vein was divided. Then #0 chromic sutures were placed around the ureter, and the ureter was divided.

At this point, a right-angle clamp was placed around any remaining tissue attaching the kidney to the retroperitoneum. The tissue was divided and the specimen removed. Following this, #0 silk sutures were placed underneath the right-angle clamp.

There was barely any bleeding and hemostasis was perfect. Estimated blood loss at this point was about 50 mL. We then closed the flank muscles in 2 layers, using interrupted #0 Vicryl sutures. The skin was then reapproximated using skin staples. The wound was cleaned. Sterile drapes were removed and the patient was extubated and taken to the recovery room in good condition.

OFFICE NOTE

PROBLEM LIST
Recurrent urinary tract infections.
Vesical dyskinesia.
Urethral syndrome.
History of urethral stricture.
Recent proteus infection.

HISTORY OF PRESENT ILLNESS
The patient returns today for further workup and evaluation because of her recurrent infections. Infections have been resistant to a large number of antibiotics. Because of her history of proteus infection, I believe it will be prudent for us to obtain x-rays of her kidneys to make sure she does not have a stone or some other anatomical abnormality.

PHYSICAL EXAMINATION
GENERAL: Well-nourished, white female, not acutely ill.
ABDOMEN: Soft, nontender, no masses. No CVA tenderness. The liver and spleen are not palpable. No hernia.
PELVIC: External genitalia: Normal general appearance without evidence of discharge or lesions, normal hair distribution. Vagina: Normal. Urethra: Without evidence of masses, tenderness, or scarring. There was no hypermobility noted. Cervix: Normal appearance and no lesions, cervical motion, tenderness, or discharge. Bladder: Tender to palpation. No fullness or palpable mass. Anus and perineum: Normal in appearance.

DATA REVIEWED
Urinalysis: pH 6.5, specific gravity 1.005. Microscopically and chemically negative on a catheterized specimen.

ASSESSMENT
1. Recurrent urinary tract infections.
2. Vesical dyskinesia.
3. Urethral syndrome.
4. History of urethral stricture.
5. Recent proteus infection.

PLAN
1. Send her for an IVP.
2. Put her on tetracycline as a suppressive.
3. Return in 3 weeks for repeat exam and to go over the results of her IVP.

OFFICE NOTE

PROBLEM LIST
Benign prostatic hypertrophy.
Bladder neck obstruction.
Hypertension.
Hypothyroidism.
Elevated PSA.
Probable prostatitis.

CHIEF COMPLAINT
Benign prostatic hypertrophy and prostatitis.

HISTORY OF PRESENT ILLNESS
The patient returns today with signs and symptoms consistent with prostatitis. He also has been found to have an elevated PSA in the past, which has been thought to perhaps be due to infection. He now comes for further workup and evaluation.

PHYSICAL EXAMINATION
GENERAL: Well-nourished, white male, not acutely ill.
PSYCHIATRIC: The patient is oriented in time, place and person x 3.
ABDOMEN: Soft, nontender, no masses. No CVA tenderness. The liver and spleen are not palpable. No hernia.
RECTAL/GENITAL: Scrotum: Without lesions, cysts, or rashes. Testes: Equal in size and symmetry and descended bilaterally, without tenderness, masses, spermatoceles, or hydroceles. Epididymides: Examination of the epididymides revealed equal size and symmetry with no masses or tenderness. Urethra: Normal urethral location and size with no lesions or discharge. Penis: Normal circumcised penis without plaques, lesions, or masses. Prostate: Symmetrical, 1+ hypertrophy with no evidence of nodularity or induration. Tender to palpation. Seminal vesicles: Symmetrical and nonpalpable with no evidence of masses. Rectal/anus: Anus and perineum are normal in appearance; normal rectal tone; no hemorrhoids or masses.

DATA REVIEWED
Catheterized urine specimen: pH 6.0, specific gravity 1.005. Microscopically shows 4-5 RBC/hpf and 4-5 WBC/hpf, but no bacteria. PSA 4.2.

ASSESSMENT
1. Benign prostatic hypertrophy.
2. Bladder neck obstruction.
3. Hypertension.
4. Hypothyroidism.
5. Elevated PSA.
6. Probable prostatitis.

PLAN
1. Give the patient Cipro 400 mg b.i.d. #56.
2. Refill Flomax.
3. Return in 6 weeks for repeat exam and be prepared to repeat his PSA at that time.

REVIEW QUESTIONS

The goal of these questions is to test your knowledge in the area of urology.

Directions: Select the correct answer for each of the multiple-choice questions provided below. *Answers are provided at the end of this chapter.*

1. TURP means:
   - A. Transurethral resection of the prostate
   - B. Transurethral reconstruction of the penis
   - C. Slang for turpentine enema
   - D. Transvaginal ultrasound and radiographs of the pelvis

2. The bilateral tubes leading from the kidneys to the bladder are the:
   - A. Urethra
   - B. Ureters
   - C. Calyces
   - D. Renal vesicles

3. The root word meaning renal pelvis is:
   - A. Pyel/o
   - B. Nephr/o
   - C. Ren/o
   - D. Cyst/o

4. The tube dissected in a vasectomy is the:
   - A. Epididymis
   - B. Seminiferous tubule
   - C. Vas deferens
   - D. Seminal vesicle

5. One medical condition justifying circumcision is:
   - A. Frenulectomy
   - B. Balanitis
   - C. Phimosis
   - D. Chordee

6. A cystoscope is used to look inside the:
   - A. Bladder
   - B. Fallopian tubes
   - C. Uterus
   - D. Prostate

7. Inflammation of the urethra is called:
   - A. Urethrectomy
   - B. Urethritis
   - C. Urethrotomy
   - D. Cystitis

8. Involuntarily urinating, such as a child wetting the bed sheets, is termed:
   - A. Enuresis
   - B. Somnambulism
   - C. Eupnea
   - D. Nocturia

9. Having to urinate at night is termed:
   - A. Enuresis
   - B. Nocturia
   - C. Nocturnal periodicity
   - D. Anuresis

10. Priapism may be a sign of:
    - A. Spinal cord injury
    - B. Balanitis
    - C. Plaque formation
    - D. Epididymitis

11. Fibrosis and chronic inflammation associated with an inability to retract the foreskin:
    - A. Phimosis
    - B. Balanitis
    - C. Hypospadia
    - D. Priapism

12. Regarding a KUB, which is true?
    - A. Gastrografin is preferred over barium as contrast
    - B. This test is used to evaluate the kidneys, ureter, and bladder
    - C. No contrast is used; this is a plain film
    - D. Both B and C

13. Emptying the bladder is termed:
   A. Expectoration
   B. Defecation
   C. Micturition
   D. Parturition

14. The tube leading from the bladder to the outside is called the:
   A. Urethra
   B. Ureter
   C. Trigone
   D. Epididymis

15. The surgical removal of the prepuce is called:
   A. Vasectomy
   B. Frenulectomy
   C. Circumcision
   D. Prostatectomy

16. Which of the following is a thiazide diuretic?
   A. HCTZ
   B. Bumex
   C. Spironolactone
   D. K-Dur

17. As part of the abdominal examination, the urologist dictates, "No CVA tenderness." In this case, CVA stands for:
   A. Cerebrovascular accident
   B. Cardiovascular accident
   C. Costovertebral angle
   D. Calculus verified on angiogram

18. A woman undergoing surgery for stress urinary incontinence might be having a procedure to adjust the:
   A. Ureterovesical angle
   B. Uterovesical angle
   C. Urethrovesical angle
   D. Urinary meatus

19. During cystoscopy on an elderly gentleman, the physician is having trouble visualizing parts of the target organ due to:
   A. Trilobar prostatic hypertrophy
   B. Obstruction by the verumontanum
   C. Inflammation of the parenchymal tissue
   D. Trifurcation of the cystic ducts

20. A condition related to chronic urinary bladder inflammation:
   A. Fasciculation
   B. Trabeculation
   C. Reticulation
   D. Collimation

21. Used to temporarily maintain patency of the ureter:
   A. Endopyelotomy stent
   B. W-J stent
   C. J-P stent
   D. Double-J stent

22. Swelling of the ureter due to bladder outlet obstruction:
   A. Ureteropathy
   B. Uritis
   C. Hydroureter
   D. Urethritis

23. A urine specific gravity result is dictated "ten-fifteen." Which of the following is the correct way to transcribe this value?
   A. 10-15
   B. 1-015
   C. 10.15
   D. 1.015

24. A patient with bladder cancer might undergo ureteroileostomy, otherwise known as a/an:
   A. LeVeen shunt
   B. Intraperitoneal shunt
   C. Ileal conduit
   D. Colovesical fistula

25. The acid-base balance of a fluid including urine is called:
   A. Electrolyte concentration
   B. Specific gravity
   C. pH
   D. PKU

26. Which of these are potassium supplements typically prescribed for patients taking loop diuretics?
   A. Kay Ciel
   B. K-Dur
   C. Slow-K
   D. All of the above

27. The medical term for undescended testicles is:
   A. Hypospadias
   B. Varicocele
   C. Cryptorchidism
   D. Testicular torsion

28. DMSO, Rimso-50, Elmiron, and Pyridium are examples of
   A. Urinary analgesics
   B. Urinary antispasmodics
   C. Urinary antibacterials
   D. Urinary antidiuretics

29. Which of the following would not be prescribed for BPH?
   A. Saw Palmetto
   B. Proscar
   C. Hytrin
   D. Caverject

30. Chronic renal failure causes:
   A. Hematuria
   B. Uremia
   C. Acute tubular necrosis
   D. Pyuria

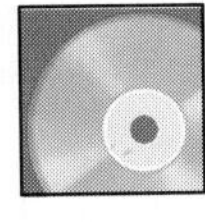

Please see the accompanying CD for additional review materials for this section.

PROOFREADING EXERCISES

These five proofreading exercises are provided to improve your skills in the areas of editing and effective identification and correction of errors in the medical record.

Directions: Identify and correct the transcription errors found in the exercises below. *Answers are provided at the end of this chapter.*

PROOFREADING EXERCISE #1

PREOPERATIVE DIAGNOSIS
Recurrent bladder tumor.

POSTOPERATIVE DIAGNOSIS
Recurrent bladder tumor.

OPERATION
Trans urethral resection of bladder tumor.

ANESTHESIA
General with mask.

INDICATIONS FOR THE PROCEDURE
The patient is an 83-year-old patient with a history of bladder cancer. He developed a recurrence, and was scheduled for surgery.

The risks and complications of the procedure were thoroughly discussed with the patient, and the patient understood and wished to proceed.

PROCEDURE IN DETAIL
The patient was taken to the operating room and under satisfactory general anesthesia, he was prepped and draped in the usual sterile fashion using Betadine. He was then placed in the supine position.

Cystoscopy was performed with the number 21-french cystic scope with the 12-degree and 70-degree angled lenses, with the findings as above noted. The urethra was dilated with van Buren signs.

(continued)

Then the rectoscope was introduced with a sheath first, and then the obturator was removed and the working element was placed.

Resection of the tumors was performed with great care not to biforate the bladder. All tumors were removed and sent for pathology. The surrounding area was carefully fulgurated. The bladder was then inspected for any remaining rumors and there were none. The bladder was then emptied, and an 18-French Foley catheter was placed; the balloon was inflated with 10 mL and the return was clear.

An examination under anesthesia was performed, which revealed a smooth, benign prostrate of approximately 30-35 grams with no palpable masses and no indurations. The bladder appeared to be fairly motile.

The patient tolerated the procedure well, and was transferred to the recovery room in good condition.

COMPLICATIONS
None.

DRAINS
An 18-French 3-way Foley connected to continuous bladder irrigation.

PROOFREADING EXERCISE #2

PREOPERATIVE DIAGNOSIS
Voluntary serialization.

POSTOPERATIVE DIAGNOSIS
Voluntary serialization.

OPERATION
Bilateral vasectomy.

ANESTHESIA
IV sedation with local installation of lidocaine, Marcaine, and bicarbonate to the spermatic chords.

FLUIDS
Crystalloids.

ESTIMATED BLOOD LOSS
Negligible.

JUSTIFICATION FOR THE PROCEDURE
This is a 45-year-old white male requesting vasectomy. He presents at this time for a vasectomy, fully understanding the risks and benefits of this type of procedure, including decannulation of the vas as well as bleeding and otalgia.

PROCEDURE IN DETAIL
After being properly identified, the patient was taken to the operating room, at which time anesthesia was administered via IV sedation and local installation of lidocaine and Marcaine to the semantic cords.

(continued)

Bilateral vasectomies were performed in the following fashion:

Using the no-scalpel vasectomy kit, each bas differens was localized using the ring clamp. The skin overlying each vas deferens was spread, and a 1-cm section of each vas differens was resected and the proximal and distal ends of each vas was cauterized using a needle-point Bovie, as well as suture ligated using 3-0 Vicryl sutures. The skin was closed bilaterally using 4-0 chromic suture in an interrupted fashion.

A notal support was applied. The patient tolerated the procedure well and was sent to the recovery room in stable condition.

PROOFREADING EXERCISE #3

CHIEF COMPLAINT
Urethral structure.

HISTORY OF PRESENT ILLNESS
This is a 40-year-old inmate who reports having been diagnosed with necrotic syndrome in June of this year prior to his incarceration. His initial creatine and bun were 2.0 and 49 respectively. The patient reports having been in a motor vehicle accident after which he was treated with analgesics and anti-inflammatories, and he feels this possibly may have caused the onset of the necrotic syndrome. He has no flank pain but does have significant 3+ distal extremity splitting edema and soreness of the souls of his feet. He also reports having had rapid weight gain from 220 pounds up to 190 pounds. All of this resolved, however, with diuretics, diet restrictions, and fluid restrictions.

PAST MEDICAL HISTORY
He reports being borderline diabetic, and he has had a history of hypertension over the past 2 years.

SOCIAL HISTORY
The patient smokes a half pack of cigarettes per day and has done so for the past 30 years. Prior to being incarcerated, he worked as a bricklayer.

FAMILY HISTORY
Positive for diabetes mellitus in his father.

MEDICATIONS
Lipitor, Calan, and Lasik.

ALLERGIES
Motrin.

PHYSICAL EXAMINATION
VITAL SIGNS: His most recent blood pressure was 154/84. The patient is awake, alert, oriented to time, place, and person.
HEENT: Grossly within normal limits.

(continued)

LUNGS: Soft inspiratory wheeze and soft rhonchi in both lungs which cleared with cough.
HEART: Regular rate and rhythm.
ABDOMEN: Soft. Bowel sounds are active, and there is no suprapubic distention or pain and no cerebrovascular accident tenderness.
GENITOURINARY: Shows an uncircumcised penis with an adequate mitis, dissented testicles, and a moderate-sized right hydro seal as well as a smaller-sized left hydro seal. Anal sphincter tone is within normal limits. The prostate is not enlarged, tender, or nodular and is of normal consistency.
EXTREMITIES: Show 3+ to 4+ pitting edema. This does not extend into the upper thigh or genital area.

IMPRESSION
History and findings consistent with nephrotic syndrome.

PLAN
1. Renal biopsy.
2. Prostrate pacific antigen.
3. Renal ultrasound.
4. A 24-hour urine collection for protean and creatinine appearance.

PROOFREADING EXERCISE #4

PREOPERATIVE DIAGNOSIS
BPH, bladder stones, urinary retention

POSTOPERATIVE DIAGNOSIS
Same.

OPERATION
Cystoscopy, urethral dilation, TERP, and electrohydraulic lithotripsy of bladder stone.

OPERATIVE PROCEDURE
The patient was brought to the operating room and placed in the subline position. He was then rolled to the left lateral decubital position. Spinal anesthesia was accomplished. After anesthesia was accomplished, the patient was placed in the dorsal lobotomy position. The genitals and peroneal area were prepped and draped in the usual sterile manner.

At this point, a #21 pan endoscopic sheath with a 12-degree lens on a short bridge was inserted into the meatus. The scope was advanced to the area of the prostatic fascia where there was noted to be trilobar obstruction of the prostatic fossa. The scope was then maneuvered past the loaves of the prostate into the bladder where the ureteral orifices were noted to be normal in size, shape, and position. The bladder was then inspected under gravity flow of normal saline with the 12-degree lens. There was no evidence of latter tumors, stones, or foreign objects. There was 1+ tribulation of the bladder wall.

A 70-degree lens was then inserted into the panendoscopic sheath. Again inspection of the bladder revealed no evidence of bladder tumors, stones, or forum objects.

(continued)

At this point, the panendoscopic sheath was removed. The meatus was dilated to a #28-French with the mail sounds. A #26-Iglesias resectoscopic unit with the Timberlake obturator was placed per ureter into the bladder. The obturator was removed and the Iglesias resectoscopic unit was placed inside the sheath. The prostate was resected down to its course circular fibers of the prostatic fossa. Bleeding points were point identified and coagulated. The scope was then pulled distally, and the apical tissue in a similar manner. The chips were evacuated with the Toomey syringe. Bleeding points were point identified and coagulated.

After evacuation of the chips, the 9-French EAL probe was inserted through the working element of the cysto urethroscope. The bladder stones were fragmented. They were evacuated through the syringe.

There were no gross bleeding or chips remaining in the bladder, and the panendoscopic unit was removed. The #24-French 3-way Foley catheter was inserted into the bladder. The balloon was instilled with 30 mL of sterile saline. The bladder was then irrigated with sterile saline until the affluent was clear. The patient was then transferred to the PAR in stable condition.

PROOFREADING EXERCISE #5

CHIEF COMPLAINT
Penile rash.

HISTORY OF PRESENT ILLNESS
This is a 44-year-old white male who has noticed a rash on the left side of his penis, which becomes reddened and irritated sometimes after inner course. There does not appear to be any lesion, and the patient has had no blistering, redness, or other signs of Hers disease or other venerable diseases.

MEDICAL HISTORY
No important medical or surgical illnesses.

CURRENT MEDICATIONS
None.

ALLERGIES
None.

REVIEW OF SYSTEMS
CONSTITUTIONAL: No weight loss, fever, chills, nausea, or vomiting.
EYES: No blurred vision or diplopia. ENT, MOUTH: No rhinitis or dysphagia.
CARDIOVASCULAR: No chest pain. RESPIRATORY: No shortness of breath.
GASTROINTESTINAL: No diarrhea or abdominal pain.
MUSCULOSKELETAL: No history of hernia. No muscular weakness, numbness, or joint pain. NEUROLOGIC: No headaches, blurred vision, or syncope.

PHYSICAL EXAMINATION
GENERAL: Well-nourished, white male, not acutely ill.
HEENT: Pupils equal and reactive to light. Cranial nerves II-XII grossly intact. Sclerae without icterus. Tongue is moist.

(continued)

NECK: Supple, no masses, no bruits.
CHEST: Clear to auscultation and percussion. No crackles or wheezes.
HEART: Regular rhythm, no murmur.
LYMPHATICS: Cervical and auxiliary nodes are normal.
ABDOMEN: Soft, nontender, no masses. No CVA tenderness. The liver and spleen are not palpable. No hernias.
GENITALIA: Reveals some roughness, scaling, and slight reddening of the skin on the left side below the glands penis. This has the appearance of yeast infection.
RECTAL: Reveals 1+, smooth, malign prostate.

DATA REVIEWED
Urine analysis: pH 60, specific gravity 10/20. Microscopically and chemically negative.

ASSESSMENT
Probable linitis.

PLAN
1. Mycology cream.
2. Drying agents.

ANSWER KEYS

REVIEW QUESTIONS ANSWER KEY

1. A
2. B
3. C
4. C
5. C
6. A
7. B
8. A
9. B
10. A
11. B
12. D
13. C
14. A
15. C
16. A
17. C
18. A
19. A
20. B
21. D
22. C
23. D
24. C
25. C
26. D
27. C
28. A
29. D
30. B

PROOFREADING EXERCISE #1 KEY

Use combining form—transurethral

PREOPERATIVE DIAGNOSIS
Recurrent bladder tumor.

POSTOPERATIVE DIAGNOSIS
Recurrent bladder tumor.

OPERATION
Trans urethral resection of bladder tumor.

ANESTHESIA
General with mask.

INDICATIONS FOR THE PROCEDURE
The patient is an 83-year-old patient with a history of bladder cancer. He developed a recurrence, and was scheduled for surgery.

The risks and complications of the procedure were thoroughly discussed with the patient, and the patient understood and wished to proceed.

PROCEDURE IN DETAIL
The patient was taken to the operating room and under satisfactory general anesthesia, he was prepped and draped in the usual sterile fashion using Betadine. He was then placed in the supine position.

Capitalize French

Incorrect format—#21

Incorrect term—sounds

Use combining form—cystoscope

Cystoscopy was performed with the number 21-french cystic scope with the 12-degree and 70-degree angled lenses, with the findings as above noted. The urethra was dilated with van Buren signs.

Incorrect term—resectoscope

Then the rectoscope was introduced with a sheath first, and then the obturator was removed and the working element was placed.

Incorrect term—perforate

Incorrect term—tumors

Incorrect term—prostate

Incorrect term—mobile

Resection of the tumors was performed with great care not to biforate the bladder. All tumors were removed and sent for pathology. The surrounding area was carefully fulgurated. The bladder was then inspected for any remaining rumors and there were none. The bladder was then emptied, and an 18-French Foley catheter was placed; the balloon was inflated with 10 mL and the return was clear.

An examination under anesthesia was performed, which revealed a smooth, benign prostrate of approximately 30–35 grams with no palpable masses and no indurations. The bladder appeared to be fairly motile.

The patient tolerated the procedure well, and was transferred to the recovery room in good condition.

COMPLICATIONS
None.

DRAINS
An 18-French 3-way Foley connected to continuous bladder irrigation.

PROOFREADING EXERCISE #2 KEY

Incorrect term—sterilization

Incorrect term—instillation

Incorrect spelling—cords

Incorrect term—re-canalization

Incorrect term—instillation

Incorrect term—spermatic

Incorrect term—orchalgia

PREOPERATIVE DIAGNOSIS
Voluntary serialization.

POSTOPERATIVE DIAGNOSIS
Voluntary serialization.

OPERATION
Bilateral vasectomy.

ANESTHESIA
IV sedation with local installation of lidocaine, Marcaine, and bicarbonate to the spermatic chords.

FLUIDS
Crystalloids.

ESTIMATED BLOOD LOSS
Negligible.

JUSTIFICATION FOR THE PROCEDURE
This is a 45-year-old white male requesting vasectomy. He presents at this time for a vasectomy, fully understanding the risks and benefits of this type of procedure, including decannulation of the vas as well as bleeding and otalgia.

PROCEDURE IN DETAIL
After being properly identified, the patient was taken to the operating room, at which time anesthesia was administered via IV sedation and local installation of lidocaine and Marcaine to the semantic cords.

Bilateral vasectomies were performed in the following fashion:

Using the no-scalpel vasectomy kit, each bas differens was localized using the ring clamp. The skin overlying each vas deferens was spread, and a 1-cm section of each vas differens was resected and the proximal and distal ends of each vas was cauterized using a needle-point Bovie, as well as suture ligated using 3-0 Vicryl sutures. The skin was closed bilaterally using 4-0 chromic suture in an interrupted fashion.

A notal support was applied. The patient tolerated the procedure well and was sent to the recovery room in stable condition.

Incorrect term—vas deferens

Incorrect term—deferens

Incorrect term—scrotal

PROOFREADING EXERCISE #3 KEY

Incorrect term—stricture

Incorrect term—creatinine

Incorrect term—nephrotic

Flag—value should be higher than 220

CHIEF COMPLAINT
Urethral structure.

HISTORY OF PRESENT ILLNESS
This is a 40-year-old inmate who reports having been diagnosed with necrotic syndrome in June of this year prior to his incarceration. His initial creatine and bun were 2.0 and 49 respectively. The patient reports having been in a motor vehicle accident after which he was treated with analgesics and anti-inflammatories, and he feels this possibly may have caused the onset of the necrotic syndrome. He has no flank pain but does have significant 3+ distal extremity splitting edema and soreness of the souls of his feet. He also reports having had rapid weight gain from 220 pounds up to 190 pounds. All of this resolved, however, with diuretics, diet restrictions, and fluid restrictions.

PAST MEDICAL HISTORY
He reports being borderline diabetic, and he has had a history of hypertension over the past 2 years.

SOCIAL HISTORY
The patient smokes a half pack of cigarettes per day and has done so for the past 30 years. Prior to being incarcerated, he worked as a bricklayer.

FAMILY HISTORY
Positive for diabetes mellitus in his father.

MEDICATIONS
Lipitor, Calan, and Lasik.

ALLERGIES
Motrin.

Incorrect term—nephrotic

Incorrect format—BUN

Incorrect term—pitting

Incorrect spelling—soles

Incorrect term—Lasix

PHYSICAL EXAMINATION

VITAL SIGNS: His most recent blood pressure was 154/84. The patient is awake, alert, oriented to time, place, and person.

HEENT: Grossly within normal limits.

LUNGS: Soft inspiratory wheeze and soft rhonchi in both lungs which cleared with cough.

HEART: Regular rate and rhythm.

ABDOMEN: Soft. Bowel sounds are active, and there is no suprapubic distention or pain and no cerebrovascular accident tenderness.

GENITOURINARY: Shows an uncircumcised penis with an adequate mitis, dissented testicles, and a moderate-sized right hydro seal as well as a smaller-sized left hydro seal. Anal sphincter tone is within normal limits. The prostate is not enlarged, tender, or nodular and is of normal consistency.

EXTREMITIES: Show 3+ to 4+ pitting edema. This does not extend into the upper thigh or genital area.

IMPRESSION

History and findings consistent with nephrotic syndrome.

PLAN

1. Renal biopsy.
2. Prostrate pacific antigen.
3. Renal ultrasound.
4. A 24-hour urine collection for protean and creatinine appearance.

Probable incorrect expansion—costovertebral angle

Incorrect term—meatus

Incorrect word—undescended

Incorrect term—hydrocele

Incorrect term—hydrocele

Incorrect terms—prostate specific

Incorrect word—clearance

Incorrect spelling—protein

PROOFREADING EXERCISE #4 KEY

PREOPERATIVE DIAGNOSIS
BPH, bladder stones, urinary retention

POSTOPERATIVE DIAGNOSIS
Same.

OPERATION
Cystoscopy, urethral dilation, TERP, and electrohydraulic lithotripsy of bladder stone.

OPERATIVE PROCEDURE
The patient was brought to the operating room and placed in the subline position. He was then rolled to the left lateral decubital position. Spinal anesthesia was accomplished. After anesthesia was accomplished, the patient was placed in the dorsal lobotomy position. The genitals and peroneal area were prepped and draped in the usual sterile manner.

At this point, a #21 pan endoscopic sheath with a 12-degree lens on a short bridge was inserted into the meatus. The scope was advanced to the area of the prostatic fascia where there was noted to be trilobar obstruction of the prostatic fossa. The scope was then maneuvered past the loaves of the prostate into the bladder where the ureteral orifices were noted to be normal in size, shape, and position. The bladder was then inspected under gravity flow of normal saline with the 12-degree lens. There was no evidence of latter tumors, stones, or foreign objects. There was 1+ tribulation of the bladder wall.

Spell out diagnosis—benign prostatic hypertrophy

Write out diagnoses

Incorrect abbreviation—TURP

Incorrect term—supine

Incorrect term—decubitus

Incorrect term—lithotomy

Incorrect term—perineal

Use combined form—panendoscopic

Incorrect term—lobes

Incorrect term—fossa

Incorrect word—bladder

Incorrect term—trabeculation

Incorrect term—foreign

Incorrect spelling—male

Incorrect term—urethra

Incorrect spelling—coarse

Use combined form—cystourethroscope

Incorrect abbreviation—EHL

Incorrect spelling—effluent

A 70-degree lens was then inserted into the panendoscopic sheath. Again inspection of the bladder revealed no evidence of bladder tumors, stones, or forum objects.

At this point, the panendoscopic sheath was removed. The meatus was dilated to a #28-French with the mail sounds. A #26-Iglesias resectoscopic unit with the Timberlake obturator was placed per ureter into the bladder. The obturator was removed and the Iglesias resectoscopic unit was placed inside the sheath. The prostate was resected down to its course circular fibers of the prostatic fossa. Bleeding points were point identified and coagulated. The scope was then pulled distally, and the apical tissue in a similar manner. The chips were evacuated with the Toomey syringe. Bleeding points were point identified and coagulated.

After evacuation of the chips, the 9-French EAL probe was inserted through the working element of the cysto urethroscope. The bladder stones were fragmented. They were evacuated through the syringe.

There were no gross bleeding or chips remaining in the bladder, and the panendoscopic unit was removed. The #24-French 3-way Foley catheter was inserted into the bladder. The balloon was instilled with 30 mL of sterile saline. The bladder was then irrigated with sterile saline until the affluent was clear. The patient was then transferred to the PAR in stable condition.

PROOFREADING EXERCISE #5 KEY

Incorrect term—herpes

Incorrect term—intercourse

Incorrect term—venereal

CHIEF COMPLAINT
Penile rash.

HISTORY OF PRESENT ILLNESS
This is a 44-year-old white male who has noticed a rash on the left side of his penis, which becomes reddened and irritated sometimes after inner course. There does not appear to be any lesion, and the patient has had no blistering, redness, or other signs of Hers disease or other venerable diseases.

MEDICAL HISTORY
No important medical or surgical illnesses.

CURRENT MEDICATIONS
None.

ALLERGIES
None.

REVIEW OF SYSTEMS
CONSTITUTIONAL: No weight loss, fever, chills, nausea, or vomiting.
EYES: No blurred vision or diplopia.
ENT, MOUTH: No rhinitis or dysphagia.
CARDIOVASCULAR: No chest pain.
RESPIRATORY: No shortness of breath.
GASTROINTESTINAL: No diarrhea or abdominal pain.
MUSCULOSKELETAL: No history of hernia. No muscular weakness, numbness, or joint pain.
NEUROLOGIC: No headaches, blurred vision, or syncope.

PHYSICAL EXAMINATION

GENERAL: Well-nourished, ~~white~~ male, not acutely ill.

HEENT: Pupils equal and reactive to light. Cranial nerves II-XII grossly intact. Sclerae without icterus. Tongue is moist.

NECK: Supple, no masses, no bruits.

CHEST: Clear to auscultation and percussion. No crackles or wheezes.

HEART: Regular rhythm, no murmur.

LYMPHATICS: Cervical and auxiliary nodes are normal.

ABDOMEN: Soft, nontender, no masses. No CVA tenderness. The liver and spleen are not palpable. No hernias.

GENITALIA: Reveals some roughness, scaling, and slight reddening of the skin on the left side below the glands penis. This has the appearance of yeast infection.

RECTAL: Reveals 1+, smooth, malign prostate.

DATA REVIEWED

Urine analysis: pH 60, specific gravity 10/20. Microscopically and chemically negative.

ASSESSMENT

Probable linitis.

PLAN

1. Mica log cream.
2. Drying agents.

No comma needed

Incorrect term—axillary

Incorrect term—glans

Incorrect term—benign

Incorrect format—6

Use combined form—urinalysis

Incorrect format—1.020

Incorrect term—balanitis

Incorrect drug—Mycolog

CHAPTER

24

Radiology/Nuclear Medicine

OBJECTIVES CHECKLIST

A prepared exam candidate will know:

- ❑ Terminology related to radiology, nuclear medicine, and radiation therapy.
- ❑ Fundamentals of x-rays and CT scans and common diagnostic techniques employed in the x-ray process, including terminology related to x-ray positioning.
- ❑ Radiographic studies that require the use of contrast media and the various types of contrast media used for this purpose.
- ❑ Fundamentals of ultrasonography, including common ultrasound studies.
- ❑ Fundamentals of MRI and MRA, including common diagnostic studies.
- ❑ Fundamentals of nuclear medicine, including terminology related to radionuclides and common diagnostic studies.
- ❑ Common radiopharmaceuticals administered to obtain scans of specific organs of the body.
- ❑ Difference between *in vitro* and *in vivo* procedures in nuclear medicine.
- ❑ Terminology and application of radiation therapy, including external-beam radiation and brachytherapy.

RESOURCES FOR STUDY

1. *The Language of Medicine*
   Chapter 20: Radiology, Nuclear Medicine and Radiation Therapy, pp. 817–847.
2. *Laboratory Tests & Diagnostic Procedures in Medicine*
   Section IV: Medical Imaging
   Chapter 10: Plain Radiography, pp. 127–132.
   Chapter 11: Contrast Radiography, pp. 133–150.
   Chapter 12: Computed Tomography, pp. 151–176.
   Chapter 13: Ultrasonography, pp. 187–198.
   Chapter 14: Magnetic Resonance Imaging, pp. 199–208.
   Chapter 15: Nuclear Imaging, pp. 209–222.
3. *The AAMT Book of Style for Medical Transcription*
   Fracture classification systems, pp. 295–297.
   Isotope nomenclature, pp. 150–151.
   Plain film x-rays, p. 317.
   Plane, p. 317.
   Radiology report, p. 450.
   Vertebra, pp. 298–299.
   X-ray, pp. 428–429.

SAMPLE REPORTS

The following five reports are examples of reports you might encounter while transcribing radiology and nuclear medicine.

PET SCAN

HISTORY
This is a 69-year-old female with a history of lung carcinoma.

TECHNIQUE
A dose of 15 mCi of fluorine-19 FDG was infused. Images were obtained from the base of the skull through the midthighs utilizing a fixed, full-ring PET scanner. Tomographic and volumetric images are reviewed.

This study is compared to a previous PET scan dated August 21, 2004, and a previous CT scan of the chest dated November 10, 2004.

FINDINGS
Again demonstrated is a stable, linear, moderate, increased metabolic activity extending from the left hilum to the left lateral chest wall. This region of increased metabolic activity measured 1.7 standard uptake value on the previous study and measures 1.8 standard uptake value on the current study. This region of abnormal linear increased metabolic activity corresponds to lung parenchyma fibrosis and scarring extending from the hilum to the lateral chest wall, demonstrated on CT scan. The remainder of the lungs demonstrates no abnormal increased metabolic activity.

The remainder of the body scan demonstrates no abnormal increased metabolic activity.

IMPRESSION
1. The stable, linear, increased metabolic activity corresponding to parenchymal scarring on CT scan in the left lung is compatible with expected uptake from parenchymal granulation and scarring.
2. There is a low probability for residual, recurrent, or metastatic lung carcinoma.
3. A 6-month interval followup PET scan is recommended to ensure continued stability.

MRI

HISTORY
The patient is a 48-year-old female with previous MRI from August 25, 2004.

TECHNIQUE
MRI of the left knee was performed at 0.7 Tesla field strength, utilizing an open-configuration magnet. Coronal T1 and fast IR, axial fat-suppressed proton-density, sagittal fat-suppressed proton-density, and fast T2 images were obtained.

FINDINGS
The examination again shows a large joint effusion with distension of the joint capsule and suprapatellar pouch. A multiloculated large cyst is seen in the popliteal fossa, more towards the medial side along the medial head of the gastrocnemius muscle. The cyst measures up to 10 cm craniocaudad, centered at the level of the joint line and up to 3.5 cm in AP diameter. Internal septations and nodularity along the wall are seen. There is some fluid intensity around the outer margins of the cystic collection, more diffusely in the soft tissues, more evident inferiorly.

Evaluation of the articular cartilage and the menisci shows no focal defects. The bone marrow signal under the weightbearing area appears normal. The collateral ligaments and cruciate ligaments appear intact. Patellar tendon and quadriceps tendon are within normal limits in dimension and signal intensity.

When compared to the previous examination, a similar appearance is noted in the contour of the popliteal cyst and also in the distribution of joint effusion. The distention of the lateral recesses of the axillary pouch appears similar. On sagittal fat-suppressed images, pericapsular soft tissue edema also appears nearly similar, with mild reduction seen on the medial aspect in the soft tissues.

IMPRESSION
1. The examination shows no significant interval change in the appearance of the left knee, showing a prominent joint effusion and nodularity along the synovial linings suggesting synovitis.
2. A large popliteal cyst with inflammatory reaction around it is seen posteromedially as described above.
3. No new areas of intraarticular abnormalities or in the periarticular soft tissues identified.

MRI

HISTORY
The patient is a 95-year-old female with dizziness and suspected CVA.

TECHNIQUE
MRI of the brain was performed at 0.7 Tesla field strength, utilizing an open-configuration magnet. Sagittal T1, coronal fast IR, axial T1, FLAIR, and fast T2 images were obtained. Also, diffusion-weighted images in the axial plane were obtained.

FINDINGS
The examination shows moderate prominence of the cortical sulci and fissures and basal cisterns. There is moderate proportionate enlargement of the ventricular system. On T2 and FLAIR images, confluent increased high-intensity signal is seen along the body of the lateral ventricles and a few scattered punctate foci are seen deeper in the white matter. No dominant focal lesions are seen at the level of the basal ganglia or thalami. A few CSF-intensity lesions are seen in the subinsular region bilaterally with tubular configuration. Also, striated T2 high-intensity areas are seen along the convexity bilaterally, consistent with dilated perivascular spaces.

No signal changes suggestive of hemorrhage are seen. There is no mass effect. No abnormal localizing extraaxial collections are seen.

The flow-related signal void in intracranial arteries and venous sinuses appears normal. Signal in the calvaria is normal. Paranasal sinuses and mastoid cells appear aerated, with some mucosal thickening seen in the ethmoid cells along the left side. No fluid levels are seen.

IMPRESSION
1. The examination shows moderate involutional changes with mild a pattern of ischemic leukomalacia.
2. No signs of mass lesion, hydrocephalus, or evidence of hemorrhage are seen.
3. Incidentally on sagittal images, advanced degenerative changes at the craniocervical juncture are seen, with erosive changes of the odontoid. Correlation with lateral plain radiographs of the cervical spine are suggested for additional assessment of bony detail.

ULTRASOUND-GUIDED BIOPSY

PROCEDURE ORDERED
Ultrasound-guided biopsy of a nodule in the left lobe of the thyroid.

CLINICAL HISTORY
This is a 70-year-old male with a history of a cold nodule in the left lobe of the thyroid.

REPORT
After the benefits (to try to obtain samples of tissue to submit to the laboratory for analysis), risks (bleeding, infection, nerve damage, and the need for emergency surgery), and alternatives (possible surgery or doing nothing) of the procedure were explained to the patient and the opportunity to ask questions given, written consent was obtained and witnessed.

The patient is anticoagulated due to a left ventricular thrombus and atrial fibrillation. The increased risk of bleeding due to the anticoagulation was also discussed with the patient. The patient was awake and alert and wished to proceed.

Using real-time sonographic imaging, the nodule in the left lobe of the thyroid was localized. The nodule is located in the mid- and lower pole of the left lobe and extends inferiorly off the supraclavicular fossa and left clavicle. The nodule measured approximately 4 cm in greatest diameter. A spot was then marked with ink on the overlying skin of the neck. The patient's neck was then prepped and draped in the usual sterile fashion. Local anesthesia was administered with 1% Lidocaine. Using sterile ultrasound gel, a sterile ultrasound probe cover, and sterile technique, a 25-gauge needle was directed into the nodule in the left lobe of the thyroid and a sample of tissue obtained and submitted to the cytotechnologist who was in attendance. This was repeated two times for a total of three passes that were made and three samples of tissue that were obtained.

At the end of the procedure, there was approximately a 1-cm hematoma in the subcutaneous tissues at the biopsy site. The patient's skin was cleansed with sterile saline and antibiotic ointment applied. A sterile overlying dressing was then applied. The patient tolerated the procedure well and left the angiography suite in good, stable condition.

IMPRESSION
Successful ultrasound-guided biopsy. Small post-procedural hematoma noted, as described above.

CT SCAN

PROCEDURE ORDERED
CT scan of the abdomen and pelvis.

TECHNIQUE
Helical imaging of the abdomen and pelvis was performed from the lung bases to the symphysis pubis with 7-mm collimation after the administration of oral and the intravenous injection of 125 mL of Visipaque. No prior cross-sectional imaging studies of the abdomen or pelvis are available at this time.

The AP scout film of the abdomen and pelvis demonstrates gas density within the wall of the urinary bladder and surgical clips projecting over the right upper quadrant of an obese patient. There are no nodules in the imaged portions of the lung bases. There is no pericardial or pleural effusion in the imaged portions of the lower thorax.

There is gas in the wall of the urinary bladder. No Foley catheter is present within the urinary bladder. There is no evidence of free intraperitoneal air or fluid. The uterus is atrophic. The abdominal aorta is nonaneurysmal, and there are no pathologically enlarged retroperitoneal lymph nodes.

Surgical clips are located in the gallbladder fossa; the gallbladder is absent. The attenuation of the liver is slightly less than that of the spleen. The hepatic and portal veins enhance with contrast, and there is no intrahepatic biliary dilatation. The spleen and adrenal glands are within normal limits. The pancreas is atrophic. The cortex of each kidney is thin. Both kidneys enhance with contrast, and there is no hydronephrosis. There is degenerative change of the lumbar spine.

IMPRESSION
1. Emphysematous cystitis.
2. Status post prior cholecystectomy.
3. Mild fatty infiltration of the liver.
4. Bilateral renal atrophy.
5. Lumbar spondylosis.

REVIEW QUESTIONS

The goal of these questions is to test your knowledge in the areas of radiology and nuclear medicine.

Directions: Select the correct answer for each of the multiple-choice questions provided below. *Answers are provided at the end of this chapter.*

1. Which of the following is not a contrast media used in radiological procedures?
   A. Isovue
   B. Omnipaque
   C. Xenon
   D. Sonolucent
2. Radiologists often refer to bodily planes when describing x-rays. The plane which cuts directly through the body vertically into right and left sides is called:
   A. Dorsal plane
   B. Transverse plane
   C. Ventral plane
   D. Midsagittal plane
3. The bodily plane separating the body in half horizontally is called the:
   A. Midsagittal plane
   B. Superior plane
   C. Ventral plane
   D. Transverse plane
4. An x-ray taken in the left decubitus position would mean the individual is:
   A. Lying with the left side up
   B. Lying on the back with legs bent
   C. Lying with the left side down
   D. Lying face up
5. A radiograph taken with the patient lying on his/her back with the head lowered by tilting the table at a 45-degree angle is termed the:
   A. Trendelenburg position
   B. Supine position
   C. Sims position
   D. Fowler position
6. Which of the following is a mammography rating system for reporting breast lesions?
   A. BIRADS
   B. Karnofsky
   C. Baume
   D. Gray scale
7. An MVA victim presents to the ER with difficulty breathing. The ER physician orders a portable PA of the chest to rule out hemothorax or pneumothorax. What does PA mean?
   A. The x-ray beam passes through the patient from front to back
   B. The x-ray beam passes through the patient from back to front
   C. The x-ray beam passes through the patient from an anterior position only
   D. The x-ray beam passes through the patient from a cephalic position
8. A patient was admitted to the hospital with a persistent cough, fever, weight loss, and one episode of blood-streaked sputum. A PA chest film did not look abnormal so a lordotic view film was ordered. What is a lordotic view?
   A. The patient lies on the left side with knees bent
   B. The patient stands erect with arms held above the head
   C. The patient stands leaning backward
   D. The patient stands leaning forward
9. On a chest x-ray, changes in the size of the heart may be seen in the:
   A. Enhanced view only
   B. Cardiac silhouette
   C. Acoustic showing
   D. M-mode only

10. Computerized tomography uses which imaging technology?
   A. X-rays
   B. Magnets and radio waves
   C. Sound waves
   D. Radioisotopes

11. A number assigned to a pixel in a CT scan which represents the amount of radiation that was absorbed by the tissue at that point in the image is called:
   A. Hounsfield unit
   B. RAD
   C. T1
   D. Sievert

12. One gray, which is a unit of measure equal to 100 rads, is abbreviated:
   A. Gr
   B. Gy
   C. Ga
   D. gr

13. Examination of the gallbladder and bile ducts by nuclear medicine scanning is termed:
   A. HIDA scan
   B. Cholescintigraphy
   C. Cholecystatony
   D. A & B

14. An upper GI series might be immediately followed by:
   A. VCUG
   B. Small-bowel follow-through
   C. Pyelography
   D. PET scan

15. Imaging of blood vessels using special sequences which enhance the signal of flowing blood and suppress that from other tissues is called:
   A. MUGA scan
   B. Magnetic resonance angiography
   C. Nuclear HIDA scan
   D. PET scan

16. Gadolinium is a commonly used contrast media for:
   A. CT scans
   B. X-rays
   C. PET scans
   D. MRI scans

17. Technetium is used extensively as a radiographic tracer in imaging studies of:
   A. Internal organs
   B. The cranium
   C. Joint spaces
   D. The fascial layers

18. Which of the following is the correct way to transcribe 40 millicuries of technetium?
   A. 40 mCi ^{99m} Tc
   B. 40 mcu Tc 99m
   C. 40 mc t_{c99}
   D. 40 mlc Tc 99

19. A T1-weighted image will have a:
   A. Bright water signal
   B. Bright bone signal
   C. Bright fat signal
   D. Bright tissue signal

20. A plain radiograph taken immediately before contrast medium is given is called a:
   A. Stress film
   B. Flat plate
   C. Scout film
   D. Spot film

21. A bone density result reported as the bone density relative to a 30-year-old female is called a:
   A. Z-score
   B. T-score
   C. C-score
   D. B-score

22. Spiral computed tomography is also known as:
   A. Collimated computed tomography
   B. Triphasic computed tomography
   C. Helical computed tomography
   D. Flow velocity computed tomography

23. An MRI technique used to enhance the T1 and T2 signals and thus improve the image is called:
    - A. Attenuation
    - B. Spin echo
    - C. Triphasic flow velocity
    - D. Signal intensity calibration

24. In an x-ray, the process of restricting and confining the x-ray beam to a given area and, in nuclear medicine, of restricting the detection of emitted radiations from a given area of interest is called:
    - A. Directed sonography
    - B. Pulse sequencing
    - C. Superconducting
    - D. Collimation

25. The location, measurement, or delineation of deep structures by measuring the reflection or transmission of high frequency sound waves is known as:
    - A. Sonography
    - B. PET
    - C. SPECT
    - D. Spin echo

26. An ultrasonic method which measures both the speed and direction of blood flow and is of diagnostic value in peripheral vascular and cardiac disease is known as:
    - A. DSA
    - B. Shadowing
    - C. Duplex Doppler
    - D. Pulse sequencing

27. An intraoral dental film adapted to show the coronal portion and cervical third of the root of the teeth in near occlusion, especially useful in detecting interproximal caries and determining alveolar septal height, is called a:
    - A. Panorex
    - B. Bitewing
    - C. Tesla
    - D. Mandibular film

28. In neuroradiology, the various sutures of the skull are often dictated. For example, the line of union between the two parietal bones is called the:
    - A. Frontal suture
    - B. Lambdoid suture
    - C. Parietal suture
    - D. Sagittal suture

29. Since plain skull films are often normal in patients with brain tumors, which study below is usually used to expeditiously diagnose a brain tumor?
    - A. MRI
    - B. Angiography
    - C. CT
    - D. MRA

30. In a radiologic description of a patient's vertebral column, the term radiolucency is used repeatedly. What does radiolucency mean?
    - A. Relatively penetrable by x-rays
    - B. Unable to be penetrated by x-rays
    - C. Relative desiccation
    - D. An area of uptake

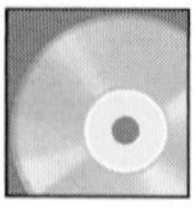

Please see the accompanying CD for additional review materials for this section.

PROOFREADING EXERCISES

These three proofreading exercises are provided to improve your skills in the areas of editing and effective identification and correction of errors in the medical record.

Directions: Identify and correct the transcription errors found in the exercises below. *Answers are provided at the end of this chapter.*

PROOFREADING EXERCISE #1

CLINICAL HISTORY
This is a 50-year-old female status post Bell palsy treated with acyclovir and prednisone in the first week of July and complaining of left-sided swelling behind the ear and blurring of vision. Rule out mass.

TECHNIQUE
Magnetic resonance imaging of the brain was performed on a 1.0 test superconducting magnet. Precontrast spin-echo T1-waited sagittal and axial, and fast-spin echo, dual-echo, and inversion-recovery axle images were obtained. After the intravenous injection of gadodiamide, post contrast enhanced spin-echo T1-waited axial and corneal images were obtained. No prior imaging studies of the brain are available at this time.

FINDINGS
There is no demonstrable mass posterior to the left article. The signal intensity of the bone marrow of the calvaria and clivus is within normal limits. The pattern of sulci and gyri are within normal limits. Located in the right centrum semiovale and the subcortical white matter of the frontal lobe are several scattered foci of dual echo and inversion-recovery high signal density. The ventricles are bilaterally symmetrical and not enlarged. There is no midline shift or evidence of an intracranial mass lesion. There is no abnormal intraaxial or extraaxial fluid collection. There is normal-appearing flow void within the demonstrated portions of the major inner cranial vessels. The imaged portions of the orbits and sinuses are unremarkable. After the administration of contrast, there are no abnormal areas of enhancement.

IMPRESSION
1. No midline lift or evidence of an intracranial mass lesion, hemorrhage, or of stroke. Additionally, there is no demonstrable mass posterior to the left oracle. If clinically indicated, directed mammography could be performed for further evaluation.
2. Minimal deep white matter ischemic changes are also noted.

PROOFREADING EXERCISE #2

CLINICAL HISTORY
This is a 67-year-old female with pain and fever.

TECHNIQUE
Helical imaging of the abdomen and pelvis was performed from the lung bases to the synthesis pubis with 7-mm culmination after the administration of oral nonionic contrast and the intravenous injection of nonionic contrast. No prior cross-sectional imaging studies of the abdomen or pelvis are available for comparison at this time.

FINDINGS
The AP scalp film of the abdomen and pelvis demonstrates surgical clips projecting over the right upper quadrant of the abdomen. There are no nodules within the imaged portions of the lung basis. There is no pericardial or pleural diffusion in the imaged portions of the lower thorax.

A 3.5-cm noncalcified soft tissue mass is located within the ascending colon (images 29–32). There is subtle extension into the adjacent paracolic fat. Trace fluid is located within the right paracolic gutter.

Numerous diverticulum protrude from the sigmoid colon and scattered diverticula protrude from the descending colon. There is no inflammatory change in the adjacent mesenteric fat.

The continuation of the liver is less than that of the spleen. The hepatic and portal veins enhance with contrast and there is no intrahepatic biliary dilatation. Surgical clips are located in the gallbladder fossa; the gallbladder is absent. The pancreas is a trophy.

The spleen, adrenal glands, kidneys, and urinary bladder are within normal limits. Using bone window settings for review, there are no demonstrable lytic or plastic lesions of the imaged portions of the spine. The abdominal aorta is nonaneurysmal, and there are no pathologically enlarged retroperitoneal lymph nodes. There is no free intraperitoneal air.

(continued)

IMPRESSION

1. A 3.5-cm soft tissue "mass" in the ascending colon which is worrisome for malignancy. Adherent stool is felt less likely. A bare minima or colonoscopy is recommended for further evaluation.
2. Trace fluid in the right paracolic gutter.
3. Colony diverticulosis without evidence of diverticulitis.
4. Minimal fatty infiltration of the liver.
5. Pancreatic atrophy.
6. Status post prior cholecystectomy.

PROOFREADING EXERCISE #3

PROCEDURE PERFORMED
Arterial, lower extremities ultrasound.

TECHNIQUE
Gray-scale, color-flow, and duplex imaging performed.

COMPARISON
No comparisons currently available.

FINDINGS
RIGHT LOWER EXTREMITY: The right common humeral and proximal superficial femoral arteries demonstrate triphasic waveforms. The remainder of the right lower extremity demonstrates biphasic waveforms. Peek systolic flow velocity within the right common femoral, superficial femoral, and popliteal arteries measures 71, 77, and 63 cm, respectively. Peak systolic flow velocity within the posterior tibial and dorsalis pedis arteries measure 49 and 22 cm, respectively.

LEFT LOWER EXTREMITY: Biphasic waveforms noted throughout the left lower extremity. Peak systemic flow velocity within the left common femoral, common superficial femoral, and popliteal arteries measures 64, 83, and 48 cm, respectively. Peak systolic flow velocity within the dorsalis pedis and posterior tibial arteries measures 30 and 47 cm, respectively.

IMPRESSION
1. Astro sclerotic change noted within the lower extremities bilaterally.
2. A definite, local high-grade stenosis not appreciated on this evaluation. If clinical concern persists, an RA evaluation could be considered.
3. Flow identified within the dorsalis pedis and anterior tibial arteries bilaterally.

ANSWER KEYS

REVIEW QUESTIONS ANSWER KEY

1. D
2. D
3. D
4. C
5. A
6. A
7. B
8. C
9. B
10. A
11. A
12. B
13. D
14. B
15. B
16. D
17. A
18. A
19. C
20. C
21. B
22. C
23. B
24. D
25. A
26. C
27. B
28. D
29. A
30. A

PROOFREADING EXERCISE #1 KEY

CLINICAL HISTORY
This is a 50-year-old female status post Bell palsy treated with acyclovir and prednisone in the first week of July and complaining of left-sided swelling behind the ear and blurring of vision. Rule out mass.

TECHNIQUE
Magnetic resonance imaging of the brain was performed on a 1.0 test superconducting magnet. Precontrast spin-echo T1-waited sagittal and axial, and fast-spin echo, dual-echo, and inversion-recovery axle images were obtained. After the intravenous injection of gadodiamide, post contrast enhanced spin-echo T1-waited axial and corneal images were obtained. No prior imaging studies of the brain are available at this time.

FINDINGS
There is no demonstrable mass posterior to the left article. The signal intensity of the bone marrow of the calvaria and clivus is within normal limits. The pattern of sulci and gyri are within normal limits. Located in the right centrum semiovale and the subcortical white matter of the frontal lobe are several scattered foci of dual echo and inversion-recovery high signal density. The ventricles are bilaterally symmetrical and not enlarged. There is no midline shift or evidence of an intracranial mass lesion. There is no abnormal intraaxial or extraaxial fluid collection. There is normal-appearing flow void within the demonstrated portions of the major inner cranial vessels. The imaged portions of the orbits and sinuses are unremarkable. After the administration of contrast, there are no abnormal areas of enhancement.

Incorrect term—tesla

Incorrect spelling—weighted

Incorrect spelling—weighted

Incorrect term—axial

Incorrect term—coronal

Incorrect term—auricle

Incorrect word—intensity

Incorrect prefix—intracranial

Incorrect word—shift

Incorrect term—sonography

Incorrect term—auricle

IMPRESSION

1. No midline lift or evidence of an intracranial mass lesion, hemorrhage, or of stroke. Additionally, there is no demonstrable mass posterior to the left oracle. If clinically indicated, directed mammography could be performed for further evaluation.
2. Minimal deep white matter ischemic changes are also noted.

PROOFREADING EXERCISE #2 KEY

CLINICAL HISTORY
This is a 67-year-old female with pain and fever.

TECHNIQUE
Helical imaging of the abdomen and pelvis was performed from the lung bases to the synthesis pubis with 7-mm culmination after the administration of oral nonionic contrast and the intravenous injection of nonionic contrast. No prior cross-sectional imaging studies of the abdomen or pelvis are available for comparison at this time.

FINDINGS
The AP scalp film of the abdomen and pelvis demonstrates surgical clips projecting over the right upper quadrant of the abdomen. There are no nodules within the imaged portions of the lung basis. There is no pericardial or pleural diffusion in the imaged portions of the lower thorax.

A 3.5-cm noncalcified soft tissue mass is located within the ascending colon (images 29–32). There is subtle extension into the adjacent paracolic fat. Trace fluid is located within the right paracolic gutter.

Numerous diverticulum protrude from the sigmoid colon and scattered diverticula protrude from the descending colon. There is no inflammatory change in the adjacent mesenteric fat.

The continuation of the liver is less than that of the spleen. The hepatic and portal veins enhance with contrast and there is no intrahepatic biliary dilatation. Surgical clips are located in the gallbladder fossa; the gallbladder is absent. The pancreas is a trophy.

Incorrect term—symphysis

Incorrect term—collimation

Incorrect term—scout

Incorrect term—bases

Incorrect term—effusion

Use plural form—diverticula

Incorrect term—attenuation

Incorrect term—atrophic

The spleen, adrenal glands, kidneys, and urinary bladder are within normal limits. Using bone window settings for review, there are no demonstrable lytic or plastic lesions of the imaged portions of the spine. The abdominal aorta is nonaneurysmal, and there are no pathologically enlarged retroperitoneal lymph nodes. There is no free intraperitoneal air.

Incorrect term—blastic

IMPRESSION

1. A 3.5-cm soft tissue "mass" in the ascending colon which is worrisome for malignancy. Adherent stool is felt less likely. A bare minima or colonoscopy is recommended for further evaluation.
2. Trace fluid in the right paracolic gutter.
3. Colony diverticulosis without evidence of diverticulitis.
4. Minimal fatty infiltration of the liver.
5. Pancreatic atrophy.
6. Status post prior cholecystectomy.

Incorrect term—barium enema

Incorrect term—colonic

PROOFREADING EXERCISE #3 KEY

Incorrect term—femoral

Incorrect spelling—peak

Incorrect term—systolic

Singular subject—measures

PROCEDURE PERFORMED
Arterial, lower extremities ultrasound.

TECHNIQUE
Gray-scale, color-flow, and duplex imaging performed.

COMPARISON
No comparisons currently available.

FINDINGS
RIGHT LOWER EXTREMITY: The right common humeral and proximal superficial femoral arteries demonstrate triphasic waveforms. The remainder of the right lower extremity demonstrates biphasic waveforms. Peek systolic flow velocity within the right common femoral, superficial femoral, and popliteal arteries measures 71, 77, and 63 cm, respectively. Peak systolic flow velocity within the posterior tibial and dorsalis pedis arteries measure 49 and 22 cm, respectively.

LEFT LOWER EXTREMITY: Biphasic waveforms noted throughout the left lower extremity. Peak systemic flow velocity within the left common femoral, common superficial femoral, and popliteal arteries measures 64, 83, and 48 cm, respectively. Peak systolic flow velocity within the dorsalis pedis and posterior tibial arteries measures 30 and 47 cm, respectively.

Incorrect term—atherosclerotic

Incorrect word—focal

Incorrect—MRA

IMPRESSION

1. Astro sclerotic change noted within the lower extremities bilaterally.
2. A definite, local high-grade stenosis not appreciated on this evaluation. If clinical concern persists, an RA evaluation could be considered.
3. Flow identified within the dorsalis pedis and anterior tibial arteries bilaterally.

CHAPTER

25

Dentistry/Oral Surgery

OBJECTIVES CHECKLIST

A prepared exam candidate will know the:

- ❑ Combining forms, prefixes, and suffixes related to the body system.
- ❑ Anatomy of the oral cavity, including identification by name and location of all teeth.
- ❑ Seven terms dentists use to describe the surfaces of the teeth.
- ❑ Inner anatomy of a tooth from crown to pulp.
- ❑ Anatomy of the cranial bones, including sutures, and the cranial musculature.
- ❑ Anatomy of the facial bones, including sinuses, and the facial musculature.
- ❑ Common signs, symptoms, and disease processes related to the oral cavity.
- ❑ Common signs, symptoms, and disease processes related to the maxillofacial area.
- ❑ Imaging studies used in the identification and diagnosis of dental and maxillofacial abnormalities, injuries, diseases, and malformations.
- ❑ Medications commonly prescribed for musculoskeletal and dental symptoms, disorders, and diseases.

RESOURCES FOR STUDY

1. *The Language of Medicine*
   Chapter 5: Digestive System (Oral Cavity), pp. 140–143.
   Chapter 15: Musculoskeletal System (Cranial Bones, Facial Bones), pp. 564–567.
2. *H&P: A Nonphysician's Guide to the Medical History and Physical Examination*
   Chapter 7: Review of Systems: Head, Eyes, Ears, Nose, Throat, Mouth, Teeth, pp. 59–70.
   Chapter 21: Examination of the Nose, Throat, Mouth, and Teeth, pp. 199–208.
3. *The AAMT Book of Style for Medical Transcription*
   Orthopedics (fracture classification systems–LeFort), p. 295.

SAMPLE REPORTS

The following five reports are examples of reports you might encounter while transcribing dentistry and oral surgery.

OPERATIVE REPORT

PREOPERATIVE DIAGNOSIS
Bilateral mandibular fractures, status post open reduction and internal fixation.

POSTOPERATIVE DIAGNOSIS
Left mandibular body nonunion.

OPERATION PERFORMED
Removal of loose orthopedic hardware from the maxilla and mandible and reapplication of arch bar for fixation of nonunion of the left mandible.

SURGEON
Mary Jones, DDS.

ANESTHESIA
General endotracheal via stoma.

ESTIMATED BLOOD LOSS
Less than 5 mL.

FLUIDS GIVEN
Crystalloid.

COMPLICATIONS
None.

CONDITION
Stable.

TECHNIQUE
The patient was brought to the operating room and positioned supine. He was placed under general anesthesia via tracheostomy stoma. He was prepped and draped in the usual manner. After he was fully asleep and paralyzed, he was examined. He had loose arch bars to the maxilla and mandible. His mandibular arch bar was segmentalized. In the left anterior mandible and the right anterior mandible in the area of the fracture sites, all of the arch bars were loose in segments and the mandible was inflamed. No abscess or fistula formation was noted. There were exposed roots of the left mandibular premolar and right mandibular premolar canine. No purulence was seen. The floor of the mouth was supple; however, the left mandibular fracture site was mildly loose and flexible. The right one was only slightly flexible and mobile.

After removal of the loose orthopedic hardware, a 1-piece arch bar from second molar to second molar was applied to the mandibular dentition and stabilized with #24-gauge circumferential wires. This effectively fixated the fracture site where there was no mobility. His occlusion was stable as his teeth were brought together.

After this procedure, he was allowed to awaken from general anesthesia with the tracheostomy stoma still in place. He was taken to the recovery room in good condition.

DISCHARGE SUMMARY

ADMITTING DIAGNOSES

1. Compound mandibular fracture.
2. Bronchospasm.

HOSPITAL COURSE

The patient was admitted with an elevated white blood count and complaint of difficulty opening her jaw. She has had pain in her jaw ever since a farm tool hit her on the side of the face. Just prior to being admitted to the hospital, she had a tooth in the line of the fracture of the left mandible removed by another oral surgeon. She was admitted in stable condition. A medical consultation was obtained and she was cleared for surgery.

The surgery performed was an ORIF of her left mandibular fracture and a right mandibular symphyseal fracture. She lost approximately 200 mL of blood and had no complications immediately postoperatively and was transferred to the medical-surgical ward.

Over the course of the next 2 days, she slowly gained use of her mouth and was able to tolerate p.o. intake. Her hospital course was unremarkable, with no acute bronchospasms or difficulties with treatment.

She was discharged in good condition, able to tolerate p.o. intake, was afebrile, vital signs were stable, and all wounds were stable and without discharge. She had no airway problems. She was discharged home with a favorable prognosis.

DISCHARGE PLAN

Plan includes soft diet for a month. Activities are to be ad lib except no contact sports for 2 months. Medications include Cleocin and Tylenol elixir with codeine. She has a followup appointment in 2 to 3 days to see Dr. Smith for radiographs and evaluation.

Future plan includes observation of the teeth in the line of the fracture, especially in the right mandibular symphyseal region, for possible necrosis of these teeth.

OPERATIVE REPORT

PREOPERATIVE DIAGNOSES

1. Osteoradionecrosis of the left mandible.
2. Periodontal disease, tooth #19.

POSTOPERATIVE DIAGNOSES

1. Osteoradionecrosis of the left mandible.
2. Periodontal disease, tooth #19.

TITLE OF OPERATION

1. Extraction of tooth #19.
2. Debridement of left mandible.

ANESTHESIA

General endotracheal anesthesia.

ESTIMATED BLOOD LOSS

10 mL.

IV FLUIDS

1300 mL crystalloid.

URINE OUTPUT

None (no Foley placed).

MEDICATIONS GIVEN

Unasyn 1.5 g IV and Decadron 8 mg.

SPECIMENS

Bony specimens of left mandible, soft tissue fibrosis, and cultures.

JUSTIFICATION FOR PROCEDURE

This is a 65-year-old male who presented to the oral-maxillofacial surgery service with a history of squamous cell carcinoma of the tongue, which was treated with radiation. The patient developed osteoradionecrosis, which required debridement. The patient underwent standard protocol of hyperbaric oxygen prior to surgery and will undergo additional hyperbaric oxygen treatments postoperatively.

The treatment options were discussed with the patient in detail, and he consented to the above procedure. All potential risks and complications were discussed, including the potential risk of mandibular fracture, nerve injury to the inferior alveolar and lingual nerves, pain, bleeding, infection, and possible need for further surgical intervention.

DESCRIPTION OF PROCEDURE

The patient was brought to operating room #8 and placed in a supine position on the table. General anesthesia was induced via the nasotracheal route without any difficulty. The patient was then padded, prepped, and draped in the usual sterile fashion.

Lidocaine 2% with epinephrine 1:100,000 was infiltrated into the area of the left buccal vestibule, and a left inferior alveolar nerve block was given. An extended mucosal incision of the ramus was made, and circular incisions were made around teeth #19, #20, and #21, with a small releasing

(continued)

incision through the attached gingiva mesial to tooth #21. The mucosa was reflected both buccally and a little bit lingually in order to gain good access to the posterior mandible and ramus. At this point, tooth #19 was extracted in a simple fashion without any difficulties.

Using a pineapple bur, the bone of the left mandible was débrided under copious irrigation with normal saline. Debridement was done to remove all dead and necrotic bone until good, healthy, bleeding bone was reached. After this was completed, the bone was checked for any sharp areas, and none were present. Any soft tissue was additionally curetted out and sent for specimen.

The wound was then thoroughly irrigated with normal saline, approximately 250 mL. The mucosal incision was closed using 3-0 Vicryl sutures in a horizontal mattress fashion. The throat pack that had been placed prior to beginning the surgical procedure was removed at the end of the surgery. The patient had Marcaine 0.25% with epinephrine 1:200,000 infiltrated into the area of the left buccal vestibule, and a left inferior alveolar nerve block was given.

The patient was suctioned out well and extubated in the operating room without any complications. The patient was taken to the recovery room in stable condition.

OPERATIVE REPORT

PREOPERATIVE DIAGNOSIS
Multiple dental caries. Child unable to cooperate in office setting.

POSTOPERATIVE DIAGNOSIS
Multiple dental caries. Child unable to cooperate in office setting.

ANESTHESIA
General.

PROCEDURE IN DETAIL
The child was escorted to the operating room and placed under general anesthesia with nasotracheal intubation in the supine position in the dental chair. He was shielded with a lead apron, covering the thyroid gland. Two radiographs were obtained. The lead apron was removed and the child was appropriately prepped and draped, and the following dental restorations were performed:

1. Tooth #B, tooth #I, and tooth #S: Sealants.
2. Tooth #L: Occlusal lingual composite resin.
3. Teeth #D, E, F, and G: Composite resin crowns.

Prophylactic and topical fluoride treatment was administered. The throat pack was removed. The oropharynx was evacuated.

The patient was then extubated and taken to the recovery room in responsive condition. Postoperative instructions were given to both parents. There were no complications with this procedure.

OPERATIVE REPORT

PROCEDURE PERFORMED
Bilateral sagittal split mandibular osteotomies with right internal fixation using 2.0-mm Leibinger bone screws, right anterior iliac bone graft to the left cleft area, palatoplasty, and augmentation of the dental alveolar process on the left side of the edentulous area of tooth #10.

PREOPERATIVE DIAGNOSES
1. Cleft palate.
2. Left maxillary hypoplasia.
3. Deficiency in bone over tooth #10 area.
4. Relative mandibular prognathism, class III malocclusion, and functional jaw deformity.

POSTOPERATIVE DIAGNOSES
1. Cleft palate.
2. Left maxillary hypoplasia.
3. Deficiency in bone over tooth #10 area.
4. Relative mandibular prognathism, class III malocclusion, and functional jaw deformity.

PROCEDURE IN DETAIL
After general anesthesia, the patient was sterilely prepped and draped, including the right anterior iliac crest, and then sterile drapes were placed around the oral cavity without touching the oral cavity. Sterile technique was used to take a right anterior iliac bone graft. A Betadine prep was done by the circulating nurse, and a Betadine paint done by myself, followed by a Betadine Tegaderm dressing over this area. A 3-cm curvilinear incision was then made over the right anterior iliac crest with a #10 scalpel blade. Dissection was carried down through the adipose tissue down to the anterior iliac crest with a Bovie in a cutting mode. Several small pieces of fat were removed from the field to gain proper access to the anterior iliac crest.

An incision was made over the periosteum of the right anterior iliac crest with a Bovie in a cutting mode, and a full-thickness subperiosteal flap was elevated on the medial aspect of the right anterior iliac crest. Using the sagittal saw, a corticocancellous chunk of bone was removed from the anterior iliac crest. This was done with ease under copious irrigation. A gouge was then used to take 2 small strips of cancellous bone from the remaining anterior iliac crest area. Excellent hemostasis was identified. Further hemostasis was achieved with bone wax. All excess bone wax was removed. Excellent hemostasis was identified prior to closure and then the layers were closed with #0 Dexon in the deep layers and 5-0 PDS subcutaneously. Good closure was identified, and benzoin, Steri-Strips, a 3 X 3 sponge, and Tegaderm dressing were infiltrated into the right iliac crest for postoperative pain control. At this time, attention was turned to the oral cavity. The bone that was taken out of the hip wound was placed in sterile saline.

Attention was turned to the oral cavity. The mouth and posterior pharynx were suctioned well. A 2-inch throat packing was placed. At this point, an incision was made in the left intraoral region for the sagittal split mandibular osteotomy, and with the Bovie in the cutting mode, a full-thickness mucoperiosteal flap was elevated. A J-stripper or coronoid retractor was used and an inferior border retractor was used. At that time, good exposure for a left sagittal split mandibular osteotomy was achieved. The sagittal split mandibular osteotomy was achieved. The sagittal split mandibular osteotomy was created with a fissure bur under copious irrigation using the Stryker TPA auto-irrigating system. This sagittal split was done with a buccal step modification. All

(continued)

osteotomies were checked for their integrity with a spatula osteotome, and then 8-mm and 10-mm straight osteotomes were used to finish the mandibular osteotomy. This was done with ease. The inferior alveolar nerve was totally in the distal segment without any evidence of direct or indirect nerve trauma.

At this time, the area was irrigated and suctioned well, and a hole was placed in the buccal step osteotomy site with a wire-passing bur under copious irrigation. A 26-gauge stainless steel wire was passed. The same procedure was done on the contralateral side, thus achieving a bilateral sagittal split mandibular osteotomy. This was done with ease without any problems. The inferior alveolar nerve was totally in the distal segment without any evidence of direct or indirect nerve trauma. A hole was placed and a stainless steel wire was placed in this area.

The mouth and posterior pharynx were suctioned well, irrigated well, and suctioned well again. The throat packing was removed, suctioned well again, and then final split was placed. The intermaxillary fixation was achieved via elastic and 26-gauge stainless steel wire. Excellent occlusion was identified. At this time, three 2.0-mm bone screws used in a contra-angle drill and a contra-angle screwdriver were placed in the superior-to-inferior alveolar nerve on both sides of the sagittal split after tightening the wire and removing some excess bone from the sagittal split because the mandible was set back. The bone only had to be removed on the right side because the mandible was asymmetric to the left for the posterior and a shifting to the right movement. There was no bone that had to be taken out to the left sagittal split.

At this time, both osteotomies were done and secured, achieving excellent stability. These areas were irrigated, suctioned well, and then they were closed with 4-0 Vicryl sutures. Good hemostasis was achieved.

An incision was made in the anterior aspect of the maxilla for the cleft site. Subperiosteal dissection was done around the cleft site of edentulous tooth #10. Serious deficiency of bone was identified, and then the corticocancellous block of bone was placed in this area, screwed in with 1.2-mm Leibinger bone screws x3, and then cancellous bone was packed around it. The soft tissue was underlined and closed with 4-0 Vicryl sutures. Excellent closure was identified. The mouth and posterior pharynx were suctioned well, and good hemostasis was identified.

The patient was brought out of anesthesia and sent to the postanesthesia care unit in satisfactory condition.

REVIEW QUESTIONS

The goal of these questions is to test your knowledge in the areas of dentistry and oral surgery.

Directions: Select the correct answer for each of the multiple-choice questions provided below. *Answers are provided at the end of this chapter.*

1. An inflammation of the gums is termed:
   A. Uveitis
   B. Gingivitis
   C. Glossitis
   D. Stomatitis
2. The medical term for bad breath is:
   A. Fetor
   B. Sprue
   C. Halitosis
   D. Dysosmia
3. A dentist who specializes in root canals is called a/an:
   A. Endodontist
   B. Odontologist
   C. Oral maxillofacial surgeon
   D. Periodontist
4. The outer surface of each tooth is called the:
   A. Pulp
   B. Dentin
   C. Enamel
   D. Cementum
5. Which of these are cancers associated with the oral mucosa?
   A. Squamous cell
   B. Melanoma
   C. Fibroma
   D. A & B
6. Surgical removal of a dental root apex is called:
   A. Odontectomy
   B. Dental extraction
   C. Pulpectomy
   D. Apicoectomy
7. The space bounded by the soft palate and tongue between the mouth and pharynx is called the:
   A. Fauces
   B. Choana
   C. Frenum
   D. Kiesselbach area
8. Which medication listed below might be used by a dentist to anesthetize a patient's mouth prior to drilling?
   A. Ketamine
   B. Etomidate
   C. Lidocaine
   D. Diprivan
9. Which piece of equipment might be used by the OMFS following a mandibular fracture?
   A. Arch bars
   B. Surgical rod
   C. Craniofacial appliance
   D. A & C
10. Nitrous oxide is sometimes used by a dentist to:
    A. Provide some pain relief
    B. Prevent intraoral bleeding
    C. Provide inhalation analgesia
    D. A & C
11. The cavity located between the teeth and the cheek is referred to as:
    A. Lingual vestibule
    B. Buccal vestibule
    C. Oropharynx
    D. Nasopharynx

12. The development of teeth is called:
    A. Odontoclast
    B. Odontodysplasia
    C. Odontogenesis
    D. Odontodynia

13. Severe, throbbing facial pain caused by a carious tooth is termed:
    A. Odontoparallaxis
    B. Odontoma
    C. Odontopathy
    D. Odontoneuralgia

14. Grinding of ones teeth, usually during sleep, is called:
    A. Odontagra
    B. Mastication
    C. Bruxism
    D. B & C

15. The definition of periodontitis is:
    A. Severe inflammation of the gums, causing the gum tissue and supporting ligaments to pull away from the tooth and alveolus
    B. Inflammation of the gums due to bacterial plaque
    C. Inflammation of the gums and oral mucosa
    D. A condition characterized by pain, fetid odor, necrosis of gum tissue, fever, and regional lymphadenopathy

16. Another term for smoker's tongue is:
    A. Leukoplakia
    B. Atrophic glossitis
    C. Glossodynia
    D. Strawberry tongue

17. A patient presents to the dentist with jaw pain, facial pain, clicking, an earache, and a headache. The likely diagnosis is:
    A. Adenotonsillitis
    B. Internal TMJ derangement
    C. Tic douloureux
    D. Wisdom tooth impaction

18. A plastic repair of the lips, often done following motor vehicle accidents, is called a:
    A. Cheiloplasty
    B. Glossoplasty
    C. Labioplasty
    D. A & C

19. A stone formation in the salivary gland is termed:
    A. Dacryolith
    B. Endolith
    C. Sialolith
    D. Cheilitis

20. Intermittent episodes of recurrent painful ulcers of the oral mucosa are called:
    A. Linguopapillitis
    B. Palatitis
    C. Aphthous stomatitis
    D. Gingivostomatitis

21. Xerostomia is the medical term for:
    A. Tears of the buccal mucosa
    B. Lacerations of the lingual mucosa
    C. Ulcerations in the oral mucosa
    D. Dry mouth

22. Which of the following are salivary ducts?
    A. Stensen
    B. Wharton
    C. Waldeyer
    D. A & B

23. An oral surgeon dictated the following, "The patient complains of dental pain and was found to have multiple carious teeth." What does carious mean?
    A. Missing
    B. Decayed
    C. Uneven
    D. Stained

24. The term alveolus dentalis is the proper medical term for:
    A. Mandibular teeth
    B. Maxillary teeth
    C. Tooth socket
    D. Tooth drilling

25. The abnormal union of a tooth with the alveolar bone is called:
   A. Dental ankylosis
   B. Perifusion
   C. Dental articulation
   D. Dental bulb

26. Gerodontology is the study of dental problems in:
   A. Anthropology
   B. Forensics
   C. Children
   D. Elderly populations

27. Confinement of a tooth in the alveolus without eruption is termed:
   A. Alveoalgia
   B. Follicle
   C. Impaction
   D. Alveolar osteitis

28. Which of these terms is not used to describe a surface of the tooth?
   A. Mesial
   B. Labial
   C. Incisal
   D. Incisional

29. Crowns, bridges, or dentures attached permanently to the jaw by means of metal anchors, most frequently titanium posts are called:
   A. Dental lamina
   B. Dental implants
   C. Dental orthopedics
   D. Dental prophylaxis

30. The medical term for a toothache is:
   A. Dentalgia
   B. Odontalgia
   C. Odontitis
   D. A & B

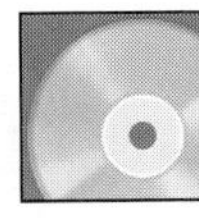

Please see the accompanying CD for additional review materials for this section.

PROOFREADING EXERCISES

These three proofreading exercises are provided to improve your skills in the areas of editing and effective identification and correction of errors in the medical record.

Directions: Identify and correct the transcription errors found in the exercises below. *Answers are provided at the end of this chapter.*

PROOFREADING EXERCISE #1

Thank you for asking me to see your patient. She is known to me do to past necrosis from radiation. She is status post laryngeal carcinoma resection with radiation to her head and neck area many years ago. Presently, she complains of left-sided fascial pain. This has been going on for the past 5 days since loosing her dentures. She complains of increased pain with opening and chewing. She is unable to chew due to the pain which is constant and worse with jaw movement. She does not complain of hypogeusia.

EXAMINATION
Her examination showed diffuse tenderness of her left temporalis, masseter, and sternocleidomastoid. No masses were seen. The skin is intact. Orally, the jaw bone appeared to be sound with no ulceration or signs of ostial radial necrosis.

DIAGNOSIS
She probably has acute muscle spasms due to loss of support in her jaws.

PLAN
Her sutures need to be replaced in order to treat this condition. She may need muscle injections if her pain continues. I have asked Dr. Smith to see the patient since he fabricated the first dentures which adequately treated her problem in the past.

PROOFREADING EXERCISE #2

PREOPERATIVE DIAGNOSIS
Odontogenic keratocyst of anterior mandible.

POSTOPERATIVE DIAGNOSIS
Same.

PROCEDURES
1. Enucleation and curettage of odontogenic keratocyst via intraaural approaches.
2. Extraction of teeth #2, #10, #13, #23-S, and #32.

ANESTHESIA
General.

ESTIMATED BLOOD LOSS
Minimal.

IV FLUIDS
1100 mL.

URINE OUTPUT
Not recorded.

SPECIMENS
1. Anterior mandibular cyst.
2. Impacted tooth #23-S.
3. Teeth #2, #10, #13, and #32.

COMPLICATIONS
None.

JUSTIFICATION FOR PROCEDURE
The patient is a 56-year-old female with biopsy-driven odontogenic keratocyst of the anterior mandible, associated with an impacted tooth, supernumerary #23. The patient has clinical evidence of buckle expansion of cortex in the anterior mandible. Diagnostic images were obtained and reviewed. All treatment options were discussed in detail. The patient was competent, and agreed and consented to nucleation and curettage of

(continued)

anterior mandibular cyst with general and local anesthesia in the operating room. The patient understood the risks and complications that were possible, and need for further surgical intervention.

DESCRIPTION OF THE PROCEDURE

The patient was brought to the operating room and placed in the prone position on the table. General anesthesia was induced without difficulty. The patient was padded, then prepped and draped in the normal sterile fashion. A time-out was taken. 10 mL of Lidocaine 2% with 1 to 100,000 epinephrine was infiltrated intraorally, and a left inferior alveolar nerve block was infiltrated in the vestibule.

A #15 blade was used to make a sulcular incision extending from the lower right first premolar area, with a vertical release at that point to the contrail lateral canine area. A full-thickness mucoperiosteal flap was elevated down to the inferior border of the maxilla. The expanded buccal cortex was visualized, along with a perforation in one area of the buccal cortex, which was probably the area of the decisional biopsy site. At this point, a #4 round burr on a Micro-100 drill was used to uncover and decorate the buccal aspect of the lesion. After the decortication, the cyst was enucleated, removed in toto, and sent as a permanent specimen.

At this point, a #702 tapered bur on a Micro-100 drill was used to expose more of the impacted supernumerary tooth #23. After sectioning of the tooth, it was elevated in 3 pieces. At this point, a pineapple bur on a Micro-100 drill was used to perform a peripheral ostectomy of the cavity. There was a small lingual perforation of the cortex. All bleeders were controlled with bruit electrocautery. The surgical area was irrigated thoroughly with normal saline. Closure of the incision was performed using 3-0 chromic interrupted sutures.

At this point, attention was turned to the upper right quadrant, where tooth #2 was extracted. In addition, teeth #10, #13, and #32 were extracted after administration of a total of an additional 5 mL of 2% lidocaine with one 2-100,000 epinephrine. Homeostasis was observed. The previously placed throat pack was removed, and the oral pharynx was suctioned.

There were no complications encountered throughout the surgery. All sponge and needle counts were correct. The patient was intubated in the operating room and taken to the recovery room in stable condition.

PROOFREADING EXERCISE #3

PREOPERATIVE DIAGNOSES
Fractures of the mandible.

POSTOPERATIVE DIAGNOSIS
Fractures of the mandible.

PROCEDURE
Closed reduction fractures of the mandible with application of dental arch bars.

ANESTHESIA
General.

PRELIMINARY NOTE
This is a 17-year-old young man involved in an alteration and reportedly was kicked in the foot by a jaw. He suffered bilateral fractures of the mandible with fractures on the right side in the middle of the body and on the left side in the angle near an unerupted moler. There was missive swelling, and he was given cold compresses. He is brought now for an attempted closed reduction with the understanding that if we are not successful, we may have to do an open procedure.

PROCEDURE
The patient was put to sleep by general endotracheal anesthesia. The face was prepared and draped in the usual manner. Manually inducing the fracture appeared to be quite satisfactory, and the teeth were in fairly good repair with excellent hygiene. Dental ark bars were applied to the mandible and the maxilla using #22 stainless steal wire. A trial of exclusions seemed satisfactory. Rubber bands will be applied once the patient is awake and alert, either later today or tomorrow.

The procedure was well tolerated and the patient was returned to the postanesthesia recovery room in satisfactory condition.

ANSWER KEYS

REVIEW QUESTIONS ANSWER KEY

1. B
2. C
3. A
4. C
5. D
6. D
7. A
8. C
9. D
10. D
11. B
12. C
13. D
14. C
15. A
16. A
17. B
18. D
19. C
20. C
21. D
22. D
23. B
24. C
25. A
26. D
27. C
28. D
29. B
30. D

PROOFREADING EXERCISE #1 KEY

Incorrect spelling—due

Incorrect spelling—facial

Incorrect word—losing

Incorrect spelling—osteoradio-necrosis

Incorrect word—dentures

Thank you for asking me to see your patient. She is known to me do to past necrosis from radiation. She is status post laryngeal carcinoma resection with radiation to her head and neck area many years ago. Presently, she complains of left-sided fascial pain. This has been going on for the past 5 days since loosing her dentures. She complains of increased pain with opening and chewing. She is unable to chew due to the pain which is constant and worse with jaw movement. She does not complain of hypogeusia.

EXAMINATION
Her examination showed diffuse tenderness of her left temporalis, masseter, and sternocleidomastoid. No masses were seen. The skin is intact. Orally, the jaw bone appeared to be sound with no ulceration or signs of ostial radial necrosis.

DIAGNOSIS
She probably has acute muscle spasms due to loss of support in her jaws.

PLAN
Her sutures need to be replaced in order to treat this condition. She may need muscle injections if her pain continues. I have asked Dr. Smith to see the patient since he fabricated the first dentures which adequately treated her problem in the past.

PROOFREADING EXERCISE #2 KEY

Type full text of diagnosis.

Incorrect term—intraoral

Incorrect term—proven

Incorrect spelling—buccal

PREOPERATIVE DIAGNOSIS
Odontogenic keratocyst of anterior mandible.

POSTOPERATIVE DIAGNOSIS
Same.

PROCEDURES
1. Enucleation and curettage of odontogenic keratocyst via intraaural approaches.
2. Extraction of teeth #2, #10, #13, #23-S, and #32.

ANESTHESIA
General.

ESTIMATED BLOOD LOSS
Minimal.

IV FLUIDS
1100 mL.

URINE OUTPUT
Not recorded.

SPECIMENS
1. Anterior mandibular cyst.
2. Impacted tooth #23-S.
3. Teeth #2, #10, #13, and #32.

COMPLICATIONS
None.

JUSTIFICATION FOR PROCEDURE
The patient is a 56-year-old female with biopsy-driven odontogenic keratocyst of the anterior mandible, associated with an impacted tooth, supernumerary #23. The patient has clinical evidence of buckle expansion of cortex in the anterior mandible. Diagnostic images were

(continued)

Needs prefix—enucleation

obtained and reviewed. All treatment options were discussed in detail. The patient was competent, and agreed and consented to nucleation and curettage of anterior mandibular cyst with general and local anesthesia in the operating room. The patient understood the risks and complications that were possible, and need for further surgical intervention.

Incorrect position—supine

DESCRIPTION OF THE PROCEDURE
The patient was brought to the operating room and placed in the prone position on the table. General anesthesia was induced without difficulty. The patient was padded, then prepped and draped in the normal sterile fashion. A time-out was taken. 10 mL of Lidocaine 2% with 1 to 100,000 epinephrine was infiltrated intraorally, and a left inferior alveolar nerve block was infiltrated in the vestibule.

Incorrect format—1:100,000

Recast sentence so it does not begin with a number

A #15 blade was used to make a sulcular incision extending from the lower right first premolar area, with a vertical release at that point to the contrail lateral canine area. A full-thickness mucoperiosteal flap was elevated down to the inferior border of the maxilla. The expanded buccal cortex was visualized, along with a perforation in one area of the buccal cortex, which was probably the area of the decisional biopsy site. At this point, a #4 round burr on a Micro-100 drill was used to uncover and decorate the buccal aspect of the lesion. After the decortication, the cyst was enucleated, removed in toto, and sent as a permanent specimen.

Incorrect term—contralateral

Incorrect term—incisional

Incorrect term—decorticate

At this point, a #702 tapered bur on a Micro-100 drill was used to expose more of the impacted supernumerary tooth #23. After sectioning of the tooth, it was elevated in 3 pieces. At this point, a pineapple bur on a Micro-100 drill was used to perform a peripheral ostectomy of the cavity. There was a small lingual perforation of the cortex.

Incorrect term—Bovie

All bleeders were controlled with bruit electrocautery. The surgical area was irrigated thoroughly with normal saline. Closure of the incision was performed using 3-0 chromic interrupted sutures.

Incorrect format—1:100,000

Incorrect term—hemostasis

At this point, attention was turned to the upper right quadrant, where tooth #2 was extracted. In addition, teeth #10, #13, and #32 were extracted after administration of a total of an additional 5 mL of 2% lidocaine with one 2-100,000 epinephrine. Homeostasis was observed. The previously placed throat pack was removed, and the oral pharynx was suctioned.

Use combined form—oropharynx

Incorrect term—extubated

There were no complications encountered throughout the surgery. All sponge and needle counts were correct. The patient was intubated in the operating room and taken to the recovery room in stable condition.

PROOFREADING EXERCISE #3 KEY

PREOPERATIVE DIAGNOSES
Fractures of the mandible.

POSTOPERATIVE DIAGNOSIS
Fractures of the mandible.

PROCEDURE
Closed reduction fractures of the mandible with application of dental arch bars.

ANESTHESIA
General.

PRELIMINARY NOTE
This is a 17-year-old young man involved in an alteration and reportedly was kicked in the foot by a jaw. He suffered bilateral fractures of the mandible with fractures on the right side in the middle of the body and on the left side in the angle near an unerupted moler. There was missive swelling, and he was given cold compresses. He is brought now for an attempted closed reduction with the understanding that if we are not successful, we may have to do an open procedure.

PROCEDURE
The patient was put to sleep by general endotracheal anesthesia. The face was prepared and draped in the usual manner. Manually inducing the fracture appeared to be quite satisfactory, and the teeth were in fairly good repair with excellent hygiene. Dental ark bars were applied to the mandible and the maxilla using #22 stainless steal wire. A trial of exclusions seemed satisfactory. Rubber bands will be applied once the patient is awake and alert, either later today or tomorrow.

The procedure was well tolerated and the patient was returned to the postanesthesia recovery room in satisfactory condition.

Missing word—reduction **of** fractures

Incorrect word—altercation

Incorrect spelling—molar

Incorrect term—arch

Incorrect term—occlusions

Words transposed—jaw by a foot

Incorrect word—massive

Incorrect term—reducing

Incorrect spelling—steel

SECTION III

English Language

CHAPTER

26

Grammar

OBJECTIVES CHECKLIST

A prepared exam candidate will know the:

- ❑ Identification and function of all eight (8) parts of speech utilized in the English language.
- ❑ Component parts of a sentence, including compound constructions.
- ❑ Identification and function of the five (5) types of phrases utilized in sentence construction.
- ❑ Identification and function of both independent and dependent clauses.
- ❑ Six types of dependent, or subordinate, clauses.
- ❑ Classification of sentences by structure.
- ❑ Classification of sentences by purpose.

RESOURCES FOR STUDY

1. *The AAMT Book of Style for Medical Transcription*
   Adjectives, pp. 12–13.
   Adverbs, pp. 14–15.
   Appositives, pp. 29–30.
   Articles, pp. 31–32.
   Clause, pp. 79–82.
   Elliptical construction, p. 160.
   Grammar, p. 196.
   Nouns, pp. 274–275.
   Phrases, pp. 314–316.
   Pronouns, pp. 334–336.
   Sentences, pp. 357–360.
   Verbs, pp. 409–413.
2. *The Gregg Reference Manual: A Manual of Style, Grammar, Usage, and Formatting*
3. *American Medical Association Manual of Style*

PART 1: PARTS OF SPEECH

There are eight (8) classes into which words are grouped according to their uses in a sentence:

1. **Noun:** the name of a person, place, object, idea, quality, or activity.
   a. **abstract noun:** the name of a quality or general idea.

      Examples: *faith, hope, love*

   b. **collective noun:** a noun that represents a group of people, animals, or things.

      Examples: *team, herd, audience*

   c. **common noun:** the name of a class of people, places, or things.

      Examples: *parent, student, teacher, dog*

   d. **predicate noun:** a word or phrase that follows a linking verb, completes the sense of the verb, and explains the subject.
      A predicate noun is also identical to the subject.

      Examples:
      Sally is our <u>*president*</u>.
      Mr. Jones was <u>*principal*</u> *of my high school.*

   e. **proper noun:** the official name of a particular person, place, or thing.

      Examples: *George Washington, Florida, Great Dane, White House.*

2. **Verb:** a word or phrase used to express action or a state of being.
   a. **helping verb:** a verb that helps in the formation of another verb.
      The primary helping verbs are *be, can, could, do, have, may, might, must, ought, shall, should, will,* and *would*. They precede other verbs to form the predicate.

      Examples:
      He <u>*might*</u> *go to the meeting.*
      I <u>*will*</u> *walk the dog later.*

   b. **transitive verb**: a verb that requires an object to complete its meaning.

      Example:
      He has cancelled the meeting (the verb *has cancelled* requires the object *meeting)*

   c. **intransitive verb:** a verb that does *not* require an object to complete its meaning.

      Examples:
      Member participation has increased.
      The wind blows.

   d. **linking verb**: a verb that connects a subject with the predicate adjective, noun, or pronoun.
      The most common linking verbs are the various forms of the verb "to be."

      Examples:
      He will be team captain. (the verb *will be* links *He* and *captain)*
      The company is happy with its growth. (the verb *is* links *company* and *happy)*

3. **Adjective:** a single word, phrase, or clause that answers the question *what kind, how many,* or *which one* and modifies the meaning of a noun or pronoun.
   The articles *(a, an,* and *the)* are also considered adjectives.

   Examples:

excellent prognosis	*eight* grandchildren
the latest results	*green* sputum
a man *of great integrity*	*silly* me
open incision	*lovely* girl

4. **Adverb:** a single word, phrase, or clause that answers the question *when, where, why, in what manner,* or *to what extent* and modifies the meaning of a verb, adjective, or another adverb.
   Hint: Adverbs often end in "ly."

   Examples:
   She spoke <u>clearly</u> when giving her instructions.
   The physician seemed <u>sincerely</u> concerned about his patients.
   The patient was <u>well</u> developed and <u>well</u> nourished.

5. **Pronoun:** a word used in place of a noun.
   Exception: Possessive pronouns function as adjectives in the sentence because they precede and modify a noun rather than replace it.

   a. **personal:** *I, you, he, she, it, we, they*

   b. **possessive**: *my/mine, his, her/hers, its, our/ours, their/theirs,* and *your/yours*

   b. **demonstrative:** *this, that, these, those*

   c. **indefinite:** *each, either, any, anyone, someone, few, all,* etc.

   d. **intensive:** *myself, yourself, himself, herself,* etc.

   e. **interrogative:** *who, which, what,* etc.

   f. **relative:** *who, whose, whom, which, that,* and compounds like *whoever, whomever,* etc.

6. **Preposition:** a word used to show the relation of a noun or pronoun to some other word in the sentence.
   A preposition always appears in a phrase (called the *prepositional phrase),* with the preposition usually at the beginning and the noun/pronoun at the end of the phrase as the *object.* Together, the preposition and noun (along with any modifiers) form a phrase that describes another word in the sentence.

Example:
The beautiful painting <u>*on the wall*</u> *is a DaVinci. (on* is the preposition, *wall* is the object, and the prepositional phrase *on the wall* describes the noun *painting)*

Commonly Used Prepositions

about	at	but (meaning "except")
above	before	by
across	behind	concerning
after	below	down
against	beneath	during
along	beside	except
amid	besides	for
among	between	from
around	beyond	in

Note: Prepositions are often directional, and the old schoolhouse hint was that prepositions were "anything an airplane could do to a cloud," meaning that the preposition describes the directional relationship between the airplane and a cloud.

7. **Conjunction:** a word or phrase that connects words, phrases, or clauses.
   a. **coordinating conjunction:** connects words, phrases or clauses of equal rank. The coordinating conjunctions are *and, but, or, nor,* and *for.*
   b. **correlative conjunction:** conjunction consisting of two elements used in pairs.

      Examples: *both. . .and, not only. . .but (also), either. . .or,* and *neither. . .nor*
   c. **subordinating conjunction:** used to join subordinate, or dependent, clauses to independent clauses; however, it does not need to link the dependent clause to the independent clause. It often can occur at the *beginning* of a sentence to introduce the subordinate clause.

      Examples:
      We stayed indoors <u>*until*</u> *the storm abated.*
      <u>*When*</u> *I take a test, I get very nervous.* (simply a recasting of the sentence, *I get very nervous* <u>*when*</u> *I take a test.)*
8. **Interjection**: a word that shoes emotion, usually without grammatical connection to other parts of a sentence.

   Examples:
   Oh! *My goodness!* *Hurry!* *Ah!* *Ouch!* *Wow!*

REVIEW EXERCISE: PARTS OF SPEECH

The following paragraph contains numbered, italicized words. For each, indicate the part of speech (noun, verb, adjective, adverb, pronoun, preposition, conjunction, or interjection). For the nouns, verbs, pronouns, and conjunctions, indicate the type.

The (1) *patient* presented to the office (2) *with* a complaint of (3) *shortness* of breath (4) *and* productive cough (5) *although* it (6) *has* been of (7) *short* duration. On (8) *my* evaluation (9) *today,* she appeared (10) *tired* and ill. (11) *Her* skin was (12) *slightly* dry, indicating (13) *some* dehydration. There was some (14) *redness* of the throat, and her nose showed moist (15) *but* congested (16) *mucous* membranes. (17) *When* I auscultated (18) *the* lungs, they were clear (19) *bilaterally,* and breath sounds were equal on (20) *both* sides.

PART 2: PARTS OF A SENTENCE

1. **Subject and Predicate**

   A sentence consists of two parts: the *subject* and the *predicate.* The *subject* of the sentence is that part about which something is being said. The *predicate* is that part which says something about the subject.

   Examples:

Subject	Predicate
Faculty and students	*planned a new class schedule.*
The beautiful woman	*kissed the handsome man.*

   a. **simple subjects and verbs**

   The whole subject is called the *complete subject,* but the *simple subject* is the principal word or group of words in the subject.

   Example:
   The old book on the table was a favorite of her grandmother's.
   Subject: *The old book on the table*
   Simple subject: *book*

   The whole predicate is called the complete predicate, but the principal word or group of words in the predicate is called the simple predicate, or the verb.

   Example:
   The teachers planned a dynamic new course curriculum.
   Predicate: *planned a dynamic new course curriculum.*
   Simple predicate, or verb: *planned*

   b. **compound subjects and verbs**

   A *compound subject* consists of two or more subjects that are joined by a conjunction and have the same verb. The usual connecting words are *and* and *or.*

   Example:
   The White House and the Pentagon called an emergency press conference.
   Compound subject: *White House and Pentagon*

   A *compound verb* consists of two or more verbs that are joined by a conjunction and have the same subject.

   Example:
   The team improved its defensive strategy and performed much better in their next few games.
   Compound verb: *improved* and *performed*

2. **Complements**

   Some sentences express a complete thought by means of a subject and verb only.

   Examples:

Subject	Verb
The girl	*cried.*
Everybody	*left.*

However, most sentences have one or more words in the predicate that complete the meaning of the subject and verb. These completing words are called *complements.*

Examples:

Subject	Verb	Complement
John and Ed	*caught*	*five wide-mouthed bass.*
She	*handed*	*me a stack of books.*
Your brother	*seems*	*very happy.*

Complements fall into two categories: *objects and subject complements.*

a. **objects**

Complements that receive or are affected by the action of the verb are called *objects.* The *direct object* of the verb receives the action of the verb or shows the result of the action. It answers the question *What?* or *Whom?* after an action verb.

Examples:
I took my lunch with me. (I took *what?*)
The patient told me she was in pain. (The patient told *whom?*)
He tried to reason with her. (He tried *what?*)

The *indirect object* of the verb precedes the direct object and usually tells *to whom* or *for whom* the action of the verb is done.

Examples:
*Fed-Ex delivered the package to me. (package—direct object; to me—*indirect object*)*
*The salesman showed me the latest arrivals. (arrivals—direct object; me—*indirect object*)*

b. **subject complements**

Complements that refer to (describe, explain, or identify) the subject are *subject complements.* A *predicate nominative* is a noun or pronoun complement that refers to the same person or thing as the subject of the verb. *It follows a linking verb.*

Examples:
Aunt Clara is my oldest relative. (relative refers to *Aunt Clara)*
He will be president next year. (president refers to *He)*

A *predicate adjective* is an adjective complement that modifies the subject of the verb. It also follows a linking verb.

Example:
The stray dog was very thin. (thin refers to *dog)*

c. **compound complements**

Two or more complements joined by a conjunction are called compound complements.

Examples:
Andrew gave David and me two tickets to the concert. (David and *me*—compound indirect object)
She was tired and hungry. (tired and hungry—compound predicate adjective*)*

REVIEW EXERCISE: PARTS OF A SENTENCE

For each of the 10 sentences below, identify the subject(s), verb(s), direct objects, indirect objects, predicate nominatives, and predicate adjectives.

1. The laboratory results showed protein in the urine.
2. The daughter and son told me the story.
3. Examination revealed exquisite tenderness and guarding of the abdomen.
4. Dr. Smith is a specialist in reproductive health and excellent with this particular problem.
5. Upon admission, the patient received fluids and oxygen and improved on this regimen.
6. Despite aggressive chemotherapy, the tumor was unaffected and continued its progression.
7. She was given at-home care directions and told to follow up with me.
8. Take the medicine with food and call me tomorrow.
9. Whatever is wrong will be determined by diagnostic testing.
10. The patient never claimed to be disoriented but did seem confused on questioning.

PART 3: PHRASES

1. **Phrase:** a group of words not containing a verb and its subject.
   Phrases are used as a single part of speech.

   a. **prepositional phrase:** a group of words beginning with a preposition and usually ending with a noun or pronoun that functions as the *object* of the preposition.
   Prepositional phrases are usually used as *adjective phrases* (modifying a noun) or as *adverb phrases* (modifying a verb). Adverb phrases answer the question *how, when, where, to what extent,* or *why.* Occasionally, prepositional phrases are used as nouns.

   Examples:
   The book on the table is mine. (on the table is an *adjective phrase* modifying the noun *book)*
   The falcon can fly at great speeds for long distances. (at great speeds and *for long distances* are *adverb phrases* modifying the verb *can fly)*
   After dinner will be too late. *(after dinner* is the subject and is used as a noun*)*

   b. **participles and participial phrases**
   A *participle* is a verb form (often identified by its present tense *-ing* ending or by its past tense *-ed, -d, -t, -en,* or *-n* endings) that is used as an adjective.

   Examples:
   The developing storm threatened to ruin the picnic.
   A watched pot never boils.
   I found him sleeping in the hammock.

   A *participial phrase* is a phrase containing a participle and any complements or modifiers it may have. The participle usually introduces the phrase, and the entire phrase acts as an adjective to modify a noun or pronoun.

   Examples:
   Michael Jordan, playing with skill, led the Bulls to victory. (phrase modifies the noun *Michael Jordan)*
   Getting up at 5 a.m., we got an early start. (phrase modifies the noun *we)*
   The firefighters arrived on the scene to find the church destroyed by fire. (phrase modifies the noun *church)*

   c. **gerunds and gerund phrases**
   A gerund is a verb form ending in *-ing* that is used as a noun.

   Examples:
   Swimming is good exercise.
   Good writing comes from much practice.
   It takes a lot of studying to pass that examination.

   A *gerund phrase* is a phrase consisting of a gerund and any complements or modifiers it may have. Like the gerund alone, the gerund phrase may be used in any place that a noun would be used.

   Examples:
   Wearing a flag pin is a great way to express patriotism. (phrase functions as the subject)
   Her idea of selling tickets to raise money is a good one. (phrase functions as the object of the preposition *of)*
   The school advises paying your registration fees by tomorrow. (phrase functions as the direct object of the verb *advises)*

d. **infinitives and infinitive phrases**

An *infinitive* is a verb form, usually preceded by the word *to*, that is used as a noun or a modifier. Sometimes the word *to* is implied in an infinitive expression.

Examples:
We want to go to the beach on Sunday.
To achieve success, a person must work hard.
To forgive is divine.
He helped me [to] do my homework.

Note: Do not confuse infinitives that begin with the word *to* with prepositional phrases that begin with *to*.

He gave the medicine to me. (prepositional phrase)
He gave the medicine to help me. (infinitive phrase)

An *infinitive phrase* consists of an infinitive and any complements or modifiers it may have. Like infinitives alone, infinitive phrases can be used as nouns or modifiers.

Examples:
We tried to reason with her. (phrase as direct object of *tried)*
To save money became her obsession. (phrase as subject)
I am too busy to go to the store with you tonight. (phrase modifies the adjective *busy)*
His plan is to go to graduate school next year. (phrase as predicate nominative)

e. **appositives**

An *appositive* is a noun or pronoun—often with modifiers—set beside another noun or pronoun to explain or identify it.

Examples:
My brother Todd is coming over for dinner.
John's father, a physician, chaired the committee last year.

An *appositive phrase* is a phrase consisting of an appositive and its modifiers. An appositive phrase usually follows the word it explains or identifies, but it may precede it.

Examples:
He donated the car, an old Volkswagen Beetle, to a local charity.
A fascinating thriller, the book is still one of my favorites.

REVIEW EXERCISE: PHRASES

The following paragraph contains numbered, italicized phrases. For each, indicate the type of phrase (prepositional, participial, gerund, infinitive, or appositive); in the case of prepositional phrases, indicate whether the phrase is used as an adjective or an adverb phrase.

As technology advances (1) *by leaps and bounds*, the healthcare industry faces the potential (2) *for great change*. One obvious way (3) *to embrace this evolving science* is (4) *to focus on advanced treatment technologies*. (5) *Looking for treatment solutions* is one way to drive the development (6) *of technology*. (7) *For years*, patients have benefited (8) *from life-saving advances* (9) *in technology*. Refined surgical instrumentation, (10) *a critical area of developing technologies*, has been one outcome of this area of scientific focus. (11) *Using statistical data based on treatment outcomes*, technology experts are able (12) *to develop advanced tools* (13) *for improving patient care*. Such tools, (14) *in the hands* of a skilled practitioner, can generate improved treatment outcomes, (15) *a desirable goal for any healthcare provider*. (16) *For many reasons*, this is good news (17) *for the industry*, (18) *pressured to lower costs and improve patient care*. The quality of patient care (19) *in the future* can only benefit from (20) *developing more advanced technology solutions*.

PART 4: CLAUSES

A *clause* is a group of words containing a subject and predicate and used as a part of a sentence. Clauses are classified according to grammatical completeness. Those that can stand alone when removed from their sentences are called *independent clauses.* Those that do not express a complete thought and cannot stand alone are called *dependent*, or *subordinate*, clauses.

1. **Independent Clauses**

   When removed from its sentence, an *independent clause* makes complete sense. When written with a capital at the beginning and a period at the end, it becomes a *simple sentence.* It is only referred to as an *independent clause* when it exists in a larger sentence with one or more additional clauses, whether independent or dependent.

   Examples:
   The patient was discharged. (simple sentence)
   Once her condition improved, the patient was discharged. (independent clause within the sentence)

2. **Dependent Clauses**

   Dependent clauses, which cannot stand alone as sentences, are used as nouns or modifiers in the same way as single words and phrases. A dependent clause is always combined in some way with an independent clause. A dependent clause, like a sentence, has a verb and a subject and may contain complements and modifiers. It is the *entire* clause that functions as the noun or modifier, and it is important not to confuse these with *independent clauses* merely because they contain a subject and verb.

   Examples:
   Whoever knows the song may join in.
   We ordered spaghetti, which everyone in the family likes.
   As she had guessed, her car was out of gas.

   a. **adjective clauses**

      Like a phrase, an *adjective clause* is a dependent clause that functions as an adjective by modifying a noun or pronoun.

      Examples:
      The house where he was born was still in very good condition. (clause modifies *house*)
      The letter, which I wrote to the editor last month, is going to be published in the next issue. (clause modifies *letter*)

      Note: Adjective clauses often begin with a relative pronoun (*who, whom, which,* or *that*) the relative adjective *whose*, or the relative adverb *where* or *when*. These refer to, or are *related* to, a noun or pronoun that has come before. The noun or pronoun to which these relative terms refer is called the *antecedent.*

      A relative pronoun, adjective or adverb does three things: (1) it refers to a preceding noun or pronoun; (2) it connects its clause with the rest of the sentence; (3) it performs a function within its own clause by serving as the subject, object, etc., of the dependent clause.

      Examples:
      Richard is a friend whom we can trust. (refers to *friend*, links the clause to the sentence and serves as the direct object of the verb *trust* within its clause)
      He is a coach whose record has been amazing. (refers to *coach*, links the clause to the sentence and serves as an adjective modifying *record*)

b. **noun clauses**

A *noun clause* is a dependent clause that is used as a noun.

Examples:

Whoever wins the election will have big shoes to fill. (clause functions as subject)
The details of what she does are not known to me. (clause functions as the object of the preposition *of*)
I know whose car this is. (clause functions as the direct object of the verb *know*)

c. **adverb clauses**

An *adverb clause* is a dependent clause that, like an adverb, modifies a verb, adjective, or adverb. Adverb clauses often begin with a *subordinating conjunction*, a conjunction that joins the clause to the rest of the sentence.

Common Subordinating Conjunctions

after	because	so that	whenever
although	before	than	where
as	if	though	wherever
as if	in order that	unless	whether
as long as	provided that	until	while
as though	since	when	

Examples:

She writes in her diary like she is in a great hurry. (how?)
She writes in her diary before she goes to sleep. (when?)
She writes in her diary wherever the light is strongest. (where?)
She writes in her diary because she enjoys it. (why?)
She writes in her diary as often as she can. (to what extent?)
She writes in her diary if she gets to bed early. (under what conditions?)

d. **elliptical clauses**

Sometimes in our writing and speaking, we do not complete the adverb clauses we use. The omitted part of the clause is implied and is said to be *elliptical*.

Examples:

I am stronger than you (are).
While (I was) *waiting for the doctor, the patient fell asleep.*

REVIEW EXERCISE: CLAUSES

Each of the following sentences contains one or more dependent clauses in italics. Indicate whether it is an adjective, noun, or adverb clause.

1. *When you draw blood from a patient,* you should wear appropriate gloves, *which can protect both you and the patient.*
2. The last chemotherapy trial worked better *than the first one did.*
3. Only children *who are under the age of two* should receive this immunization.
4. He had no explanation for *what he was doing.*
5. *Whatever the patient says* has to be clinically correlated *so that we can accurately document the present illness.*
6. She is confident *that her test results will be negative.*
7. I know *where she lives,* and *driving there* will take awhile.
8. The brace *that I gave her on her last visit* has greatly improved her symptoms, *which were rather severe at that time.*
9. Patients *whose symptoms are unrelieved by steroid injection* will likely not respond well to surgical intervention.
10. He works for the clinic *where you had your previous surgery.*

PART 5: SENTENCE CLASSIFICATION

1. **Sentences Classified by Structure**
   Classified according to their structure, there are four kinds of sentences: *simple, compound, complex,* and *compound-complex.*

   a. **simple sentence**
   A *simple sentence* is a sentence with one independent clause and no dependent clauses.

   Examples:
   Great literature stirs the imagination.
   Great literature stirs the imagination and challenges the intellect. (compound predicate in a simple sentence)

   b. **compound sentence**
   A *compound sentence* is a sentence composed of two or more independent clauses but no dependent clauses.

   Example:
   Great literature stirs the imagination, and <u>it</u> challenges the intellect. (two independent clauses joined by the conjunction *and)*

   c. **complex sentence**
   A *complex sentence* is a sentence that contains one independent clause and at least one dependent clause.

   Example:
   Great literature, which stirs the imagination, also challenges the intellect. (single independent clause with an interruptive dependent clause)

   d. **compound-complex sentence**
   A *compound-complex sentence* is a sentence that contains two or more independent clauses (compound) and at least one dependent clause (complex).

   Example:
   Great literature, which challenges the intellect, is sometimes difficult, but it is also rewarding. (two independent clauses joined by the conjunction *but,* with an interruptive dependent clause in the first independent clause)

2. **Sentences Classified by Purpose**
   Classified according to their purpose, there are four kinds of sentences: *declarative, imperative, interrogative,* and *exclamatory.*

   a. **declarative sentence**
   A *declarative sentence* is a sentence that makes a statement.

   Examples:
   In 1492, Columbus discovered the Americas.
   The dog was sleeping on the back porch.

   b. **imperative sentence**
   An *imperative sentence* is a sentence that gives a command or makes a request.

   Examples:
   Stop talking and finish eating your supper.
   Please give me a chance to explain.
   Don't ride a motorcycle without a helmet.

c. **interrogative sentence**
An *interrogative sentence* is a sentence that asks a question.

Examples:
Which medication did you take?
Are you going to the theater on Friday night?

d. **exclamatory sentence**
An *exclamatory sentence* is one that expresses a strong feeling.

Examples:
How amazing!
It's a miracle!
Freeze!

REVIEW EXERCISE: SENTENCE CLASSIFICATION

For each of the following sentences, indicate the classification by structure and purpose.

1. According to the patient, she has had a long history of urinary tract infections, and she is used to taking antibiotics periodically for these.
2. After you spent all those years in college, why would you decide to become a bartender?
3. We really needed her help in developing a new strategy for membership growth and marketing our benefits.
4. The patient complained of severe restrictive chest pain, but we ruled out an MI with EKG and cardiac enzymes.
5. If you touch me, I will call the police!
6. Let me have your order tomorrow if you can.
7. Despite her mild improvement on this regimen, I am going to try her on a different protocol, and we'll see if we get better result.
8. Watch out!
9. Take this medication, which I'm giving you a prescription for, and be sure to call me if your symptoms don't improve.
10. How much longer do we have to wait for the doctor to arrive?

ANSWER KEYS

REVIEW EXERCISES ANSWER KEY

Part 1: Parts of Speech

1. noun (common)
2. preposition
3. noun (abstract)
4. conjunction (coordinating)
5. conjunction (subordinating)
6. verb (linking)
7. adjective
8. pronoun (possessive) *Note: Adjective is also an acceptable answer.*
9. adverb
10. adjective
11. pronoun (possessive) *Note: Adjective is also an acceptable answer.*
12. adverb
13. adjective
14. noun
15. conjunction (coordinating)
16. adjective
17. conjunction (subordinating)
18. adjective
19. adverb
20. adjective

Part 2: Parts of a Sentence

1. *results* (subject), *showed* (verb), *protein* (direct object)
2. *daughter* and *son* (compound subject), *told* (verb), *me* (indirect object), *story* (direct object)
3. *Examination* (subject), *revealed* (verb), *tenderness* and *guarding* (compound direct object)
4. *Dr. Smith* (subject), *is* (verb), *specialist* (predicate nominative), *excellent* (predicate adjective)
5. *patient* (subject), *received* and *improved* (compound verb), *fluids* and *oxygen* (compound direct object of *received*)
6. *tumor* (subject), *was unaffected* and *continued* (compound verb), *progression* (direct object of *continued*)
7. *She* (subject), *was given* and *told* (compound verb), *directions* (direct object of *was given*) and *to follow up with me* (direct object of *told*)
8. *You* (implied subject), *take* and *call* (compound verb), *medicine* (direct object of *take*) and *me* (direct object of *call*)
9. *Whatever is wrong* (subject), *will be determined* (verb)
10. *patient* (subject), *claimed* and *seemed* (compound verb), *to be disoriented* (direct object of *claimed*), *confused* (predicate adjective)

Part 3: Phrases

1. prepositional (adverb)
2. prepositional (adjective)
3. infinitive
4. infinitive
5. gerund
6. prepositional (adjective)
7. prepositional (adverb)
8. prepositional (adverb)
9. prepositional (adjective)
10. appositive
11. participial
12. infinitive

13. prepositional (adjective)
14. prepositional (adverb)
15. appositive
16. prepositional (adverb)
17. prepositional (adjective)
18. participial
19. prepositional (adverb)
20. gerund

Part 4: Clauses

1. adverb, adjective
2. adverb
3. adjective
4. noun
5. noun, adverb
6. adverb
7. noun, noun
8. adjective, adjective
9. adjective
10. adjective

Part 5: Sentence Classification

1. compound-complex, declarative
2. complex, interrogative
3. simple, declarative
4. compound, declarative
5. complex, exclamatory
6. complex, imperative
7. compound-complex, declarative
8. simple, exclamatory
9. compound-complex, imperative
10. simple, interrogative

CHAPTER

27

Punctuation Rules

OBJECTIVES CHECKLIST

A prepared exam candidate will know the:

- ❑ Identification and function of the three forms of terminal punctuation.
- ❑ Rules and exceptions governing the use and placement of colons.
- ❑ Rules and exceptions governing the use and placement of semicolons.
- ❑ Rules and exceptions governing the use and placement of commas.
- ❑ Difference between commas that separate and commas that set off.

RESOURCES FOR STUDY

1. *The Gregg Reference Manual: A Manual of Style, Grammar, Usage and Formatting*
2. *The AAMT Book of Style for Medical Transcription*
   Colons, pp. 85–87.
   Commas, pp. 87–91.
   Periods, pp. 310–311.
   Punctuation, p. 340.
   Semicolons, pp. 354–356.

OVERVIEW

As with all other areas of usage and style, the goal of punctuation in formal documentation is to promote clarity and consistency throughout the record. Punctuation, particularly commas and semicolons, should be applied with reasonable and prudent consideration for the standards that govern their usage. They should never be applied in random or haphazard fashion, without a sense of purpose or reasonable function. The "rules" that exist in language texts of authority (such as *The Gregg Reference Manual*) and those summarized in *The AAMT Book of Style* outline specific and concrete definitions for either including or omitting a particular form of punctuation. To attempt to delineate them all here would be exhaustive, but a great many of the itemized rules for commas, for example, can be summarized in some general statements about usage that will enable the MT to graduate to a more consistent application of these standards based on knowledge.

TERMINAL PUNCTUATION

Terminal punctuation, or the punctuation that ends a sentence, should always be included throughout the document and should be chosen to express tone and purpose. For most sentences in a medical report, obviously, the terminal punctuation is going to be a *period*. Rarely does a physician request or even dictate in a tone that implies the need for an *exclamation point* or *question mark*. It is important to note here, however, that often dictators will provide direct quotes from the patient or other involved parties, in which a question mark or other punctuation might often be included. Always remember that terminal punctuation should fall within the quotation marks, regardless of its function within the quote itself.

Examples:
The patient was brought to the ER by ambulance.
The patient was repeatedly crying out "Why me?" and complaining of unrelenting pain.
She says the symptoms "have been coming and going."

INTERNAL PUNCTUATION

Internal punctuation exists *within* a sentence and is used primarily to set off or separate one word or phrase from another.

A. Colons

1. Between Independent Clauses

Use a colon between two independent clauses when the second clause explains or illustrates the first clause and there is no coordinating conjunction or transitional expression linking the two clauses.

Example:
I have two goals in this year: lose 50 pounds and remodel my kitchen.

2. Before Lists and Enumerations

a. Place a colon before such expressions as *for example, namely,* and *that is* when they introduce words and phrases.

Example:
Visa provides identity-theft insurance; for example, if someone steals your card, you are protected from the charges incurred by that individual.

b. When a clause contains an anticipatory expression (such as *the following, as follows, thus,* and *these*) and directs attention to a series of explanatory words, phrases, or clauses, use the colon between the clause and the series.

Example:
The following items will be deleted from our website menu: Events, News, and Contacts.

3. In Expressions of Time or Proportions

a. When hours and minutes are expressed in figures, separate them with a colon.

Example: *6:35 p.m.*

b. Use a colon to represent the word *to* in ratio expressions.

Examples: *2:1, epinephrine 1:250,000*

4. In References to Books/Publications

a. Use a colon to separate the title and the subtitle of a book or article.

Example:
Meg Cox wrote *The Heart of the Family: Searching America for New Traditions that Fulfill Us.*

b. Use a colon to separate volume number and page number in footnotes and references.

Example: *8:763–766*

B. Commas

While the incorrect placement of a comma in a medical document is rarely quality-critical, the *correct* placement of them and a thorough understanding of their grammatical implications reflect a skill set that should be the goal of any quality-driven MT. In most instances, these standards rely on a fundamental understanding of and ability to identify both *independent* phrases and clauses and *dependent* phrases and clauses. In those examples below, the independent (or stand-alone) clauses are underlined to differentiate them from the dependent clauses in the sentences.

1. Commas That Separate

a. Two or more adjectives describing the same noun.

Example:
It was a long, hot summer.

b. Two or more items in a simple series.

Examples:
Temperature was 98.6, pulse 80, respirations 22, and blood pressure 132/74.

The area was prepped with Betadine, draped with sterile drapes, and completely anesthetized.

c. Lines of a full address when listed horizontally and/or within a sentence.

Example:
The clinic address is 2152 Park Street, Jacksonville, Florida, 99999.

d. A person's name from his/her credential or title.

Examples:
John A. Smith, Jr., MD
Lea M. Sims, CMT

e. Two or more independent clauses.

Examples:
She was evaluated in triage, and she was found to be hypotensive.
A bladder flap was created, and upon identification of the fundus, a transverse incision was made and widened with blunt dissection.
The abdomen was insufflated with CO_2 gas, and a trocar inserted into both ports under direct visualization.

2. Commas That "Set Off"

a. Nonessential words or phrases that introduce an independent clause.

Examples:
After discussion of her case with the tumor panel, it was felt that she would best benefit from a course of chemotherapy and concomitant radiation treatment.
About a week ago, the patient suffered a fall from the stairs.
Without consent from the parent, I felt we could not move forward with surgery.

b. Nonessential words or phrases that interrupt the flow from subject to verb or from verb to object within an independent clause.

Examples:
The problem, if I remember correctly, was related to the patient's diet.
We made an incision, careful not to damage the underlying structures, with a #11 blade.
The alternative, as I told the patient, is to let this heal in by secondary intention.

c. Nonessential words or afterthoughts that occur at the end of an independent clause.

Example:
There is very little we can offer her at this point, unfortunately.

d. Appositives or Direct Address

Examples:
I have requested a consult with a pulmonologist, Dr. Jones, *for respirator management.*
Thank you, John, *for allowing me to participate in this patient's care.*

e. Nonessential or dependent clauses within an independent clause.

Examples:
The patient, whom I have seen in consultation before, was admitted by Dr. Smith for exacerbation of COPD. (nonessential)
The mass, which was biopsied in September, is unchanged on today's exam. (nonessential)
The mass that was biopsied in September is unchanged on today's exam. (essential)
She was seen by a cardiologist who was on call for the ER. (essential)
She was seen by Dr. Smiley, who was on call for the ER. (nonessential).
The area was thoroughly explored for hemostasis, with no evidence of bleeding or hemorrhage noted. (nonessential)
The area was infiltrated using Marcaine 5% with epinephrine. (essential)

f. Month, day, and year when all three are written.

Example:
On July 1, 1998, she underwent successful CABG.

g. Full-sentence quotations from the rest of the independent clause.

Example:
The patient's husband stated, "I found her on the kitchen floor unresponsive and not breathing."

C. Semicolons

1. To Separate Clauses

Semicolons are often misunderstood and either over-utilized or erroneously applied in documentation. They should serve to occasionally separate two closely related sentences, particularly when the second sentence contains a transitional word or phrase (like *however* or *therefore*). When in doubt about their application, it is always safer to separate the two sentences with a period.

Examples:
She was told not to return to work at this time; we will re-evaluate that on her next visit.
He was given an aggressive course of IV antibiotics; however, his condition did not improve.

2. In a Complex Series

The second instance of utilizing a semicolon is to separate items in a complex series. A *simple series*, whose examples were provided above, is one whose items are separated by commas. A *complex series* is one in which at least one of the items contains an internal comma or commas, thereby making it necessary to separate the items themselves with alternate punctuation, namely a semicolon.

Example:
The patient has older twin sisters, one of whom died of breast cancer in 1998; a brother that died of rectal cancer earlier this year; and a younger sister who is alive and in good health.

REVIEW EXERCISES

Given the information provided in this chapter, can you correctly punctuate the following sentences? These were taken from in-the-trenches, real dictation, but be careful. Not all of them need correction.

1. "I explained to her and her daughter the severity of this injury and that her wrist would never function the same."
2. "She was admitted and monitored and no neurological injury was found."
3. "This is an 81-year-old male with whom I am quite familiar who has an underlying problem of a more serious nature which is diabetes that has caused him to have premature atherosclerotic heart disease."
4. "The red cells appeared normal with a rare fragmented cell seen."
5. "The patient is a pleasant 51-year-old black male who presented to the office of his new primary care physician Dr. Williams on the day of admission complaining of an episode of chest pain and palpitations which occurred about a week earlier."
6. "He complained of palpitations and to rule out cardiac dysrhythmia a consultation with a cardiologist was obtained."
7. "Over the past few months she has had episodic left-sided abdominal pain and pain behind her left breast which became severe and eventually she states she collapsed."
8. "Again in light of the fact that she has been on corticosteroids it would be somewhat unusual to develop pneumonitis and an atypical infection should also be in our differential."
9. "He became combative violent and abusive and security had to be involved in subduing the patient and haloperidol 5 mg and Ativan 2 mg IM was used to help control the patient."
10. "We then made a lateral incision beginning at the greater trochanter and extending distally and carried it down through the deeper subcutaneous tissues."

ANSWER KEY

REVIEW EXERCISES

1. No commas needed.
2. monitored,
3. male,
   familiar,
   nature,
   diabetes,
4. normal,
5. physician,
   Williams,
   (no comma after “palpitations”; phrase that follows is essential because it relates to onset/duration of symptoms)
6. palpitations,
   dysrhythmia,
7. months, (optional)
   severe,
   eventually,
   states,
8. Again,
   corticosteroids,
   pneumonitis,
9. combative,
   violent, (optional)
   abusive,
   patient,
10. incision,
    distally,

CHAPTER 28

English Usage

OBJECTIVES CHECKLIST

A prepared exam candidate will know the:

- ❑ Rules and exceptions related to agreement, both for subjects/verbs and pronouns/antecedents.
- ❑ Rules and exceptions governing the use and placement of interrogative and relative pronouns.
- ❑ Correct use of modifiers, both adjective and adverb forms, including compound modifiers.
- ❑ Principles related to diction and the most commonly confused words encountered in English usage.

RESOURCES FOR STUDY

1. *The Gregg Reference Manual: A Manual of Style, Grammar, Usage and Formatting*
2. *The AAMT Book of Style for Medical Transcription*
   Compound modifiers, pp. 91–98.
   Pronouns, pp. 334–336.
   Subject-verb agreement, pp. 376–378.
   Who, whom, p. 422.
3. Appendix 2: Medical Soundalikes (*found at the end of this text*)

PART I: AGREEMENT

A. SUBJECTS AND VERBS

1. **Rule of Agreement.** A verb must agree with its subject in number and person.

Examples:
I know that he is my friend.
She is coming to spend the weekend with me.

Note: A plural subject is always required after the use of the word *you*, whether *you* is singular or plural.

Examples:
You alone have made it possible to complete this project.
You both have been on my mind all day.

2. **Subjects joined by *and*.**

If the subject consists of two or more words connected by *and* or by *both . . . and*, the subject is plural and requires a plural verb.

Examples:
The teacher and her students have been working hard on the play.
The sales projections and the estimated costs are reasonable.

Use a singular verb when two or more subjects connected by *and* refer to the same person or thing.

Example:
Our President and committee chair is Lisa Smith.

Use a singular verb when two or more subjects connected by *and* are preceded by *each, every, many a*, or *many an*.

Examples:
Every member has a right to a vote.
Each puppy needs a good home.

3. **Subjects joined by *or*.**

If the subject consists of two or more *singular* words connected by *or, either. . . . or, neither. . . . nor*, or *not only. . . . but also*, the subject is singular and requires a singular verb.

Example:
Either May or June is a good month for the wedding.

If the subject consists of two or more *plural* words that are connected by *or, either. . . . or, neither . . . nor*, or *not only. . . . but also*, the subject is plural and requires a plural verb.

Example:
Neither dogs nor cats like cold weather.

If the subject consists of both singular and plural words connected by *or, either. . . . or, neither . . . nor*, or *not only. . . . but also*, the verb agrees with the nearer, or closest, subject.

Example:
Neither the board members nor the Executive Director is in favor of spending money on that project.

Note: When establishing agreement between subject and verb, ignore any intervening, and potentially distracting, phrases or clauses.

Examples:
The order for new textbooks is on the table.
The key consideration in this argument, the budgetary feasibility of the project, is not being given sufficient weight in the analysis.

B. PRONOUNS AND ANTECEDENTS

Rule of Agreement. A pronoun agrees with its antecedent in number and gender. The antecedent of a pronoun is the word to which the pronoun refers, either in the same sentence or in a previous one.

Examples:
He should have thought of that himself.
Mary is devoted to her career.

The words *each, neither, either, one, everyone, everybody, no one, nobody, anyone, anybody, someone, somebody* are referred to by a singular pronoun—*he, him, his, she, her, hers, it,* and *its.* Intervening phrases do not change the number of the antecedent.

Example:
Each of the women had removed her shoes.

Two or more singular antecedents joined by *or* or *nor* should be referred to by a singular pronoun.

Example:
Neither Greg nor John had his keys with him.

Two or more antecedents joined by *and* should be referred to by a plural pronoun.

Example:
Greg and John had their keys in their pockets.

REVIEW EXERCISE: AGREEMENT

For each of the following sentences, indicate correct subject/verb or pronoun/antecedent agreement by selecting the word or phrase in parentheses that completes the sentence.

1. One out of every 20 patients (*respond/responds*) to this medication.
2. Each of the women told the reporter what (*she/they*) had seen.
3. Neither of the proposed amendments (*was/were*) accepted in their entirety.
4. Each of the articles featured in JAAMT (*was/were*) good.
5. (*Has/Have*) either of the orders been sent?
6. Neither the nursing home nor the paramedics (*has/have*) the patient's DNR papers.
7. Neither Jeremy nor Paul used (*his/their*) tickets to the show.
8. Many an at-home medical transcriptionist (*has/have*) felt isolated.
9. The frequency of fatal traffic accidents (*is/are*) rising.
10. A certain degree of privacy and security (*seem/seems*) appropriate.

PART 2: INTERROGATIVE AND RELATIVE PRONOUNS

A. *WHO* AND *WHOM; WHOEVER* AND *WHOMEVER*

All four of these pronouns are both *interrogative* when they are used in asking questions and are *relative* when they are used to relate to or refer to a noun in the main clause.

Examples:
Who is going to the party?
My sister is the one who is going to the party.
To whom should I send this bill?
Dr. Smith, whom I have never met, runs that program.

These pronouns may be either singular or plural in meaning.

Examples:
Who is speaking?
Who are going?

Who (or *whoever*) is the nominative (or subjective) form. Use *who* whenever *he, she, they, I,* or *we* could be substituted in the *who* clause.

Examples:
Who is arranging the meeting next month?
Who did they say was presenting to the group?
The matter of who to appoint to the task force was not addressed.
Mary is the one who can best do the job.

Whom (or *whomever*) is the objective form. Use *whom* whenever *him, her, them,* or *me* could be substituted as the object of the verb or object of the preposition in the *whom* clause.

Examples:
Whom did you meet yesterday?
To whom did you write your letter?
I will hire whomever I believe will get the job done.
It depends on whom they elect to office.

B. *WHO, WHICH,* AND *THAT*

Who and *that* are used when referring to persons. Select *who* when referring to an individual person or individuality of a group, and select *that* when referring to a class, species, or type.

Examples:
He is the only person in my family who understands how I feel.
She is the kind of boss that employees really respond to.

Which and *that* are used when referring to places, objects, and animals. *Which* is used to introduce nonessential clauses (set off by commas) and *that* is usually used to introduce essential clauses (no commas).

Examples:
Bonnie's report on membership benefits, which I read on the website, should be of some help.
The report that I told you about is now up on the website.

REVIEW EXERCISE: INTERROGATIVE AND RELATIVE PRONOUNS

For each of the following sentences, indicate the pronoun's correct form by selecting the word in parentheses that completes the sentence.

1. In *Romeo and Juliet*, the two characters (*who/whom*) I loved the most were Tybalt and Mercutio.
2. If I had known (*who/whom*) you were referring to, I could have given you that information.
3. Next month's issue will feature (*whoever/whomever*) the editor selects.
4. Since I did not know (*who/whom*) the member wanted to speak to, I took a message.
5. Everybody (*who/whom*) receives Plexus will get the poster insert in May.
6. Only the members (*who/whom*) have paid their dues are allowed to vote.
7. She was one of those (*who/whom*) the politicians could not influence.
8. No one has figured out to (*who/whom*) the anonymous letter was referring.
9. The association is looking for someone (*who/whom*) it can appoint to chair this committee.
10. You may tell anyone (*who/whom*) you think is interested that the group is having an informational meeting next Friday.

PART 3: COMPOUND MODIFIERS

A compound modifier consists of two or more words that act as a unit modifying a noun or pronoun. The use of hyphens to join these words varies depending on the type of compound modifier, as indicated below.

Some compound modifiers are so commonly used together, or are so clear, that they are automatically read as a unit and do not need to be joined with hyphens.

Examples:
dark brown lesion
deep tendon reflexes
1st trimester bleeding
jugular venous distention
left lower quadrant
low back pain
ST-T wave abnormality
3rd degree burn

A. ADJECTIVE ENDING IN -LY

Use a hyphen in a compound modifier beginning with an adjective that ends in *-ly*. (This requires distinguishing between adjectives ending in *-ly* and adverbs ending in *-ly.)* Do not use a hyphen with compound modifiers containing an adverb ending in *-ly*.

Example:
scholarly-looking patient
<u>but</u> *quickly paced steps*

B. ADJECTIVE-NOUN COMPOUND

Use a hyphen in an adjective-noun compound that precedes and modifies another noun.

Examples:
second-floor office
<u>but</u>
The office is on the second floor.

C. ADJECTIVE WITH PREPOSITION

Use hyphens in most compound adjectives that contain a preposition.

Example: *finger-to-nose test*

D. ADJECTIVE WITH PARTICIPLE

Use a hyphen to join an adjective to a participle, whether the compound precedes or follows the noun.

Examples:
good-natured, soft-spoken patient
The patient is good-natured and soft-spoken.

E. ADVERB WITH PARTICIPLE OR ADJECTIVE

Use a hyphen to form a compound modifier made up of an adverb coupled with a participle or adjective when they precede the noun they modify but not when they follow it.

Examples:
well-developed and well-nourished woman
but
The patient was well developed and well nourished.
fast-acting medication
but
The medication is fast acting.

F. ADVERB ENDING IN -LY

Do not use a hyphen in a compound modifier to link an adverb ending in *-ly* with a participle or adjective.

Examples:
recently completed workup
moderately acute pain
financially stable investment

G. ADVERB PRECEDING A COMPOUND MODIFIER

Do not use a hyphen in a compound modifier preceded by an adverb.

Example: *somewhat well nourished patient*

H. VERY

Drop the hyphen in a compound modifier with a participle or adjective when it is preceded by the adverb *very*.

Example: *very well developed patient*

I. DISEASE-ENTITY MODIFIERS

Do not use hyphens with most disease-entity modifiers even when they precede the noun. Check appropriate medical references for guidance.

Examples:
cervical disk disease
oat cell carcinoma
pelvic inflammatory disease
sickle cell disease
urinary tract infection
but
insulin-dependent diabetes mellitus and non-insulin-dependent diabetes mellitus

J. EPONYMS

Use a hyphen to join two or more eponymic names used as multiple-word modifiers of diseases, operations, procedures, instruments, etc.

Do not use a hyphen if the multiple-word, eponymic name refers to a single person.

Use appropriate medical references to differentiate.

Examples:
Osgood-Schlatter disease (named for US orthopedic surgeon Robert B. Osgood and Swiss surgeon Carl Schlatter)
Chevalier Jackson forceps (named for Chevalier Jackson, US pioneer in bronchoesophagology)

K. EQUAL, COMPLEMENTARY, OR CONTRASTING ADJECTIVES

Use a hyphen to join two adjectives that are equal, complementary, or contrasting when they precede or follow the noun they modify.

Examples:
anterior-posterior infarction
physician-patient confidentiality issues
His eyes are blue-green.

L. FOREIGN EXPRESSIONS

Do not hyphenate foreign expressions used in compound adjectives, even when they precede the noun they modify (unless they are always hyphenated).

Examples:
in vitro experiments
carcinoma in situ
cul-de-sac (always hyphenated)
ex officio member

M. HIGH- AND LOW-

Use a hyphen in most *high-* and *low-* compound adjectives.

Examples:
high-density mass
low-frequency waves
high-power field

N. NOUN-ADJECTIVE COMPOUND

Use a hyphen to join some noun-adjective compounds (but not all). Check appropriate references (dictionaries and grammar books). When a hyphen is appropriate, use it whether the noun-adjective compound precedes or follows the noun it is modifying.

Examples:
It is a medication-resistant condition.
The condition was medication-resistant.
This is a symptom-free patient.
The patient was symptom-free.
Stool is heme-negative.

O. NOUN WITH PARTICIPLE

Use a hyphen to join a noun and a participle to form a compound modifier whether it comes before or after a noun.

Examples:
bone-biting forceps
She was panic-stricken.
mucus-coated throat (the throat was coated with mucus, not mucous)
callus-forming lesion (the lesion was forming callus, not callous)

P. NUMERALS WITH WORDS

Use a hyphen between a number and a word forming a compound modifier preceding a noun.

Examples:

3-week history
5 x 3 x 2-cm mass
2-year 5-month-old child
8-pound 5-ounce baby girl

Q. PROPER NOUNS AS ADJECTIVE

Do not use hyphens in proper nouns even when they serve as a modifier preceding a noun.

Examples:
John E Kennedy High School
New Mexico residents

Do not use hyphens in combinations of proper noun and common noun serving as a modifier.

Example: *Tylenol capsule administration*

R. SERIES OF HYPHENATED COMPOUND MODIFIERS

Use a suspensive hyphen after each incomplete modifier when there is a series of hyphenated compound modifiers with a common last word that is expressed only after the final modifier in the series.

Examples:
10- to 12-year history
3- to 4-cm lesion
full- and split-thickness grafts

If one or more of the incomplete modifiers is not hyphenated, repeat the base with each, hyphenating or not, as appropriate.

Example: *preoperative and postoperative diagnoses (not pre- and postoperative diagnoses)*

S. TO CLARIFY OR TO AVOID CONFUSION

Use a hyphen to clarify meaning and to avoid confusion, absurdity, or ambiguity in compound modifiers. The hyphen may not be necessary if the meaning is made clear by the surrounding context.

Example: *large-bowel obstruction* (*obstruction of the large bowel,* not *a large obstruction of the bowel*)

T. HYPHENATED COMPOUND MODIFIERS

Use a hyphen or en dash to join hyphenated compound modifiers or a hyphenated compound modifier with a one-word modifier.

Example:
non-disease-entity modifier
or
non–disease-entity modifier

Use a hyphen or en dash to join two unhyphenated compound modifiers.

Example:
the North Carolina-South Carolina border
or
the North Carolina–South Carolina border

Use a hyphen or en dash to join an unhyphenated compound modifier with a hyphenated one.

Example:
beta-receptor-mediated response
<u>or</u>
β-receptor–mediated response

Use a hyphen or en dash to join an unhyphenated compound modifier with a one-word modifier.

Example:
vitamin D-deficiency rickets
<u>or</u>
vitamin D–deficiency rickets

REVIEW EXERCISE: COMPOUND MODIFIERS

The following sentences contain potential compound modifiers. Identify the sentences that are correct with a "C" and the sentences that are incorrect with an "I."

1. He smiled at the lovely looking lady in the front row.
2. She responded with an ear-to-ear grin.
3. She noticed that he was well-groomed and well-dressed.
4. The patient had a recently acquired hesitation in his gait.
5. Exam revealed a very well-developed female.
6. She complained of a 2–3 day headache.
7. He indicated that he spent the weekend doing back-breaking activities, like moving furniture for a friend.
8. X-rays revealed an area of small bowel distention.
9. He gave a 3-week history of decreased appetite and fatigue.
10. The patient was pain free after the procedure.

ANSWER KEYS

REVIEW EXERCISES ANSWER KEY

Part 1: Agreement

1. responds
2. she
3. was
4. was
5. Has
6. have
7. is
8. his
9. is
10. seems

Part 2: Interrogative and Relative Pronouns

1. whom
2. whom
3. whomever
4. whom
5. who
6. who
7. whom
8. whom
9. who
10. who

Part 3: Compound Modifiers

1. I
2. C
3. I
4. I
5. I
6. I
7. C
8. I
9. C
10. I

SECTION IV

The Healthcare Record

CHAPTER

29

Medicolegal Issues

OBJECTIVES CHECKLIST

A prepared exam candidate will know the:

- ❑ Basic tenets of health information privacy and security, including the roles of HIM professionals within the documentation domain.
- ❑ Role of risk management in the healthcare setting and the correlation between documentation and risk management.
- ❑ Role and function of the Joint Commission on Accreditation of Healthcare Organizations (JCAHO) in establishing standards at the acute care provision level.
- ❑ Fundamental legal terms encountered in healthcare delivery, particularly as they pertain to patient privacy, safety, and security of health information.
- ❑ Purpose and principles associated with the Health Insurance Portability and Accountability Act (HIPPA).
- ❑ Seven patient rights as defined by HIPAA.
- ❑ Fundamentals of HIPAA compliance as they pertain to medical transcription and the patient care documentation process.
- ❑ Definitions related to covered entities and business associates, as well as the provisions and stipulations related to each.

RESOURCES FOR STUDY

1. *HIPAA for MTs*
2. *Legal Aspects of Health Information Management*
3. *Glencoe Law and Ethics for Medical Careers*

OVERVIEW

Information is one of the healthcare industry's most important resources. Health information management professionals serve the healthcare industry and the public by managing, analyzing, and utilizing data that is necessary for patient care, including transcription, statistics, birth data, death statistics, coding (reimbursement), tumor registry, and correspondence. Once transcribed, reports are charted on the patient's medical record. This is done on a daily basis to provide continuity of care. Confidentiality of patient records is an important aspect of HIM. The HIM director is the first line of defense in maintaining the integrity of the patient's protected health information (PHI). With the enactment of HIPAA, the role of the HIM Director, in conjunction with the Information Systems Director, has become more vital to managing confidential patient information. The HIM Department is also an integral member of the team when the hospital undergoes JCAHO review.

The Risk Management Department works closely with the HIM Department. The Department of Risk Management has the responsibility of identifying, analyzing, evaluating, and reducing or eliminating the risk of possible injury to patients, visitors, staff, and the institution itself. The Risk Manager has duties including liability claims management, participating in safety and security programs, and monitoring loss prevention and reduction. This department is also involved in risk management education for its employees.

The Joint Commission on Accreditation of Healthcare Organizations (JCAHO) evaluates and accredits more than 15,000 healthcare organizations and programs in the United States. An independent, not-for-profit organization, the Joint Commission is the nation's predominant standard-setting and accrediting body in healthcare. The review is used internally by health care organizations to support performance improvement and externally, to demonstrate accountability to the public. Participation in Joint Commission accreditation is voluntary at for profit hospitals, but mandatory for all government hospitals. Participation in Joint Commission Accreditation is mandatory for those hospitals receiving reimbursement from Medicare/Medicaid. Accreditation standards are published in the Accreditation Manual for Hospitals (AMH).

Joint Commission standards address the organization's level of performance in key functional areas, such as patient rights, patient treatment, and infection control, and the standards focus not simply on an organization's ability to provide safe, high-quality care, but on its actual performance as well. Standards set forth performance expectations for activities that affect the safety and quality of patient care. If an organization does the right things and does them well, there is a strong likelihood that its patients will experience good outcomes. The Joint Commission develops its standards in consultation with healthcare experts, providers, measurement experts, purchasers, and consumers.

MEDICOLEGAL TERMS

As medical transcriptionists, we are familiar with the terminology that relates specifically to our profession—disease processes, anatomy and physiology, diagnoses, treatments, etc., but how familiar are we with some of the terms and concepts in our medicolegal system?

When looking at the legal and medical professions, probably the first area of law that comes to people's minds is that of medical malpractice. Medical malpractice is a controversial topic and becomes a highly debated political issue especially at election time. Another area in the legal field that has come into its own in recent years is that of health law. The increasing costs of healthcare, financing this care, care for the uninsured and indigent, privacy, confidentiality, and security of patient care have given rise to many new laws.

GLOSSARY OF TERMS

Abuse (as in Medicare/Medicaid fraud and abuse): incidents or practices that may directly or indirectly cause financial losses to government health programs, beneficiaries, or recipients.

Advance directive: power of attorney that gives someone decision-making powers upon the person's incompetence.

ADA: Americans with Disabilities Act.

Common law: body of law made up of judicial opinions and precedents as opposed to legislatively created laws or statutes.

Damages: money compensation paid through the courts to persons who have suffered an injury or detriment due to the negligence or omission of another.

DNR (Do Not Resuscitate Order): this order specifies what efforts should or should not be taken in order to revive a patient who has experienced cardiac or pulmonary arrest and what level of care should be provided in the case of an arrest.

Electronic signature: a symbol, a process used to sign a document.

ERISA: an abbreviation for Employee Retirement Security Income Act—covers employee benefit plans such as health plans and pensions.

Ethical behavior: behavior that conforms to accepted professional standards of conduct.

Ethics: a set of moral principles or behavior.

Family and Medical Leave Act (FMLA): the Family and Medical Leave Act of 1993 entitles a covered employee to take up to 12 weeks of leave in a 12-month period for the birth or adoption of a child, or the serious health condition of the employee or the employee's child, spouse, or parent.

Fraud: an "intentional" misrepresentation or deception that an individual knows to be false and could result in unauthorized benefit to himself or some other person. A criminal intent to defraud is when the misrepresentation or deception is made willingly. (An example would be Medicare fraud—charges knowingly submitted for treatment not provided.)

Good Samaritan Acts: according to the 7th edition of Black's Law, this is "A statute that exempts from liability a person (such as an off-duty physician) who voluntarily renders aid to another in imminent danger but negligently causes injury while rendering aid." This type of legislation is passed on a state-by-state basis.

Grandfather clause: a provision of law that exempts certain persons or pre-existing conditions from the scope of a regulation or requirement.

Healthcare directive: any statement made by a competent individual about preferences for future medical treatment in the event that the patient is unable to make decisions at the time of treatment.

Indemnification: the act of compensating for loss or damage.

Independent contractor: an individual who is hired to complete a specific project but who is free to do that work as he or she wishes; it is not based on how the person is paid, how often the person is paid, or whether the person works part-time or full-time. An independent contractor is not an employee, thus cannot sue an employer for a wrongful act or injury suffered on the job. The independent contractor will receive a 1099 form for tax reporting purposes.

Informed consent: a person's agreement to allow something to happen after the person has been informed of all the risks involved and the alternatives.

Life-sustaining procedure: a medical procedure that uses mechanical or artificial means to sustain a person's vital functions and basically just serves to postpone a person's death.

Malpractice: negligence or incompetence on behalf of an individual, usually applied to professionals such as attorneys or physicians.

Medicaid: a program that helps pay for medically necessary medical services for needy and low-income persons. It uses state and federal government money. Covered under Social Security Act Title XIX.

Medicare: a federal insurance program for people age 65 and older and certain disabled people. The Centers for Medicare & Medicaid Services (CMS) operates Medicare. The Medicare program consists of two parts, Medicare Part A (hospital insurance) and Medicare Part B (supplemental medical insurance). Covered under Social Security Act Title XVIII.

Negligence: the most common cause of action in medical malpractice cases. It will arise where injury results from a failure of the wrongdoer to exercise due care.

Occupational Safety and Health Act (OSHA): the federal occupational safety and health agency. It enforces the Occupational Safety and Health Act (the OSH Act), which provides the legal framework for the work of OSHA. OSHA has established federal health and safety rights for all workers in the U.S. whether or not they are United States citizens.

Pain and suffering: includes the loss of physical abilities, such as the use of your hand or foot, and physical discomfort, such as chronic backache or stiffness in your neck. The term also includes any emotional pain you might suffer, such as worry, anxiety, embarrassment, and the loss of the pleasures and enjoyment of life.

Risk management: in healthcare, this is preventive medicine. This calls for identifying problems and forestalling incidents that could lead to claims. Accurate and proper documentation of healthcare provided is vital in risk management. Often what is omitted from the medical record can be more harmful to the healthcare provider than what is included.

Sexual harassment definition: Title VII of the Civil Rights Act of 1964 makes it unlawful for an employer to discriminate against any individual with respect to compensation, terms, conditions, or privileges of employment, because of such individual's sex.

Standard of care: the standard of care used in malpractice cases has been stated as "A physician is bound to bestow such reasonable and ordinary care, skill, and diligence as physicians and surgeons in good standing in the same neighborhood, in the same general line of practice, ordinarily have and exercise in like cases."[1]

Statutory employee: workers deemed to be employees by statute. A home-based worker performing work on materials or goods furnished by the employer could be considered a statutory employee. Statutory employees receive W2 Form from the employer. Statutory employees are not liable for self-employment tax because their employers must treat them as employees for social security tax purposes.

Tort: a tort occurs when someone deliberately or through carelessness causes harm or loss to another person or their property.

References

1. 61 Am. Jur. 2d *Physicians and Surgeons* #205 (1981).
2. Garner BA (ed.). *Black's Law Dictionary*, 7th Edition. Eagan, MN: West Publishing Company, 1991.
3. Hall MA, Ellman IM. *Health Care Law and Ethics in a Nutshell*. Eagan, MN: West Publishing Company, 1990.
4. Southwick AF. *The Law of Hospital and Health Care Administration*, 2nd Edition. Chicago: Health Administration Press, 1988.

HIPAA

To provide effective treatment, healthcare providers must have comprehensive, accurate, and timely medical information. The automation of medical information permits the collection, analysis, storage, and retrieval of vast amounts of medical information that is not only used but also shared with other providers at remote locations. The increasing demand for access to medical information by providers and others, such as insurance companies, has led to increasing concern about patient privacy and confidentiality, resulting in the enactment of the privacy and security provisions of the Health Insurance Portability and Accountability Act of 1996 (HIPAA).

There are seven Patient Rights under HIPAA. They are:

1. Right to a notice of privacy practices.
2. Right to access PHI.

3. Right to request amendment to PHI.
4. Right to request alternative means of communicating PHI.
5. Right to request restrictions on PHI.
6. Right to an accounting.
7. Right to complain about our privacy practices.

The privacy rule regulates the use and disclosure of "protected health information" (PHI) by certain entities. Protected health information is information transmitted or maintained in any form—by electronic means, on paper, or through oral communications—that: (1) relates to the past, present, or future physical or mental health or condition of an individual, the provision of health care to an individual, or the past, present, or future payment for the provision of health care to an individual; and (2) identifies the individual or with respect to which there is a reasonable basis to believe the information can be used to identify the individual. Information that has been de-identified in accordance with the rule's stringent de-identification criteria is not considered protected health information and is not subject to the rule.

The Life of a Medical Report

It may help to understand how the privacy rule relates to medical transcription by examining the life of a transcribed report as it moves through the healthcare system. It begins with a patient encounter. Whether that encounter occurs in a hospital, a physician office, or an outpatient clinic, health information is collected to create the transcribed report; this information is **protected health information**, according to HIPAA. The healthcare provider collecting the information is a **covered entity**. Once the information has been collected by the provider, it is transmitted in some form for transcription. This is considered a permitted **disclosure** of the information, as long as only the minimum amount of information necessary for transcription is disclosed. If the information has been transmitted from a provider to an MT business for transcription for the covered entity, that MT business is considered a **business associate** of the **covered entity** (the healthcare provider).

Organizations *directly* subject to the HIPAA privacy rule are those that typically generate individually identifiable patient health information and therefore have primary responsibility for maintaining the privacy and confidentiality of such information. These **covered entities**, as defined by HIPAA, are: (1) most health plans; (2) healthcare clearinghouses; and (3) healthcare providers that transmit any health information in electronic form in connection with certain administrative transactions related to payment for health care. Employees of covered entities generally are not themselves covered entities but effectively must comply with the rule because improper uses and disclosures of information by employees may be imputed to employers. Thus, medical transcriptionists who work as employees of hospitals, clinics, private physician offices, and other covered entities should follow the policies and procedures established by those organizations with respect to the handling of protected health information.

As a general matter, a covered entity may use or disclose protected health information only: (1) with an individual's written "consent" for treatment, payment, and healthcare operations; (2) with an individual's written "authorization" for purposes unrelated to treatment, payment, or healthcare operations; and (3) without consent or authorization for certain purposes enumerated by the rule, such as research and public health, if specified conditions are met. Except for disclosures made to healthcare providers for treatment purposes and certain other disclosures identified by the rule, a covered entity may use or disclose only the minimum protected health information necessary to accomplish the intended purpose. The rule generally requires covered entities to grant individuals access to records containing protected health information about them, as well as the opportunity to request amendments to such records. Covered entities also must comply with a host of administrative requirements intended to protect patient privacy. For instance, each covered entity must appoint a privacy officer who is responsible for ensuring that the entity develops and implements written policies and procedures designed to safeguard individuals' privacy.

The HIPAA privacy rule also applies *indirectly* to **business associates** of covered entities. Business associates are individuals and organizations who are not employees of covered entities but who provide services on behalf of covered entities, which involve the receipt or disclosure of protected health information. An MT business that provides transcription services for a covered entity is a business associate of that covered entity. The privacy rule requires covered entities to enter into a written agreement with each business associate—known as a "business associate agreement"—that limits the latter's ability to use and disclose the protected health information and that includes numerous other provisions. Significantly, the business associate may not use or disclose the protected health information other than as permitted or required by the business associate agreement or as required by law. Thus, an MT business generally may not use or disclose protected health information for a purpose unrelated to the provision of transcription services–unless the covered entity authorizes the MT business through the agreement to make uses or disclosures for that purpose. The specific requirements of business associate agreements are discussed further below.

Medical transcriptionists who are *employees* of healthcare providers or other HIPAA "covered entities" are affected by HIPAA, but they should go to their employers for guidance regarding HIPAA compliance. However, even these MTs should also be aware of the issues, in case they consider going into business for themselves, even on a part-time basis, at some point in the future. Consider the fact that "doing a little work on the side" makes one an independent contractor and thus a business owner.

MTs who are *subcontractors* to MT businesses will be required to agree contractually to essentially the same restrictions and conditions that apply to MT businesses with respect to handling patient information and, therefore, may also find this document useful.

REVIEW EXERCISES

REGULATORY REQUIREMENTS & JCAHO

1. Abbreviations and symbols can only be used when:
   A. The dictator identifies them
   B. Abbreviations and symbols are never used
   C. They are found in a medical dictionary
   D. They have been approved for the medical staff policy and procedure manual
2. Accreditation by JCAHO is voluntary for private and not-for-profit hospitals and is:
   A. Required in all states
   B. Unnecessary
   C. Conducted annually
   D. Required for reimbursement for certain patient groups
3. Which of the following is required for confidentiality purposes?
   A. Sprinkler system
   B. Adequate lighting
   C. Paper shredder
   D. Special "trash" receptacles
4. JCAHO defines authentication as:
   A. Proof of authorship
   B. A complete clinical record
   C. A complete consultation report
   D. Recording a clinical event as soon as possible
5. Identification of authors cannot be accomplished by:
   A. A written signature
   B. Identifiable initials
   C. A computer key
   D. A check mark at the signature line
6. Which one of the below is incorrect? JCAHO states that approved abbreviations and symbols:
   A. Must have an explanatory legend available to those authorized to make entries and to those who must interpret the entries
   B. May have more than one meaning
   C. Must be completely spelled out
   D. Must be approved by medical staff rules and regulations
7. Which is most applicable? JCAHO states that when economically feasible and appropriate, medical entries should be typed to assist in:
   A. Legibility
   B. Timeliness
   C. Completeness
   D. Clinical pertinence
8. JCAHO Accreditation is important because:
   A. Accreditation meets Medicare conditions of participation for reimbursement
   B. The government requires all hospitals to undergo accreditation.
   C. The public demands it
   D. Physicians have requested it
9. JCAHO means:
   A. Joint Commission Association of Healthcare Organizations
   B. Joint Commission on Accreditation of Healthcare Organizations
   C. Joint Commissioners Association of Healthcare Organizations
   D. Joint Commission on Acute Healthcare Organizations
10. Joint Commission grants accreditation for a maximum of:
    A. One year
    B. Three years
    C. Two years
    D. Eighteen months

HIPAA

1. HIPAA stands for:
   A. Health Insurance Portability and Accident Act
   B. Health Information Portability and Accountability Act
   C. Health Insurance Portability and Accountability Act
   D. Health Information Portability and Insurance Act

2. A breach in confidentiality of patient information can occur:
   A. When a report is being transcribed on a digital system
   B. When a doctor dictates a patient's health information into the transcriptionist's answering machine
   C. When a transcriptionist uses a headset to play back information
   D. When a doctor sees a patient

3. Organizations that have the primary responsibility for protecting individually identifiable patient health information are called covered entities. Which below would constitute an example of a covered entity?
   A. Business associate
   B. Hospital administrator
   C. Personal friend
   D. Health plan

4. Medical transcriptionists who are employees of a covered entity must follow:
   A. The HIPAA regulations
   B. The people involved in billing for healthcare
   C. Business associate agreement with the healthcare provider
   D. The policies and procedures established by the organization with respect to the handling of protected health information

5. Failure of a covered entity to comply with HIPAA standards can result in:
   A. Civil monetary penalties of up to $200 for each accidental violation
   B. Civil monetary penalties of up to $100 for each accidental violation
   C. Imprisonment for 20 years for selling PHI
   D. Civil monetary penalties of up to $250,000 per year

6. A medical transcriptionist working as an independent contractor should have which of the below:
   A. A list of all social security numbers for patients
   B. Direct access to the U.S. Government HIPAA clearinghouse
   C. A Business Associate agreement with accounts, policies, and procedures on maintaining confidential information and access to information necessary to do the job
   D. A list of all business associates for healthcare providers

7. HIPAA requires an MT business, as a business associate, to have these components in an emergency contingency plan. One of these is:
   A. Ability to electronically transmit transcribed data
   B. Disaster recovery plan
   C. Exit strategy
   D. Notice of confidentiality

8. AAMT recommends that MT businesses retain protected health information only as long as it is necessary to do business; that is, no longer than it is necessary to:
   A. Verify records and authenticate by originator
   B. Verify information, distribute, and bill for services provided
   C. Provide information to patients
   D. Complete billing and transmission back to healthcare provider

9. When physically transporting protected health information, an MT business would be violating confidentiality by:
   A. Using a bonded commercial courier for transport and having them sign a confidentiality agreement

B. Leaving PHI in an unprotected location for pick up, such as in a mailbox or front door
C. Delivering documents personally in a sealed, tamper-proof container
D. Covering patient identifiable information that is visible on the outside of the envelope

10. Ways to protect identifiable patient information when faxing include all of the following except:
    A. Having a cover sheet informing recipient of confidentiality of information being faxed and providing a warning to any recipient not authorized to have access to such information
    B. Maintaining the fax machine in an easily visible and accessible location
    C. Preprogramming frequently used fax numbers to avoid mistakes
    D. Keeping the fax machine in a secure area of the business to prevent access by unauthorized individuals

11. In the HIPAA privacy rule, PHI generally refers to:
    A. Individually identifiable health information
    B. A patient's social history
    C. How many times a patient has been in the hospital
    D. A business associate

12. Protected health information is information that is transmitted or maintained in any form—by electronic means, on paper, or through oral communications. Which group is subject to the rule?
    A. Relates to information that has been de-identified in accordance with the rule's stringent de-identification criteria
    B. Relates to hospital risk management policies
    C. Relates to the past, present, or future payment for the provision of healthcare to an individual
    D. Relates to information release policies and procedures

13. For the home-based MT, the computer used for work needs to be secure. The computer is not secure if:
    A. The computer is password protected
    B. The computer is kept in a locked, secure room to prohibit access
    C. The computer is used by all family members
    D. The password is changed every 30 days

14. According to HIPAA regulations, which one of the following is incorrect?
    A. All inpatients must be listed in the patient directory
    B. Psychotherapy notes that document or analyze the contents of conversation during a counseling session are kept separate from the rest of the patient's medical record
    C. Information such as address, age, social security number, and phone number is protected health information
    D. Passwords should include both letters and numbers or other special characters

15. One of the patient's rights under HIPPA is:
    A. Right to change their PHI
    B. Right to access their PHI
    C. Right to eliminate their PHI
    D. Right to change physicians

RISK MANAGEMENT

1. Which function is not included in a risk manager's main duties?
    A. Liability claims management
    B. Participating in safety and security programs
    C. Loss prevention and reduction
    D. Medical staff evaluation

2. If a policy and procedure manual does not reflect current practices, this can be referred to risk management because:
    A. Time is wasted in correcting the manual
    B. New personnel will not be trained properly
    C. The manual represents the normal course of business

D. Changes must be cleared by the risk manager

3. Dictated information that indicates potential risk to the patient or to the institution, including personnel, should be reported to:
   A. The director of health information management (medical records)
   B. The risk manager
   C. The CFO
   D. The appropriate institutional personnel, as identified in the institution's program policies

4. AAMT recommends that independent MTs and MT businesses retain any healthcare records for a period of:
   A. Six months
   B. Only as long as is necessary for verification, distribution, and billing purposes
   C. Two weeks
   D. Seven years (the legal standard)

5. Risk management is defined as:
   A. Healthcare institution activities designed to prevent patients suing the hospital and reducing financial loss
   B. Healthcare institution activities that identify, analyze, evaluate, reduce, or eliminate the risk of possible injury and loss to patients, visitors, staff, and the institution itself
   C. Activities to monitor medical transcriptionists as to the quality of work submitted
   D. Protecting the hospital's reputation

6. The doctor dictating an operative report on the right knee changes to the left knee in the middle of the report. The transcriptionist would:
   A. Type as the doctor dictated
   B. Type as the doctor dictated and make a note of it
   C. Type as dictated and send to quality assurance for review
   D. Flag the report and bring to the attention of the supervisor or the report's originator for resolution

7. Professional liability insurance is also called:
   A. Malpractice insurance
   B. Licensing insurance
   C. Errors and omission insurance
   D. Loss prevention insurance

8. There are three basic objectives that a healthcare organization risk management program must have. Which of the below is not one of the objectives?
   A. To create and maintain a safe, healthy environment and enhance the quality of care
   B. To protect the physicians from malpractice suits
   C. To minimize risk of medical or accidental injuries and losses
   D. To provide cost-effective techniques to ensure against financial loss

9. Audit trails contribute to risk management and are also known as:
   A. Paper trails
   B. Documentation trails
   C. Cookie trails
   D. Sample trails

10. A comprehensive risk management program contains three components. They are:
    A. Risk identification, risk control, and risk financing
    B. Risk identification, continuity of care, and risk financing
    C. Providing safe environments, medical staff credentialing, and risk identification
    D. Infection control reports, risk control, and risk financing

ANSWER KEY

REVIEW EXERCISES

REGULATORY REQUIREMENTS & JCAHO

1. D
2. D
3. C
4. A
5. D
6. B
7. A
8. A
9. B
10. B

HIPAA

1. C
2. B
3. D
4. D
5. B
6. C
7. B
8. B
9. B
10. B
11. A
12. C
13. C
14. A
15. B

RISK MANAGEMENT

1. D
2. C
3. D
4. B
5. B
6. D
7. C
8. B
9. B
10. A

Appendices

APPENDIX 1

Normal Lab Values

Background

The laboratory consists of two major sections: Clinical Pathology and Surgical Pathology. Within Clinical Pathology, there are three major departments: Microbiology, Hematology, and Chemistry, as well as specialty areas within each department. Surgical Pathology includes the histology department.

The entire laboratory is directed by a pathologist who is a medical doctor specializing in laboratory medicine. The lab is staffed by technologists and technicians, histologists, phlebotomists, and clerks.

A full-service laboratory will process many types of specimens, the most common being blood, urine, sputum, and stool, but also any other body fluid or tissue obtained through aspiration, biopsy, excision, or amputation.

Blood is drawn into specialized tubes which come in various sizes and shapes. Most blood collection tubes contain an anticoagulant which prevents the blood from clotting. The tops of the collection tubes are color-coded to indicate the type of anticoagulant. For example, green-top tubes contain sodium heparin, purple-top tubes contain EDTA, and blue-top tubes contain sodium citrate. Samples drawn with an anticoagulant will never clot (if properly collected). Tubes with red tops or red and black "tiger" tops do not contain an anticoagulant, and the blood will immediately begin to clot within the tube. It is important that the blood sample be collected in the tube specified for the test, because the wrong anticoagulant can interfere with the test results.

Tests are performed on either whole blood, serum, or plasma. In order to separate the cells from the liquid portion of the blood, the tubes are placed in a centrifuge for 5–10 minutes, forcing the cells and platelets to the bottom of the tube. The watery portion of the sample is called "plasma" if the sample has been anticoagulated and "serum" if the sample has been allowed to clot. Plasma appears slightly cloudy because it still contains clotting factors (proteins). Serum, on the other hand, is normally clear and straw-colored, since the clotting proteins form fibrin strands that entrap cells and platelets in the clot and therefore are no longer a component of the watery portion of the blood.

Common Laboratory Studies

The following tests are the most common laboratory tests performed. Most test results must be evaluated in the context of other laboratory studies and physical findings, as one test is rarely diagnostic for any one disease. For convenience and diagnostic purposes, tests are often grouped together as panels or profiles to assess a particular body system or disease, but these categories are not strict and there is much overlap.

The tables below include only the most common reasons for abnormal test results. Also, each laboratory sets their own reference (normal ranges) based on the methodology being used. These ranges will vary slightly from one laboratory to the next. Normal values for many tests also vary according to age and gender. If values vary, those listed here are for adult males.

Electrolytes and Acid/Base Balance

Sodium, potassium, chloride, and bicarbonate interact to help the body maintain normal fluid levels in the intracellular and extracellular spaces, maintain acid-base balance, and maintain muscle contractility. The kidneys, and to a certain extent the lungs, play the most critical roles in maintaining proper concentrations of these positively and negatively charged molecules, although many metabolic disorders and diseases can disrupt electrolyte balance.

TEST NAME	COMMENT	NORMAL RANGE	NORMAL RANGE (SI)
Na+ (sodium)	Elevated levels are indicative of dehydration. Hyponatremia may be caused by excessive fluid retention (dilutional effect) or by sodium loss through sweating, vomiting, or renal disease.	136 to 145 mEq/L	136 to 145 mmol/L
K+ (potassium)	Decreased levels associated with some diuretics, renal disease, or GI loss through diarrhea or vomiting. Increased levels are seen in renal disease or from rapid breakdown of muscle or red cell lysis.	3.5 to 5 mEq	3.5 to 5 mmol/L
Cl^- (chloride)	Elevated levels seen in dehydration or renal disease. Decreased levels result from fluid retention (dilutional effect) or from increased excretion from renal disease, diuretic therapy, or vomiting.	100 to 106 mEq/L	100 to 106 mmol/L
HCO_3 (bicarbonate)	May also be referred to as CO_2 because bicarbonate is measured indirectly by measuring CO_2 levels. Bicarbonate buffers the blood to maintain pH. Abnormal levels must be evaluated in the context of other electrolyte levels and physical symptoms.	24 to 30 mEq/L	24 to 30 mmol/L
pH	Normal range must be maintained through buffering system of bicarbonate and electrolytes.	7.35 to 7.45	7.35 to 7.45
CO_2	High levels indicate ingestion/retention of bicarbonate or excessive loss of acids as in vomiting or hypoventilation. Decreased levels seen in diabetic acidosis, renal failure, or diarrhea.	22–26 mEq/L	22–26 mmol/L
Anion Gap	Used to assess metabolic acidosis and indirectly measures the total of anions from sulfates, phosphates, proteins, ketones, and lactic acid using the equation $Na - (Cl + HCO_3)$	12 to 20 mEq/L	12 to 20 mmol/L

Minerals

Minerals such as calcium, magnesium, and phosphorus (in the form of phosphates) are critical for maintaining bones and teeth. Phosphorus also plays an important role in energy utilization, red cell function, and overall metabolism. Calcium and magnesium play an important role in muscle contraction, and calcium is an integral component of the coagulation system. Calcium and phosphorous levels are inversely proportional and are primarily under the control of the parathyroid glands. Excretion and retention of these minerals is controlled by the kidneys. These minerals have some electrolytic activity but traditionally are not considered a part of an "electrolyte panel."

TEST NAME	COMMENT	NORMAL RANGE	NORMAL RANGE (SI)
Ca (calcium)	Elevated levels may indicate hyperparathyroidism, acute or chronic bone disease (e.g., metastasis), or renal disease. Hypocalcemia may result from parathyroid disease, malabsorption, or renal failure.	8.2 to 10.2 mg/dL	2 to 2.5 mmol/L
Mg (magnesium)	Elevated levels, if not caused by over-ingestion (e.g., milk of magnesia) are often due to renal failure. Decreased magnesium may indicate chronic alcoholism.	1.5 to 2.3 mg/dL	0.6 to 1.0 mmol/L
P (phosphorus)	Phosphates are abundant in foods, so typically decreased levels are due to over-excretion by the kidneys. Elevated levels may be due to release from injured bones.	2.5 to 4.5 mg/dL	0.8 to 1.5 mmol/L

Studies Related to Iron Metabolism

Iron is an integral part of hemoglobin and myoglobin molecules which the body uses to bind and transport oxygen. Iron is absorbed from the intestine and carried through the blood to the bone marrow bound to transferrin. Iron is stored bound to a protein called ferritin. The iron binding capacity represents the amount of iron that the body is capable of transporting through the blood by way of transferrin.

TEST NAME	COMMENT	NORMAL RANGE	NORMAL RANGE (SI)
Fe (iron)	Serum iron is decreased with malabsorption and/or malnutrition or with chronic blood loss. Elevated serum iron may be due to excessive dietary intake or hemochromatosis, pernicious anemia, or hemolytic anemia.	50 to 160 mEq/dL	9.0 to 28.8 mcmol/L
Ferritin	Ferritin levels are indicative of stored iron. Decreased levels are typically due to chronic iron deficiency. Levels may be elevated in liver disease, iron overload, infection, or inflammation.	20 to 200 ng/mL	20 to 200 mcg/L
TIBC (total iron binding capacity)	Increased in anemia caused by hemorrhage or iron deficiency. TIBC is decreased in hemochromatosis, nephrotic syndrome, or liver disease.	250 to 350 mcg/dL	45 to 63 mcmol/L
Transferrin	Decreased levels may be due to inadequate production because of liver damage. Elevated levels are common in severe iron deficiency as the body tries to capture more iron.	250 to 425 mg/dL	2.5 to 4.2 g/L

Studies Related to Kidney Function

The kidneys are responsible for filtering water-soluble waste products from the blood as well as maintaining the correct level of electrolytes, proteins, and glucose for fluid balance throughout the body. Water naturally passes through membranes toward higher concentrations of sodium and other dissolved molecules; therefore the proper osmolality (concentration) is needed to keep fluid levels balanced between the intracellular and extracellular spaces. Kidney disease is marked by an inability to properly regulate levels of minerals, proteins, glucose, and nitrogenous wastes.

Blood enters the kidney and is first filtered by the glomeruli, where all but cells, platelets, and large protein molecules are allowed to pass through the glomerular membrane. The filtrate passes through the renal tubules which reabsorb the necessary amounts of glucose and electrolytes, and excrete the excess molecules as well as the wastes into the urine.

BUN is used to assess glomerular filtration because BUN is not reabsorbed by the tubules. Whatever amount passes through the glomerulus is excreted in the urine. Creatinine is also used to assess glomerular function in the same way, only it is considered a more accurate assessment. The GFR (glomerular filtration rate) is dependent upon blood pressure, blood volume, and the resistance of the glomerular membrane.

TEST NAME	COMMENT	NORMAL RANGE	NORMAL RANGE (SI)
BUN (blood urea nitrogen)	Increased in renal disease or impaired blood flow to the kidneys due to decreased blood volume/pressure and also due to renal obstruction. BUN is decreased in severe protein deficiencies.	5 to 20 mg/dL	1.8 to 7.1 mcmol/L
Creatinine	Metabolic production of creatinine remains fairly constant, so increases in creatinine are almost always due to renal impairment or decreased blood pressure/volume passing through the kidneys.	0.6 to 1.2 mg/dL	50 to 100 mcmol/L
24-hour creatinine clearance-measure of glomerular filtration rate	Calculated by comparing creatinine excreted in the urine over 24 hours relative to blood levels of creatinine. GFR is decreased in shock, obstruction of blood flow to kidneys, or kidney disease.	90 to 135 ml/min/1.73m^2	0.86 to 1.3 ml/sec/m^2

Studies Related To Liver Function (LFTs)

The liver performs many metabolic tasks, including detoxification and protein production. The liver is responsible for manufacturing albumin, which is needed to maintain proper osmolality, and many of the carrier proteins (globulins) needed to transport non-water-soluble molecules through the blood. The liver also clears the blood of drugs, environmental chemicals, and metabolic wastes. Liver disease shows up in three ways: increased levels of liver enzymes found in the plasma due to spillage from damaged liver cells; decreased plasma proteins due to impaired ability manufacture needed molecules; and increased waste products (e.g. ammonia, bilirubin, drugs) in the blood due to inability to detoxify and metabolize.

TEST NAME	COMMENT	NORMAL RANGE	NORMAL RANGE (SI)
ALT (SGPT)	Enzyme spills into blood when cells are damaged. Increased levels are seen in liver disease or degenerative muscle diseases.	8 to 45 U/L	8 to 45 U/L
AST (SGOT)	Enzyme spills into blood when cells are damaged. Increased in active liver disease and pancreatitis. May also be increased with damage to myocardial or skeletal muscle damage.	<35 U/L	<35 U/L
Alkaline phosphatase ("alk phos")	Increased in biliary obstruction, hepatic and bone disease, including metastasis.	20 to 120 U/L	20 to 120 U/L

TEST NAME	COMMENT	NORMAL RANGE	NORMAL RANGE (SI)
Total protein	Includes all serum proteins but mostly albumin and globulins. Decreased in malnutrition, chronic disease, and with liver diseases which impair protein production.	6.4 to 8.3 g/dL	64 to 83
Albumin	Decreased in liver disease, malnutrition, and chronic infection.	3.5 to 5.0 g/dL	35 to 50 g/L
Globulin	Includes carrier proteins such as ceruloplasmin, haptoglobin, transferrin, lipoproteins, and the immunoglobin class of proteins (e.g. IgG, IgM, etc.)	1.5 to 3.0 g/dL	15 to 30 g/L
A/G ratio (albumin/ globulin ratio)	Ratio is reversed when albumin is decreased and globulin is increased.	1.5 to 3.0	1. to 3.0
Ammonia (NH_3)	Byproduct of protein metabolism which is normally converted to urea by the liver. Ammonia increases in hepatic failure.	15 to 45 mcg/dL	11 to 32 mcmol/L
Total bilirubin	Bilirubin is the breakdown product of hemoglobin. Increased levels are seen in hemolysis, newborns, and liver disease.	0.2 to 1.3 mg/dL	3.4 to 22.1 mcmol/L
Direct bilirubin	Measures bilirubin which has been processed by the liver to be excreted in the bile. Increased levels indicate obstruction in the biliary system.	0.1 to 0.4 mg/dL	1.7 to 6.8 mcmol/L
Indirect bilirubin	Measures bilirubin which has not been processed by the liver. Increased levels indicate liver impairment or hemolysis causing bilirubin levels to rise faster than the liver can process.	0.1 to 0.9 mg/dL	1.7 to 15.3 mcmol/L
GGT	Increased in biliary obstruction, liver disease, pancreatitis, and alcoholism.	<65 U/L	<65 U/L
Haptoglobin	Protein molecule which transports hemoglobin when not bound within the red cell. Levels are decreased in liver disease (impaired production) and increased in cases of chronic hemolysis.	40 to 180 mg/dL	0.4 to 1.8 g/L
LH (LDH, lactate dehydrogenase)	Enzyme found in liver cells and red cells. Increased levels in serum due to hepatitis or hemolytic anemia.	<110 U/L	<110 U/L

Tests Related to Glucose Metabolism

Glucose is the primary form of energy used by all cells. Insulin is required to move glucose from the blood into the cells. Elevated glucose levels stimulate the release of insulin. Abnormal glucose levels may result from too little insulin, too much insulin, or from resistance to the effects of insulin.

TEST NAME	COMMENT	NORMAL RANGE	NORMAL RANGE (SI)
Glucose	Elevated in diabetes, metabolic syndrome, or chronic states of stress. Decreased in acute inflammation, diabetic crisis, starvation/ fasting, or reactive hypoglycemia.	60 to 115 mg/dL (fasting)	3.3 to 6.4 mmol/L
Insulin	Increased levels seen in hyperglycemia and hyperinsulinism.	5 to 25 mcU/mL	24 to 172 pmol/L
Hemoglobin A_{1c} (glycosylated hemoglobin)	Increased in states of sustained elevation of blood glucose over previous 4–6 weeks.	4 to 7%	4 to 7 %

Nonspecific Tests for Inflammation

Inflammation causes an increase in serum proteins, including albumin, globulins, and C-reactive protein. The sedimentation rate, i.e., the time it takes for red cells to fall out of solution, is affected by the increased levels of inflammatory proteins.

TEST NAME	COMMENT	NORMAL RANGE	NORMAL RANGE (SI)
ESR (erythrocyte sedimentation rate) Westergren and Wintrobe methods	Elevated values are associated with inflammation and autoimmune disorders.	Westergren method 0 to 20 mm/hr Wintrobe method 0 to 15 mm/hr	
CRP (C-reactive protein)	Elevated levels associated with states of inflammation.	<0.5 mg/dL	<5 mg/L

Arterial Blood Gas Studies

(Compare to studies above which evaluate venous blood.) These tests are evaluated together to assess the pulmonary gas exchange in patients with respiratory or circulatory disease. Because gases can be compressed, it is difficult to measure gases in terms of volumes, so they are measured according to the amount of pressure they exert (torr) and/or, the percent saturation. You may also hear the term "partial pressure" since each individual gas exerts a "part" of the overall gas pressure.

TEST NAME	COMMENT	NORMAL RANGE	NORMAL RANGE (SI)
pH (hydrogen ion concentration)	Respiration cannot occur outside this strict pH range.	7.35 to 7.45	7.35 to 7.45
HCO_3(bicarbonate ion)	Controlled by the kidneys and acts as a buffer to maintain strict pH range.	22 to 26 mEq/L	22 to 26 mmol/L
sO_2 or O_2 sat (oxygen saturation)	Indicates percentage of hemoglobin molecules bound with oxygen.	94% to 100 %	0.94 to 1
pO_2 or PaO_2 (pressure of oxygen)	Measures the lungs' ability to oxygenate the blood.	80–100 mmHg	10.6 to 13.3 kPa
pCO_2 or $PaCO_2$ (pressure of carbon dioxide)	Measures the lungs' ability to exchange O_2 for CO_2.	35 to 45 mmHg	4.7 to 5.3 kPa

Cardiovascular/Cerebrovascular Risk or Disease

Cardiovascular tests can be separated into two major categories, those that assess risk of disease and those that diagnose disease and/or trauma. Cholesterol and lipid studies are used to assess a patient's risk of atherosclerotic disease of the heart (myocardial infarction, angina), brain (stroke), or peripheral arteries (peripheral vascular disease). Several other studies which evaluate inflammation and metabolic traits also add to risk assessment. Enzyme studies as well as other biologically active proteins which appear in the blood as a result of cardiac damage are used to assess a recent or acute infarction.

Cholesterol and lipids (fatty acids) are not water soluble, so they must be carried in the blood bound to protein molecules called lipoproteins. Elevated levels in the blood cause deposits to form within arterial walls called plaques, which narrow the lumen of the arteries, reducing or even obstructing flow.

Enzymes and other intracellular components are released into the blood when muscle cells are damaged. Rates of liberation of intracellular components vary, and the patterns of rising and falling levels are diagnostic. When cardiac muscle damage is suspected, serial blood evaluations are performed at defined time intervals.

TEST NAME	COMMENT	NORMAL RANGE	NORMAL RANGE (SI)
Total cholesterol	Total of all cholesterol fractions. Elevated levels are a risk factor for atherosclerosis.	<200 mg/dL	<520 mmol/L
LDL (low density lipoprotein)	Elevated levels are associated with higher risk of atherosclerosis.	40–130 mg/dL, less than 70 mg/dL	1–3 mmol/L
HDL (high density lipoprotein)	"Favorable" form of cholesterol. Higher levels reduce risk of atherosclerosis.	35–80 mg/dL	1–2 mmol/L
VLDL (very low density lipoprotein)	Elevated levels are associated with higher risk of atherosclerosis.		
Triglycerides	Elevated levels increase risk of atherosclerosis.	<160 mg/dL	<1.8 mmol/L
Homocysteine	Elevated levels are associated with increased risk of atherosclerosis.	<1.6 mg/dL	<12mcmol/L
hsCRP (high sensitivity C-reactive protein)	Elevated levels indicate vascular inflammation, increasing risk of atherosclerosis.	0.02 to 0.8 mg/dL	0.2 to 8.0 mg/L
BNP (brain natriuretic peptide)	Mildly elevated levels seen immediately following MI; grossly elevated levels indicative of damage to left ventricle as in congestive heart failure.	<50 pg/mL	<50 ng/L
troponin I	Elevated levels are seen early after myocardial infarction.	<1.5 ng/mL	<1.5 mcg/L
CK (CPK, creatine phosphokinase)	Levels increase with skeletal or cardiac muscle damage.	15 to 105 U/L 0 to 7 ng/mL	15 to 105 U/L 0 to 7 mcg/L
CK-MB	Isoenzyme specific for cardiac muscle damage. Levels increase in the first 24 hours following MI.		
Myoglobin	Levels elevated with muscle damage, not specific for cardiac muscle.	14–51 mcg/L	0.8–2.9 mil/L
LH (LDH, lactate dehydrogenase)	Serum levels rise after muscle damage, although not specific for cardiac muscle.	100 to 190 U/L	100 to 190 U/L

Thyroid-Related Studies

The thyroid gland secretes hormones which regulate metabolism. These hormones have far-reaching effects on many body systems. Thyroid hormones are regulated by feedback loops. A decrease in T_3 or T_4 causes thyroid-stimulating hormone levels to rise, increasing T_3 and T_4. As levels rise, TSH goes back down. Of the two, T_3 is more metabolically active than T_4, but it binds loosely to TBG so it is quickly removed from the blood. T_4 binds more tightly to thyroid-binding globulin (TBG) so it survives in the blood for a longer period, but very little is "free" to exert an effect on cells.

TEST NAME	COMMENT	NORMAL RANGE	NORMAL RANGE (SI)
T_4 (thyroxine)	Increased in Graves disease and acute thyroiditis.	4.5 to 12 mcg/dL	58 to 154 nmol/L
Free T_4	Decreased in iodine deficiency and chronic disease.	0.8–2.7 ng/dL	10.3–35 pmol/L
T_3	Elevated levels indicative of hyperthyroidism; decreased in hypothyroidism when TBG is normal.	70–190 ng/dL	1.1 to 2.9 nmol/L
Free T_3	Not bound to TBG, metabolically active form of T_3	260 to 480 pg/dL	4.0 to 7.4 pmol/L
TSH (thyroid-stimulating hormone)	Increased in primary hypothyroidism. Decreased in primary hyperthyroidism.	0.4 to 4.2 mcU/mL	0.4 to 4.2 mU/L
T_3 uptake	Used to indirectly measure TBG (thyroid-binding globulin).	25 to 38%	0.25 to 0.38
Antithyroid antibodies	Elevated in Hashimoto thyroiditis.	None	
TBG (thyroid- binding globulin)	Abnormal levels affect metabolically active fraction of T_3 and T_4.	1.25 to 2.5 mg/dL	12 to 25 mg/L

Parathyroid Studies

The parathyroid glands maintain the balance of calcium, magnesium, and phosphorous between the blood and bones.

TEST NAME	COMMENT	NORMAL RANGE	NORMAL RANGE (SI)
PTH (parathyroid hormone)	Increased PTH results in hypercalcemia, and conversely decreased PTH causes hypocalcemia and increased serum phosphorus.	11 to 54 pg/mL	1.2 to 5.6 pmol/L

Immune System

Tests of the immune system include assays for cell markers, complement levels, and antibodies. For example, white blood cells have specific proteins on the outer surface. These proteins can be used to identify white cells. Antibodies are reported in ratios or titers, which are determined by testing serial dilutions (concentrations) and reporting the end point (the smallest dilution that shows a reaction.) Also, since antibodies are very specific, they work well for tagging proteins so they can be measured. This concept is the basis of ELISA and fluorescent antibody tests.

TEST NAME	COMMENT	NORMAL RANGE	NORMAL RANGE (SI)
CD4	Used to monitor HIV infection. Decreased CD4 levels correlate with increased viral activity.	5 to 1500 cells/mm^3	0.5 to 1.5 $\times$ 10^9 cells/L

TEST NAME	COMMENT	NORMAL RANGE	NORMAL RANGE (SI)
ANA (antinuclear antibodies)	Increased levels of antibodies against nuclear elements are common in autoimmune diseases such as SLE.	Negative	
Anti-ds-DNA (antibodies against double-stranded DNA)	Increased levels of antibodies against DNA are seen in autoimmune diseases.	Negative	
RF (rheumatoid factor)	Seen in 80% of patients with rheumatoid arthritis	Negative	

Cancer Markers

Cancer markers include serum proteins and genetic markers which are expressed in some forms of cancer. The serum markers are used to screen for disease and then to monitor remission or progression of confirmed disease. Genetic markers are used to screen for risk of disease or to characterize known disease.

TEST NAME	COMMENT	NORMAL RANGE	NORMAL RANGE (SI)
PSA (prostate specific antigen)	Levels increase in prostatitis and prostate cancer.	<4 ng/mL	<4 mcg/L
CEA (carcinoembryonic antigen)	Elevated values may indicate carcinoma of the lung, digestive tract, or pancreas.	<5.0 ng/mL	<5.0 mcg/L
AFP (alpha-fetoprotein)	Elevated levels seen in hepatocellular cancer, hepatic disease, embryonal cancers, and in the maternal serum of a fetus with a neural tube defect (e.g., spinal bifida).	<15 ng/mL	<15 mcg/L
CA-125	Elevated levels associated with ovarian and digestive tract carcinomas	<35 U/mL	<35 kU/L
CA-19-9	Elevated values associated with digestive tract carcinomas.	<37 U/mL	<37 kU/L
BRCA-1, BRCA-2	Genetic markers associated with breast, prostate, and ovarian cancer		

Hematology

Samples used by the hematology lab are collected into purple-top tubes (also called lavender-top) and are not allowed to clot or separate from the serum as in most chemistry tests. Whole blood with intact cells is needed in order to obtain accurate cell counts and platelet counts. A small portion of the sample may be centrifuged in a microcentrifuge in order to determine the hematocrit, although this value is most often calculated indirectly using red cell counts and indices.

CBC (Complete Blood Count)

The CBC is one of the most common tests ordered, yet a diagnosis is rarely made based on the results of a CBC alone. A CBC must be interpreted along with other diagnostic and physical findings.

A CBC enumerates the formed elements of the blood, including white cells, red cells, and platelets. A CBC also includes specific information about the size and composition of red cells, called indices (MCV, MCH, MCHC, RDW). Platelets are actually small, extruded fragments of megakaryocytes and therefore are not actually cells. Platelets are integral to coagulation as they release factors which initiate clot formation as well as physically create barriers for sealing cuts and abrasions.

TEST NAME	COMMENT	NORMAL RANGE	NORMAL RANGE (SI)
WBC	Mild to moderate elevations seen in infection, pregnancy. Moderate to severe elevations can indicate leukemoid reaction, severe infection, or leukemia. Decreased levels seen in overwhelming infection, viral infection, bone marrow suppression, and immunodeficiency disease and status post chemotherapy and radiation therapy.	5000 to 10000/mm^3	5 to 10 $\times$ 10^9 cells/L
RBC	Increased in polycythemia vera, pulmonary disease and to compensate for high altitudes. Decreased levels seen in acute or chronic hemorrhage, decreased hemoglobin synthesis, aplastic anemia, bone marrow suppression, leukemia, and status post chemotherapy and radiation therapy.	4.8 to 5.6 $\times$ 10^6/mm^3	4.8 to 5.6 $\times$ 10^{12}/L
Hgb (hemoglobin)	Elevated levels are seen in polycythemia vera, dehydration, and compensation for reduced oxygen concentration in higher altitudes. Levels are reduced in malnutrition, iron deficiency, thalassemia, hemorrhage, leukemia, and anemia of chronic disease.	12 to 16 g/dL	7.5 to 10 mmol/L
Hct (hematocrit)	The percentage of whole blood composed of red blood cells. Reduced values coincide with reduced RBC. Normally, the hematocrit will be equal to roughly 3 times the hemoglobin value.	40% to 48%	40% to 48%
MCH (mean corpuscular hemoglobin)	Average weight of hemoglobin contained per red cell.	27 to 31 pg/cell (picogram)	27 to 31 pg/cell (picogram)
MCHC (mean corpuscular hemoglobin concentration)	Average concentration of hemoglobin per red cell. Decreased levels (hypochromia) associated with iron-deficiency anemia, hereditary anemias, chronic blood loss.	32 to 36 g/dL	320 to 360 g/L
MCV (mean corpuscular volume)	A measure of the size of red cells. Decreased values (microcytosis) are associated with iron deficiency and/or chronic blood loss (and many other conditions). Higher values (macrocytosis) may be due to B12 and/or folic acid deficiency or liver disease.	82 to 92 mcm^3	82 to 92 fL (femtoliter)

TEST NAME	COMMENT	NORMAL RANGE	NORMAL RANGE (SI)
RDW	A measure of the degree of variation in the size of red cells (anisocytosis). The higher the number, the less uniformity, indicating stress on the bone marrow. Seen in many conditions and diseases.	<15%	<15%
Platelets	Increased levels are seen in essential thrombocytosis, some forms of leukemia, and polycythemia vera. Reduced numbers (thrombocytopenia) seen in idiopathic thrombocytopenia (autoimmune disease), adverse drug reactions, aplastic anemia, disseminated intravascular coagulation (DIC), bone marrow suppression (e.g. chemotherapy and radiation).	150,000 to 400,000/mm^3	150 to 400 $\times$ 10^9/L

Differential

The differential separates the white cells into their various subtypes and reports each subtype as a percentage of the total. Traditionally, a differential is performed by staining a smear of peripheral blood and evaluating a total of 100 white cells under a microscope, reporting the percentage of each type of cell seen. The names of the white cell subtypes are based on their staining characteristics using a Wright stain. The granulocytes were so named because the granules contained within the cells stain various shades of pink, purple, and blue. Eosinophils have the typical small granules and also large granules which stain darkly with eosin, an intense red dye. Basophils likewise have large granules which stain heavily with the basic dye (dark bluish purple) contained in the Wright stain. Although many differential counts are still performed on stained blood smears, automated cell counters are also used to count white cell subtypes. An absolute count of each white cell is determined by multiplying the percentage in the differential by the total white count.

TEST NAME	COMMENT	NORMAL RANGE	ABSOLUTE COUNT
Granulocytes	Includes segmented neutrophils (mature), band neutrophils (less mature), basophils, and eosinophils.		
Segmented neutrophils ("segs"), also called polymorphonuclear leukocytes ("polys")	Increased in bacterial infection, pregnancy, some forms of leukemia. Decreased in some cases of poisoning, some viral infections, some leukemias, and status post chemotherapy and radiation.	40% to 70%	2000 to 6500/mm^3
Bands, also called stabs	Elevation in band neutrophils may also be referred to as a "left shift." Elevations seen in acute and severe infections.	4% to 8%	200 to 800/mm^3
Basophils	Increased in chronic myelogenous leukemia and polycythemia. Decreased in hyperthyroidism and bone marrow suppression.	0–1%	40 to 60/mm^3
Eosinophils	Increased in allergic reactions, parasitic infections, and chronic myelogenous leukemia.	0–5%	100 to 400/mm^3
Monocytes	Increased in some viral infections, monocytic leukemia, and some collagen diseases. Decreased in bone marrow suppression.	5% to 8%	200 to 600/mm^3

TEST NAME	COMMENT	NORMAL RANGE	ABSOLUTE COUNT
Lymphocytes	Usually increased in viral infections or some forms of leukemia. Greater than 10% atypical lymphocytes are characteristic of infectious mononucleosis. Decreased counts are seen in AIDS and autoimmune disorders.	25% to 40%	1250 to 4000/mm^3
Blasts	Very immature white cells. Diagnostic for leukemia when seen in the peripheral blood.	None	

Abnormal Red Cells Seen On Peripheral Smear

Reticulocytes (immature red cells) can be noted on a Wright-stained peripheral smear but are more accurately counted and reported as a percent of total red cells using a methylene blue stain. Red cell morphology (shape) can be indicative and sometimes even diagnostic for certain diseases (e.g. sickle cells). The presence of these various red cell types are graded 1+ (10% of cells affected) through 4+ (greater than 75% of cells affected).

TEST NAME	COMMENT	NORMAL RANGE
Reticulocytes ("retics")	Elevated numbers are seen during recovery of severe anemia or in chronic anemia, as the stressed bone marrow pushes red cells into the peripheral blood prematurely.	None to 1+
Macrocytes	Large red cells, correlate with elevated MCV.	None to 1+
Microcytes	Small red cells, correlate with decreased MCV.	None to 1+
Nucleated RBC (nRBC) (normoblast)	Very immature red cells still containing remnants of a nucleus. Seen in some leukemias or severe anemias where the bone marrow is stressed to produce adequate RBCs.	None
Polychromasia	Seen as larger, more purplish red cells on Wright stain. Correlate with elevated reticulocyte count and elevated MCV.	None to 1+
Sickle cells	Sickle-shaped cells seen in sickle-cell disease, caused by abnormal hemoglobin molecules which distort the normal cell shape.	None
Poikilocytosis (subtypes tear drop, dacryocyte, elliptocyte, acanthocyte)	Variation in shape of red cells. Especially seen in thalassemia, liver and kidney disease, but this is a nonspecific finding seen in many conditions.	None to 1+
Anisocytosis	Variation in size of red cells. Correlates with RDW on CBC. Nonspecific finding seen in many conditions.	None to 1+
Schistocytes	Remnants of destroyed red cells, indicative of mechanical "shredding" of the red cell membrane (prosthetic heart valves), or from hemolytic anemia (uremia, disseminated intravascular coagulation).	None
Target cells	Named for their characteristic "target" appearance. Associated with hemoglobinopathies, especially thalassemia, and liver disease. May be a nonspecific finding.	None to 1+
Spherocytes	Spherical red cells which have lost their typical concave shape. Can be a nonspecific finding. Large numbers indicative of hereditary spherocytosis or spherocytic anemia.	None to 1+

Coagulation Studies

Coagulation studies are used to diagnose coagulopathies and monitor anticoagulation therapy. In contrast to many laboratory studies, PT and PTT tests do not measure actual concentrations of coagulation factors; rather, these tests measure their activity. Abnormalities in PT or PTT may lead to further studies to diagnose deficiencies of one of the many factors making up the coagulation system.

TEST NAME	COMMENT	NORMAL RANGE	NORMAL RANGE (SI)
PT (prothrombin time or "pro time")	Measures the time required for a clot to form. Prolongation may indicate hepatic disease, deficiency in vitamin K, Factor V, Factor VII, Factor IX, or fibrinogen. Also prolonged by coumarin therapy.	11 to 13 seconds	11 to 13 seconds
PTT (partial thromboplastin time)	Also measures the time required for a clot to form. Prolongation may indicate deficiency of fibrinogen or Factor IX, X, XI or XII.	21 to 35 seconds	21 to 35 seconds
INR (International Normalized Ratio)	The potency of thromboplastin used to perform the PT varies from one batch to another, so each batch of thromboplastin is assigned a sensitivity index value. The PT result is multiplied by the index value to arrive at a standarized number which can be interpreted the same regardless of the laboratory, methodology, or test reagents. The INR is important for monitoring coumarin therapy.	Normal ratio is 1. Target ranges for INR vary according to the underlying disease. DVT prophylaxis 1 to 1.5. Recurrent DVT 3 to 4. Atrial fibrillation 2 to 3.	
D-dimer	Product of clot lysis (breakdown). Values are elevated in DIC, MI, venous thrombosis.	<250 mcg/L	<1.37 nmol/L
FSP (fibrin split product or fibrin degradation product)	Breakdown product of fibrin clot. Elevated levels are indicative of DIC.		
Fibrinogen	Fibrinogen is converted to fibrin by clot initiation factors. Levels decrease with active clot formation. Fibrinogen is also an acute phase protein and is elevated in infection and inflammation.	200 to 400 mg/dL	2 to 4 g/L

Urinalysis

A urinalysis is much like a CBC in that it is used to screen for abnormalities, but rarely can a diagnosis be made on the results of a urinalysis alone. The urinalysis has three major components: the dipstick, macroscopic examination, and microscopic examination.

The macroscopic examination is simply observing the urine for color and clarity and any sediment large enough to be seen by the naked eye. Urine is normally straw colored to dark yellow and clear. Abnormal colors include brown, red, amber, or even very dark yellow. Drug metabolites may change the color of urine to bright orange or even green. Elevated proteins or large numbers of white or red cells or drug metabolites may cloud the urine.

Dipstick Test

The dipstick is a narrow plastic strip with as many as 10 different test pads. Each test pad reacts by changing colors, and the color and intensity are indicative of the results. After the stick is dipped into a urine sample, it is placed on a reader which detects the color changes.

TEST NAME	COMMENT	NORMAL RANGE
pH	Decreased (acidosis) in diabetic ketosis, UTI. Alkaline urine (increased pH) is seen with UTI, chronic renal failure, vomiting, and hyperventilation.	4.6 to 8.0
Protein	Protein appears in the urine in renal disease, diabetes mellitus, and infection.	None
Glucose	Glucose is normally reabsorbed by the renal tubules, but elevated blood glucose can overwhelm the kidneys, causing glucose to spill into the urine. Glucose may also appear in the urine in liver disease, impaired tubular reabsorption, and uncontrolled diabetes mellitus.	None
Ketones	Ketones are an end-product of fat metabolism. Ketones appear in the urine in diabetic ketoacidosis, low-carbohydrate diets, and starvation.	None
Blood	Blood may be detected in the urine as intact cells or as hemoglobin. Hematuria (intact cells in the urine) may result from infection, malignant hypertension, or trauma. Hemoglobinuria is present in burn victims, transfusion reactions, intravascular hemolysis, and DIC.	None
Bilirubin	Bilirubin appears in the urine under any circumstance that causes increased RBC destruction, with liver impairment, or biliary obstruction.	None
Urobilinogen	Bilirubin is acted on in the gut by bacteria to produce urobilinogen, which is reabsorbed and metabolized by the liver. It appears in the urine when bilirubin is increased.	None
Nitrite	Nitrates, normally excreted in the urine, are converted to nitrites by bacteria. Positive nitrite is indicative of bacterial UTI.	None
Leukocyte esterase	Leukocyte esterase is detectable in the urine when the urine contains white cells. Typically, a positive esterase test indicates a UTI.	None.
Specific gravity	This is a measure of the kidneys' ability to concentrate urine. The value is decreased (dilute urine) in diabetes insipidus, glomerulonephritis, and renal damage. Elevated values (concentrated urine) may be seen in dehydration, diabetes mellitus, and congestive heart failure.	1.005 to 1.030

Microscopic Examination

The microscopic part of the examination involves centrifuging the urine sample and placing a drop of the concentrated sediment under a microscope to examine the specimen for formed elements. Results are reported as the average number of elements seen in either the low-power or high-power field of the microscope (written *hpf* for high-power field and *lpf* for low-power field).

TEST NAME	COMMENT	NORMAL RANGE
WBC	Intact white cells may be seen in the urine sediment, indicating an infection within the urinary tract.	0 to 4 cells/hpf (should correlate with dipstick results)
RBC	Intact red cells may originate from anywhere within the urinary tract. See above for possible implications.	0 to 3 cells/hpf (should correlate with dipstick results)
Epithelial cells	Epithelial cells throughout the urinary tract slough off and appear in the urine under normal circumstances. Very large numbers may indicate trauma within the urinary tract.	Renal tubule epithelial cells: 0 to 3 cells/hpf Bladder and squamous epithelial cells are normal.
Bacteria	Very small numbers of bacteria may be seen in urine when the sample is contaminated during collection. Large numbers indicate infection.	

TEST NAME	COMMENT	NORMAL RANGE
Casts (red cell, white cell, hyaline, granular, waxy, broad, or fatty)	Clumps or masses of cells (red, white, or epithelial cells) or proteins that form in the renal tubules are called casts. They are seen in cases of renal tubular disease or glomerular disease.	None
Crystals	Crystals may form in the urine as metabolites crystalize under acidic or alkaline conditions. Many have little to no clinical significance, but some form as a result of increased levels of metabolites in the urine. Calcium oxalate and triple phosphate are the most common abnormal crystals seen.	Amorphous urates, sodium urate, calcium carbonate, ammonium biurate, calcium phosphate, amorphous phosphates are reported when present. Any number is considered abnormal.

APPENDIX 2

Medical Soundalikes

FREQUENTLY CONFUSED TERMS

ABDUCT to move away from	**ADDUCT** to move toward
AIDE an assistant	**AID** to provide assistance
ADE a drink (lemonade)	
ANATOMIC relating to the human anatomy or body location	**ATOMIC** nuclear particles
ANTERIOR before	**INTERIOR** within
APPRAISED to determine the value (property appraisal)	**APPRISED** to inform (the patient was apprised of her diagnosis)
ASCITIC a collection of fluid in the abdomen	**ACIDIC** an acid-like substance
ATOPIC relating to atopy (allergy)	**ECTOPIC** out of place (ectopic pregnancy)
AURA subjective symptoms often occurring prior to a seizure or migraine	**ORA** plural of os (mouth)
AWL instrument for making holes	**ALL** the whole, everybody, everything
AXIS a line through the center of an organ	**ACCESS** to obtain entrance into
CAROTID the artery in your neck	**PAROTID** the gland in your jaw
CARRIES he carries books to school	**CARIES** decayed teeth (carious)

CIRCUMSCRIBED bound by line, limited or confined (well-circumscribed border)	**CIRCUMCISED** excision of penile foreskin (diagnosis: phimosis)
CIRRHOSIS interstitial inflammation of an organ, especially the liver	**XEROSIS** abnormal dryness, especially of the hands or feet
COLLABORATE to work jointly with others	**CORROBORATE** to support with evidence
COMPLEMENT lab test	**COMPLIMENT** kind remark
CONSTIPATION difficulty passing stools	**OBSTIPATION** extreme constipation
CONTRACTIONS rhythmic muscle movements (contractions during labor)	**CONTRACTURES** retraction of muscles (from disuse/deconditioning)
CORD long rope-like structure (vocal cord, etc.)	**CHORD** musical note which combines more than one individual note
CORNEAL pertaining to the cornea of the eye	**CORNUAL** pertaining to an area of the fallopian tube
COURSE his course was uneventful	**COARSE** lungs revealed coarse rales
CREATINE occurs in muscle tissue as phosphocreatine (high in urine suggests MD)	**CREATININE** a component of urine (final product of creatine catabolism)
DISCREET showing good judgment (ability to be silent)	**DISCRETE** distinct separation (as in a discrete lesion)
DIVERTICULUM singular	**DIVERTICULA** plural
DYSPHAGIA difficulty swallowing	**DYSPHASIA** difficulty speaking
EFFECT to cause to happen	**AFFECT** to produce an effect upon (influence) psych: a flat affect
EFFUSION collection of fluid in tissue	**INFUSION** introduction of fluid into a vein
ELUDE evade or escape notice **ELUTE** to give off (drug-eluting silent)	**ALLUDE** to refer indirectly
EMIGRATE to leave one country to settle in another	**IMMIGRATE** to come into a country to take up residence

ETIOLOGY cause of disease	**IDEOLOGY** a belief system
FACIAL pertaining to the face or facial region	**FASCIAL** a band of fibrous tissue
FISSURE a cleft or groove	**FISHER** usually a surname or "one who fishes"
FORNICATION illicit sexual coitus	**FORMICATION** sensation of insects crawling on the skin
FOSSA general term for a hollow or depressed area (plural = fossae)	**FOCI** plural of focus (more than one point of convergence)
GATE an opening in a fence	**GAIT** walking stride
HABITUS physical characteristics	**HABITAT** region in which a species lives
HEAL to make well	**HEEL** posterior portion of the foot
HEROIN an illicit drug	**HEROINE** female star in an action film
ILIUM hip bone	**ILEUM** intestine
ILLICIT illegal	**ELICIT** to obtain
INCISE to cut into	**EXCISE** to cut out
INCISION to cut into or through	**EXCISION** to cut out or remove
INSTALLATION to induct into office	**INSTILLATION** to impart gradually
INSURE to provide insurance for or to underwrite	**ENSURE** to make certain (ensure compliance)
JOULES dynamic equivalent of heat (300 joules delivered)	**JEWELS** diamonds, rubies, etc.
LAY to put or place (lay the book on the table)	**LIE** to recline or to speak an untruth (lie down on the table)
LOOP a circle of suture	**LOUPE** a magnifying instrument
LUHR mandibular plating system	**LUER** brand name of curet, forceps, needles, retractors, rongeurs, etc.
MARSHAL like Marshall Dillon	**MARTIAL** martial law was instituted

MELENIC dark stools due to presence of blood	**MELANOTIC** skin affected by melanoma
MUCOUS membrane that produces mucoid material	**MUCUS** material produced by the mucous membrane
OPPOSED providing resistance to an idea	**APPOSED** fitted together (as in edges of wounds)
ORAL pertaining to the mouth	**AURAL** pertaining to the ear
OS an opening in a cavity	**OZ** where the Wizard lives
OVERT obvious behavior	**EVERT** to turn out (evert a suture line)
PEELING to strip off (as in peeling skin or peeling back a catheter)	**PEALING** loud ringing of bells (think of Big Ben)
PERFUSE to cause blood to flow (through an artery or lumen of a tube)	**PROFUSE** pouring forth abundantly (diaphoresis)
PERINEAL relating to the perineum area between the thighs and the coccyx	**PERONEAL** relating to the lateral fibula and the muscles attached thereto
PLAIN ordinary (an x-ray without contrast)	**PLANE** a location on the body (sagittal, coronal, etc.)
PLURAL more than one	**PLEURAL** pertaining to the lungs
PROSTHETIC artificial (prosthetic heart valves, penile implants) **PROSTRATE** to lie prone in adoration	**PROSTATIC** male prostate gland
REFLEX an involuntary response to external stimuli (patellar reflex)	**DEFLEX** repositioning of an infant's head to aid vaginal delivery
REGIMENT squadrons of military personnel **REGIME** a form of government	**REGIMEN** course of medical treatment
RHONCHI a transmitted chest sound heard on auscultation	**BRONCHI** plural for bronchus

ROOT base of a problem (portion of a tooth inside the gum line)	**ROUTE** a planned method of travel (method of drug delivery)
SACK a bag to carry things	**SAC** a structure in the body
SEAMEN U.S. Navy personnel (men on the sea)	**SEMEN** male ejaculate
SEEDING radioactive seed placement (treatment for prostate CA)	**SEATING** designated seating (as in a theater)
SERIAL in a series (e.g., serial EKGs)	**CEREAL** Frosted Flakes, oatmeal, etc.
SHOTTY feels like buckshot (shotty lymph nodes)	**SHODDY** unkempt
SITE a place or location (operative site)	**SIGHT** the ability to see (her sight was adequate)
SPICULATION small spike-like projections	**SPECULATION** to think or wonder about
TETANIC marked muscular contractions (heard in OB/GYN reports)	**TITANIC** a big boat on the bottom of the North Atlantic ocean
THECAL pertaining to the thecal sac	**FECAL** pertaining to feces
TICK a blood-sucking animal	**TIC** an involuntary movement (as in Tourette's syndrome)
TINEA fungal infection of the skin	**TENIA** tapeworm
TRACT a pathway (urinary tract)	**TRACK** mark or series of marks (needle tracks in IVDA)
TRIAL as in a trial of medication	**TRAIL** a path to follow
TYMPANIC relating to the tympanic membrane	**TYMPANITIC** a sound quality (as in striking a tympany drum) (a tympanitic abdomen)
UNKEMPT lacking neatness (unpolished)	**UNKEPT** no such word, according to Webster
VARICOSE veins that are dilated or thrombosed	**VERY CLOSE** something in close proximity to another

VENOUS pertaining to veins rather than arteries	**VENUS** fourth planet or a sculpture without arms
VERSUS one or the other	**VERSES** lines in a poem
VESICAL pertaining to the bladder	**VESICLE** any sac-like structure
VILLOUS a projection, especially from the a mucous membrane	**VILLUS** shaggy, covered with villi
WANT to need or require	**WONT** accustomed to, inclined, or apt
WAVE to motion with hands or a swell on the surface of the water	**WAIVE** to give up claim to
WAVER to fluctuate one's opinion	**WAIVER** a document declaring giving up claim
WHEAL a raised area of skin from an intradermal injection	**WHEEL** round tool invented by cavemen

APPENDIX 3

Pharmacology

GENERIC DRUG IDENTIFIERS

Did you know that many generic drugs contain prefixes and suffixes that identify them by type or action? Knowing these suffixes can assist you in readily identifying a drug with which you may not be familiar. A number of brand names also retain the identifiable suffix, enabling you to determine their use as well. *Examples:* Accupril, Xylocaine, Streptase, Compazine, Norpramin, Wycillin, Cefotan, Retrovir.

GENERIC SUFFIX	DRUG TYPE	EXAMPLES
-ane	inhalational anesthetic	halothane isoflurane sevoflurane
-ase	thrombolytic (enzyme)	anistreplase streptokinase urokinase
-azepam	benzodiazepine	diazepam halazepam lorazepam
-azine	phenothiazine antipsychotic	fluphenazine prochlorperazine thioridazine
-azole	antifungal	econazole ketoconazole oxiconazole
-azosin	$alpha_1$ blockers	doxazosin prazosin terazosin
-barbital	barbiturate	butabarbital pentobarbital phenobarbital
-caine	local/regional anesthetic	benzocaine lidocaine bupivacaine procaine

GENERIC SUFFIX	DRUG TYPE	EXAMPLES
-cillin	penicillin	amoxicillin ampicillin cloxacillin methicillin penicillin
-curium, - curonium	neuromuscular blocking agent	doxacurium mivacurium pancuronium vecuronium
-cycline	tetracycline antibiotic	doxycycline methacycline tetracycline
-floxacin	fluoroquinolone antibiotic	ciprofloxacin levofloxacin norfloxacin
-iazide	thiazide diuretic	chlorothiazide hydrochlorothiazide polythiazide
-ipine	calcium channel blocker	amlodipine nicardipine nifedipine
-micin, -mycin	aminoglycoside or macrolide antibiotic	gentamicin streptomycin tobramycin azithromycin erythromycin
-olol	beta blocker	atenolol metoprolol propranolol
-olone	corticosteroid	clocortolone fluocinolone triamcinolone
-onide	corticosteroid	amcinonide desonide halcinonide
-phylline	bronchodilator	aminophylline dyphylline oxtriphylline theophylline
-pramine	tricyclic antidepressant	desipramine imipramine trimipramine
-pril	ACE inhibitors for CHF	captopril enalapril lisinopril
-profen	NSAID	fenoprofen ibuprofen ketoprofen
-sone	corticosteroid	betamethasone dexamethasone hydrocortisone

GENERIC SUFFIX	DRUG TYPE	EXAMPLES
-terol, -terenol	bronchodilator	albuterol isoproterenol metaproterenol pirbuterol salmeterol
-tidine	H2 blocker for PUD	cimetidine famotidine ranitidine
-triptyline	tricyclic antidepressant	amitriptyline nortriptyline protriptyline
-tropin	gland-stimulating hormone	follitropin gonadotropin menotropin urofollitropin
-vir	antiviral	acyclovir indinavir ganciclovir

Resource: *Understanding Pharmacology for Health Professionals, 3rd Edition, Susan M. Turley, Prentice Hall, 2002.*

APPENDIX 4

JCAHO Dangerous Abbreviations

EFFECTIVE JANUARY 1, 2004

ABBREVIATION	POTENTIAL PROBLEM	PREFERRED
U (for unit)	Mistaken as zero, four, or cc	Write "unit"
IU (for international units)	Mistaken as IV or 10	Write "international unit"
O.D. or Q.O.D.	Mistaken for each other. The period after the Q can be mistaken for an "I" and the "O" can be mistaken for "I"	Write "daily" and "every other day"
Trailing zero (x.0 mg) (Note: Prohibited only for medication-related notations); Lack of leading zero (.X mg)	Decimal point is missed	Never write a zero by itself after a decimal point (X mg), and always use a zero before a decimal point (0.X mg)
MS MSO_4 $MgSO_4$	Confused for one another. Can mean morphine sulfate or magnesium sulfate	Write "morphine sulfate" or "magnesium sulfate"
µg	Mistaken for mg (milligrams) resulting in one thousand-fold dosing overdose	Write "mcg"
H.S. (for half-strength or Latin abbreviation for bedtime)	Mistaken for either half-strength or hour of sleep (at bedtime), q.H.S. mistaken for every hour. All can result in dosing errors.	Write out "half-strength" or "at bedtime"
T.I.W. (for three times a week)	Mistaken for three times a day or twice weekly resulting in an overdose	Write "3 times weekly" or "three times weekly"
S.C. or S.Q. (for subcutaneous)	Mistaken as SL for sublingual, or "5 every"	Write "Sub-Q," "subQ," or "subcutaneously"
D/C (for discharge)	Interpreted as discontinue whatever medications follow (typically discharge meds)	Write "discharge"
c.c. (for cubic centimeter)	Mistaken for U (units) when poorly written	Write "mL" for milliliters
A.S., A.D., A.U. (Latin abbreviation for left, right, or both ears)	Mistaken for OD, OD, and OU, etc.	Write "left ear," "right ear," or "both ears"

NOTE: The trailing zero is omitted for all medication orders and other medication-related documentation. However, in reporting laboratory values and in certain other numeric notations, the precision of the numeric value is indicated by the digits after the decimal point, even when that trailing digit is a zero. For example, a serum potassium level might be reported as 4.0 mEq/Liter, not 4 mEq/Liter. Similarly, sizes for endotracheal tubes and other clinical equipment are often specified numerically with one place after the decimal point. This is acceptable, even when the number after the decimal point is a zero.

JCAHO also recommends using the above-noted abbreviations whether the abbreviations are typed in capital letters, lower case letters, with or without periods between the letters.

The safety of the patient comes first. As a long-term objective, ambiguous and otherwise dangerous forms of notation should be eliminated from all health care documentation.

FINALLY: Please refer to the Institute for Safe Medication Practices (ISMP) website at http://www.ismp.org/ for a complete list of dangerous abbreviations relating to medication use that it recommends be explicitly prohibited.

Also, refer to *The AAMT Book of Style for Medical Transcription*, 2nd Edition, pp. 461 to 464. This listing contains the ISMP recommendations as of 2001.

Sources: http://www.ismp/org/ and http://www.jcaho.org/accredited+organizations/patient+safety/04+npsg/04_faqs.htm#abbreviations

APPENDIX 5

How to Take a Test/ Test-Taking Tips

During the learning process, the brain still controls all bodily functions including reason, thinking, movement, sensory perception, and our emotions. The cerebral cortex controls the brain's highest-level functions such as sight, hearing, memory, and thought. In preparing to study for a test, it is important to understand these processes as well as the process of critical thinking and how it is used to process information.

Diet

The mind-body connection is of critical importance. Maintaining good health allows you to learn more efficiently. Maintaining a well-balanced diet and an appropriate amount of fluids and electrolytes is critical. Preparing for the CMT exam is no time to go on a restrictive diet. Your brain needs amino acids to repair and replace tissues, neurons, and chemicals in the brain. It needs glucose for energy, and it needs vitamins and minerals to keep neurotransmitter activity healthy. Here are a few guidelines regarding "brain food."

Vitamin B_1 (thiamine) is important because a deficiency can cause confusion, depression, fatigue, or memory loss. Severe deficiency can cause irreversible brain damage.

Vitamin B_2 (riboflavin) is important because a deficiency can cause depression and lethargy.

Vitamin B_6 (pyridoxine) is vital because low levels can worsen premenstrual tension, cause depression, irritability, fatigue, and poor serotonin (a neurotransmitter that promotes relaxation) production.

Vitamin B_{12} (cobalamin) is critical because a deficiency can contribute to bipolar disorder, chronic fatigue, confusion, insomnia, irritability, memory loss, paranoia, phobias, and restlessness.

Vitamin C deficiency can cause anxiety, depression, excitability, fatigue, and hysteria.

A lack of **folate** (folic acid) can result in depression and lethargy. A **niacin** deficiency can cause anxiety, depression, fatigue, or memory loss. A short-term lack of **calcium** can cause tremors and/or confusion. Difficulties in learning or comprehending can result from an **iron** deficiency. Low levels of **magnesium** in the brain can result in agitation, confusion, irritability, or tremors, and low levels of **zinc** in the brain can impair memory.

In the weeks prior to sitting for the CMT exam, it is recommended that you eat a variety of foods every day, including vegetables, fruits, grains, and low-fat proteins. Choose low-fat foods, especially those low in saturated fat, trans-fats, and cholesterol. Use sugars, salts, and vegetable oils in moderation, and drink plenty of water to maintain proper hydration and flushing out of impurities.

Research has found that no single food can boost your brainpower, but high-carbohydrates, such as pasta, can help improve your mood, thus putting you in the best state of mind for learning. Carbohydrates are easily converted into glucose, which is a simple sugar that provides energy to the brain. Glucose in turn triggers the production of serotonin, which strongly affects mood and emotions. Serotonin helps you stay calm and relaxed and improves your ability to concentrate. Conclusion: Eating pasta can help improve your studying skills.

Learning Styles

There are various styles of learning, including visual, auditory, and kinesthetic. If you are an individual who learns best by watching how something is done or by reading about it, you are a visual learner. To make the most of this learning style, read everything you can find in preparation for the exam (see *Appendix 6: References for Further Study*). You can also make yourself flash-cards and get your family involved in your learning process or leave notes to yourself regarding difficult concepts on your bathroom mirror, refrigerator, etc. You can also watch medical documentaries on TV or browse Internet medical sites for additional information.

If you learn best by hearing things, then you are an auditory learner. To make the most of this learning style, use as much auditory information as possible. Dictate sample questions into your own tape recorder and play them back in your car or join a study group that meets regularly to share ideas. You can also attend medical lectures in your community and play dictation tapes in your car or on your tape recorder. (*Note: Dictation tapes from previous CMT exams can be purchased directly from AAMT.*)

If you prefer to jump right in and learn by doing, you are a kinesthetic learner. To make the most of this style of learning, you should attend workshops, go on field trips, participate in group projects, tutor, mentor, or teach others. You can definitely learn by teaching others. If you have difficulty speaking in front of a group of people, try mentoring on a one-to-one basis. Share your knowledge with another MT less experienced than yourself, and you, in turn, will improve your knowledge as well.

Attitude and Motivation

Other important factors in learning are attitude and motivation. The approach you take to a particular task is your attitude, and your interest in a particular task or how meaningful it is to you is reflected in your attitude. If you have set a goal for yourself to sit for and pass the CMT exam, then your attitude is positive toward the task at hand. Now you need to develop the strategies necessary to see this goal become a reality. One teacher relates that there are invariably a few people in each new MT class whose attitude starts out as defeatist. One particular, otherwise intelligent, professional woman left the first class in tears saying, "I am not smart enough to learn this!" Of course, I convinced her she was indeed smart enough. She just needed to take it one step at a time. She needed to break down the tasks at hand into manageable forms and learn them (not memorize). When all of the individual tasks are put together as a whole and critical thinking is added, the "big picture" emerges and a new medical language specialist is created.

Motivation can be looked at as the proverbial "light at the end of the tunnel" that inspires you to keep going, no matter how difficult the process seems, until you reach your goal of becoming a certified medical transcriptionist. There are two types of motivation: intrinsic and extrinsic. Intrinsic includes a general desire to learn, a sense of curiosity, a willingness to take risks, an interest in the subject to be studied, and the desire to excel at something. Extrinsic motivation includes the desire for improved self-esteem, a sense of fulfillment, increased competence, reaching one's goal, valuable credentials on your resume, and hopefully a better job with a higher salary.

Concentration and Memory

Let's talk about concentration and memory. In order to adequately concentrate on the task at hand (studying for the CMT exam), you must keep distractions to a minimum. Try to clear your mind of external influencing factors, which prevent you from concentrating as you study. Turn off that television and put the children to bed (and your significant other too, if necessary). Use earplugs if needed to create a silent study cocoon for yourself, if this is what you need to optimize your concentration and learning. Make sure you are not hungry, angry, tired, or sad. Use a comfortable chair, but not too comfortable—you don't want to fall asleep—and be sure you have task lighting if needed.

It is important that you study when the time is right for you. Everybody is different. Some people are morning people and some are late night people. Find a study time that fits your work and life schedule. Study in a familiar place, utilizing incandescent light rather than fluorescent light, which can cause eyestrain. Of course, you can study outside in natural sunlight if this fits your lifestyle and climate. Set realistic goals for your study session, make a "to-do list" if it helps you stay centered, and focus on one topic at a time. Drink water throughout your study session to maintain hydration, take short breaks every 45 minutes to 1 hour, and vary your study activities by reading some, taking a few notes, or quiet thinking about what you have just read to keep your study process active rather than passive. Some individuals like "white noise" in the background when studying. This "noise" is a low-level background sound that masks outside distractions. This could include soft music, which obliterates the sound of a clock ticking or a noisy air conditioner. Earplugs will work here, too.

Many people report the benefits of "power napping" wherein one takes a short nap of 5 to 15 minutes (but no longer), saying this rejuvenates the body and mind. Other people prefer cardiovascular exercise like brisk walking, StairMaster, treadmill, etc., prior to a study session to get their juices flowing. Still others prefer yoga or a Pilates-type exercise (low impact) to "center" the body prior to a period of prolonged concentration. Each person is different, and you need to know yourself and what works for you.

Once you have improved your concentration abilities, now you need to commit what you are learning to memory. How your brain processes information determines what you remember and what you forget. There are three basic stages involved in information processing. These are registration, short-term memory, and long-term memory.

In registration, information is received and may eventually be understood and selected to be remembered. This process involves reception, perception, and selection. In reception, you sense something but you do not recognize what it means. For instance, you might auscultate someone's heartbeat but not be able to describe it accurately. In perception, you recognize what you have heard and attach a meaning to it. Now, when hearing that same heartbeat, you are able to determine if the beats are those of sinus rhythm and perhaps even hear a murmur. The final phase is registration, and this involves choosing to remember information so that the next time you hear the same heartbeat you will recognize what it is and what it means.

When new information is selected to be remembered, it automatically goes into short-term memory, which can last a little as 15 seconds. Research has determined that short-term memory can hold five to nine bits of information, depending on how well that information is grouped. For example, we've all heard dictated, "Recall was 5 out of 5 after 1 minute, and 3 out of 5 after 5 minutes." This means the patient's short-term memory is working just fine but his/her long-term memory is deficient. A good memory is a skill that can be developed through practice.

Long-term memory is stored in an organized manner in the brain, but its duration there depends on how completely the information has been processed and how long you use it. An example here might be an individual who learns conversational Spanish. If he uses it on a daily basis he will not only retain that knowledge but will advance it as well. However, should that same individual stop using this skill on a regular basis, over a period of time the skill can be lost completely.

Therefore, learning medical language and utilizing medical language on a daily basis is critical to being able to retrieve that knowledge when needed, as in a testing situation. Make medicine a part of your whole life, not just during your work time each day. Watch medically based television shows, converse with other MTs, attend AAMT functions locally and nationally, and immerse yourself in your profession.

Summary
The skill set required to be a successful, certified medical transcriptionist encompasses much more than just typing, as we all know, and certification tells the world that you are indeed a professional. Your CMT credential means you are a goal-directed individual who takes pride in your profession and expects to be paid as such.

Therefore, the evening before your scheduled exam, get a good night's sleep, eat a healthy breakfast (containing carbohydrates and protein), take your vitamins, drink plenty of water, drive yourself to the testing center, and complete your CMT exam comfortable in the knowledge that you have done everything you can to make your dream of being a certified medical transcriptionist a reality.

We take the liberty of adding our CONGRATULATIONS to all those who understand what it takes to reach this goal and how important it is, not only to you, but to our profession as a whole.

Source: Some material from *Studying & Test Taking Made Incredibly Easy*. Philadelphia: Lippincott Williams & Wilkins, 1999.

APPENDIX 6

References for Further Study

Berkow R. *The Merck Manual of Diagnosis and Therapy*, 16th ed. Whitehouse Station, NJ: Merck & Co., 1992.

Blauvelt CT, Nelson FRT. *A Manual of Orthopaedic Terminology*. Philadelphia: C.V. Mosby, 1998.

Boegli EH. *Prentice Hall Health's Complete Review of Surgery Technology*, 2nd ed. Upper Saddle River, NJ: Prentice Hall Health, 2005.

Chabner D-E. *The Language of Medicine*, 7th ed. Philadelphia: Saunders, 2004.

Crowley LV. *An Introduction to Human Disease: Pathology and Pathophysiology Correlations*. Boston: Jones and Bartlett, 2001.

Dirckx JH. *H & P: A Nonphysician's Guide to the Medical and History Examination*. Modesto, CA: Health Professions Institute, 2001.

Dirckx JH. *Human Diseases*. Modesto, CA: Health Professions Institute, 2003.

Dirckx JH. *Laboratory Tests & Diagnostic Procedures in Medicine*. Modesto, CA: Health Professions Institute, 2004.

Dorland's Illustrated Medical Dictionary, 30th ed. Philadelphia: W.B. Saunders Company, 2004.

Drake R, Drake E. *Saunders Pharmaceutical Word Book*. Philadelphia: Saunders, 2005.

Fetrow CW, Avila JR. *Professional's Handbook of Complementary & Alternative Medicines*, 3rd ed. Philadelphia: Lippincott Williams & Wilkins, 2003.

Goldberg B. *Alternative Medicine: The Definitive Guide*. Fife, Washington: Future Medicine Publishing, Inc., 1995.

Hamann B. *Disease: Identification, Prevention and Control*, 2nd ed. New York: McGraw Hill, 2001.

HIPPA for MTs. American Association for Medical Transcription (www.aamt.org), 2002.

Hughes P (ed). *The AAMT Book of Style for Medical Transcription*, 2nd ed. Modesto: AAMT, 2002.

Judson K, Hicks SB. *Glencoe Law & Ethics for Medical Careers*, 3rd ed. New York: McGraw-Hill, 2002.

Lance LL. *Quick Look Electronic Drug Reference*. Baltimore: Lippincott Williams & Wilkins, 2005.

Levien DH. *Introduction to Surgery*, 3rd ed. Philadelphia: W.B. Saunders, Co., 1999.

Lunsford AA. *The St. Martin's Handbook*, 5th ed. New York; Bedford/St. Martin's, 2003.

Marieb, EN. *Essentials of Human Anatomy & Physiology*. San Francisco: Benjamin-Cummings, 2002.

McWay DC. *Legal Aspects of Health Information Management*, 2nd ed. Clifton Park, NY: Thomson Delmar Learning, 2002.

Merriam Webster's Collegiate Dictionary, 10th ed. Springfield, MA: Merriam-Webster, 1997.

Murray M, Pizzorno J. *Encyclopedia of Natural Medicine*. New York: Prima Publishing, 1998.

Novelline RA. *Squire's Fundamentals of Radiology*, 6th ed. Cambridge, MA: Harvard, 2004.

Phillips N. *Berry & Kohn's Operating Room Technique*, 10th ed. Philadelphia: C.V. Mosby, 2003.

Sabin WA. *The Gregg Reference Manual*, 10th ed. Burr Ridge, IL: McGraw-Hill/Irwin, 2004.

Shaw DL. *Anatomy and Physiology Glossary*. Thorofare, NJ: Slack, 1990.

Sheldon H. *Boyd's Introduction to the Study of Disease*. Philadelphia: Lippincott Williams & Wilkins, 1992.

Stedman's Abbreviations, Acronyms & Symbols, 3rd ed. Baltimore: Lippincott Williams & Wilkins, 2003.

Stedman's Alternative & Complementary Medicine Words, 2nd ed. Baltimore: Lippincott Williams & Wilkins, 2005.

Stedman's Anatomy & Physiology Words, 2nd ed. Baltimore: Lippincott Williams & Wilkins, 2002.

Stedman's Cardiovascular & Pulmonary Words, 4th ed. Baltimore: Lippincott Williams & Wilkins, 2004.

Stedman's Dermatology & Immunology Words, 3rd ed. Baltimore: Lippincott Williams & Wilkins, 2005.

Stedman's Emergency Medicine Words. Baltimore: Lippincott Williams & Wilkins, 2003.

Stedman's Endocrinology Words. Baltimore: Lippincott Williams & Wilkins, 2001.

Stedman's GI & GU Words, 4th ed. Baltimore: Lippincott Williams & Wilkins, 2005.

Stedman's Guide to Idioms. Baltimore: Lippincott Williams & Wilkins, 2005.

Stedman's Illustrated Dictionary of Dermatology Eponyms. Baltimore: Lippincott Williams & Wilkins, 2005.

Stedman's Internal Medicine & Geriatric Words. Baltimore: Lippincott Williams & Wilkins, 2002.

Stedman's Medical & Surgical Equipment Words, 4th ed. Baltimore: Lippincott Williams & Wilkins, 2004.

Stedman's Medical Dictionary, 27th ed. Baltimore: Lippincott Williams & Wilkins, 2000.

Stedman's Medical Eponyms, 2nd ed. Baltimore: Lippincott Williams & Wilkins, 2005.

Stedman's Medical Terminology Flashcards. Baltimore: Lippincott Williams & Wilkins, 2005.

Stedman's Medical Terms and Phrases. Baltimore: Lippincott Williams & Wilkins, 2004.

Stedman's Neurology & Neurosurgery Words, 3rd ed. Baltimore: Lippincott Williams & Wilkins, 2003.

Stedman's OB/GYN & Pediatric Words, 4th ed. Baltimore: Lippincott Williams & Wilkins, 2005.

Stedman's Oncology Words, 4th ed. Baltimore: Lippincott Williams & Wilkins, 2003.

Stedman's Ophthalmology Words, 3rd ed. Baltimore: Lippincott Williams & Wilkins, 2004.

Stedman's Organisms & Infectious Disease Words. Baltimore: Lippincott Williams & Wilkins, 2001.

Stedman's Orthopaedic & Rehab Words, 4th ed. Baltimore: Lippincott Williams & Wilkins, 2002.

Stedman's Pathology & Lab Medicine Words, 3rd ed. Baltimore: Lippincott Williams & Wilkins, 2002.

Stedman's Plastic Surgery/ENT/Dentistry Words, 3rd ed. Baltimore: Lippincott Williams & Wilkins, 2003.

Stedman's Plus Spellchecker 2004. Baltimore: Lippincott Williams & Wilkins, 2004.

Stedman's Psychiatry Words, 3rd ed. Baltimore: Lippincott Williams & Wilkins, 2002.

Stedman's Radiology Words, 4th ed. Baltimore: Lippincott Williams & Wilkins, 2003.

Stedman's Surgery Words, 2nd ed. Baltimore: Lippincott Williams & Wilkins, 2002.

Stedman's Medical Word of the Day Calendar. Baltimore: Lippincott Williams & Wilkins, 2005.

Tamparo CD, Lewis MA. *Diseases of the Human Body*. Philadelphia: F.A. Davis, 2000.

Tessier C. *The Surgical Word Book*, 3rd ed. Philadelphia: Saunders, 2004.

Turabian KL. *A Manual for Writers of Term Papers, Theses, and Dissertations*. Chicago: University of Chicago Press, 1996.

Turley SM. *Understanding Pharmacology for Health Professionals*. Upper Saddle River, NJ: Prentice Hall Health, 2002.